Marijuana in America

Marijuana in America

Cultural, Political, and Medical Controversies

James Hawdon, Bryan Lee Miller, and
Matthew Costello, Editors

BLOOMSBURY ACADEMIC
NEW YORK • LONDON • OXFORD • NEW DELHI • SYDNEY

BLOOMSBURY ACADEMIC
Bloomsbury Publishing Inc, 1359 Broadway, New York, NY 10018, USA
Bloomsbury Publishing Plc, 50 Bedford Square, London, WC1B 3DP, UK
Bloomsbury Publishing Ireland, 29 Earlsfort Terrace, Dublin 2, D02 AY28, Ireland

BLOOMSBURY, BLOOMSBURY ACADEMIC and the Diana logo are trademarks of Bloomsbury Publishing Plc

First published in the United States of America by ABC-CLIO 2022
Paperback edition published by Bloomsbury Academic 2026

COVER PHOTO: Marijuana field. (Nastasic/iStockphoto)

Library of Congress Cataloging-in-Publication Data
Names: Hawdon, James, editor. | Miller, Bryan Lee, editor. | Costello, Matthew, editor.
Title: Marijuana in America : cultural, political, and medical controversies / James Hawdon, Bryan Lee Miller, and Matthew Costello, editors.
Description: Santa Barbara, California : ABC-CLIO, [2022] | Includes bibliographical references and index.
Identifiers: LCCN 2021054470 (print) | LCCN 2021054471 (ebook) | ISBN 9781440869631 (hardcover) | ISBN 9781440869648 (ebook)
Subjects: LCSH: Marijuana—United States—History. | Marijuana—Political aspects—United States—History. | Marijuana—Social aspects—United States—History. | Marijuana—Economic aspects—United States—History. | Marijuana abuse—United States—History. | BISAC: SELF-HELP / Substance Abuse & Addictions / Drugs | MEDICAL / Public Health
Classification: LCC HV5822.M3 M2925 2022 (print) | LCC HV5822.M3 (ebook) | DDC 362.29/50973—dc23/eng/20211228
LC record available at https://lccn.loc.gov/2021054470
LC ebook record available at https://lccn.loc.gov/2021054471

ISBN: HB: 978-1-4408-6963-1
PB: 979-8-2164-9471-3
ePDF: 978-1-4408-6964-8
eBook: 979-8-2161-1484-0

To find out more about our authors and books visit www.bloomsbury.com and sign up for our newsletters.

Contents

Introduction

People have sought and found a vast supply of substances with which to alter their consciousness over the centuries. They have used these drugs in their religions, as their medicines, and in their celebrations. They have found new drugs, novel ways to use old drugs, different combinations of drugs, and a myriad of reasons to use drugs. They have applied technology to make more potent drugs, and they have found ways to produce and distribute them more widely, quickly, and efficiently. While people have used a variety of drugs for eons, some have been more central to the human experience than have others. One of the longest and most used drugs in human existence is cannabis, or marijuana. Marijuana's use is as old as it is varied, as humans have used marijuana as a fiber, in religious practices, as medicine, as food, and for recreational purposes for centuries. Today, marijuana is by far the most commonly used illegal drug on the planet, and it is the most widely used illegal drug in every region of the world—even as laws decriminalizing or even legalizing marijuana production, sale, possession, and use are proliferating in the United States and some other nations.

Marijuana is truly an amazing substance. When one considers how marijuana has symbolized so many divergent and contradictory things, it is little wonder it has been studied by so many people from so many perspectives. If we think about what marijuana symbolizes or has symbolized, it becomes apparent how embedded in the social fabric it is. Depending on the reference group and setting of use, marijuana symbolizes or has symbolized hope or despair, freedom or enslavement, health or illness, and conformity or deviance. It has been described as both a key to reality and an escape from reality. It has been demonized as "the assassin of youth" but also considered a holy sacrament. When we think of all the ways people have thought of and used marijuana over the course of history, it is little wonder why it is referred to in such diverse writings as holy scriptures, medical texts, and criminal codes and why millions of pages have been devoted to its alleged properties, benefits, and dangers. Given its influence and presence in so many realms of life, it is understandable why marijuana is a prominent feature in popular culture, including fiction and nonfiction literature, songs, movies, and television shows.

What we hope to provide with *Marijuana in America* is a reference resource for those interested in learning more about the drug and its impact on American society. We believe this resource is particularly needed now, as the nation moves toward widespread legalization of medical marijuana and increasingly widespread legalization of recreational marijuana use. We are undertaking a great social experiment, and while numerous groups of people have used cannabis in its many forms for centuries, its legal use in modern societies is relatively new. Since rates of use will very likely increase as more states legalize recreational marijuana use, it becomes ever more important to have a better understanding of the drug, its history, its uses, its dangers, and the laws that regulate its place in American life.

Marijuana in America does not include entries on every conceivable topic related to the drug, however tenuously. But this work covers a far greater range of topics than is often found in reference materials, and it reflects a focus on illuminating the most important issues, trends, and events related to marijuana use in the United States and elsewhere. We provide coverage of topics ranging from the chemistry of marijuana to patterns of use around the globe. We include chapters on the health impacts of marijuana consumption and its use for medicinal purposes. We devote chapters to marijuana's impact on areas of everyday life ranging from sexual activity to driving under its influence. We also include entries addressing depictions and use of marijuana in religion and popular entertainment and important legal and political developments pertaining to marijuana over the years. We thus offer a wide breadth of topics to provide the reader with a sense of just how varied the plant's uses are and how embedded into our culture it has become.

Although the entries are presented alphabetically, the book's contents reflect five main topical areas: (1) types and forms of marijuana and marijuana use, (2) health and physiological effects of marijuana use, (3) the history of marijuana, (4) marijuana and society, and (5) marijuana and popular culture. Our coverage of types and forms of marijuana includes entries on the botany of marijuana, including chapters on various forms of the cannabis plant (e.g., indica, sativa, hemp). We also include entries on the chemistry of marijuana that provide information about some of its active ingredients and novel forms, as well as chapters devoted to various delivery methods, including inhalation methods (e.g., dabbing and joints) and oral and topical methods (e.g., edibles and oils).

The second main area of focus concerns the various effects of marijuana use. This coverage is divided into entries that discuss marijuana's effect on the body and mind and those focused on marijuana's uses as medicine. Entries are dedicated to the use of marijuana in treating both mental and physical illnesses.

We then move to the more social aspects of marijuana and the history of marijuana. This category includes entries that discuss the use of marijuana in religions and contemporary patterns of use in various regions of the world. We also illuminate important figures and organizations in the history of marijuana, including several U.S. presidents and their administrations and a number of law enforcement agencies. We also include a number of entries dedicated to the most important laws that regulate marijuana use in the United States at both the state and federal levels. Additional entries explore linkages between marijuana and crime as well as law enforcement efforts to combat its production, distribution, and use.

The encyclopedia also includes a number of entries examining marijuana and society. We provide entries on marijuana and the various institutions of society (e.g., marijuana and the family, military, workplace, sports) as well as the marijuana subculture. We also provide insights into the marijuana economy and the characteristics of marijuana users. We also include several entries that summarize several leading theories of marijuana use, ranging from the biosocial to the sociological.

Finally, this encyclopedia provides illuminating glimpses into the intersections of marijuana and pop culture. It includes entries about movies and television shows that are either dedicated to marijuana or in which marijuana assumes a central place in the plot. Recognizing marijuana's almost sacred place in the world of rock and hip-hop, we also discuss some of the most influential marijuana-promoting musicians and bands. Our coverage even includes entries on magazines dedicated to marijuana.

As we hope you can see from the wide range of topics covered, our goal is to offer a resource that can both answer many questions people may have about marijuana and stimulate interest in the myriad of ways marijuana can be studied. We hope you find the encyclopedia to be interesting and useful; we hope you find the breadth of topics covered to be thought provoking; and we hope we have piqued your interest in a plant whose use dates back to the earliest human civilizations. We hope you enjoy consulting *Marijuana in America* as much as we enjoyed researching, editing, and writing its contents.

James Hawdon, Bryan Lee Miller, and Matthew Costello

Chronology

Cannabis is a truly global plant with a variety of identities. It is believed to be one of the first cultivated plants; it is known by many names: cannabis, marijuana, hemp, ganja, and bhang to name just a few. It has a long and storied history, and its use as a food, fuel, and fiber dates to perhaps 8,000 BC. It has been used for medicinal, spiritual, and recreational reasons for at least 5,000 years. Indigenous to Hindu Kush Mountains and Central Asia, its use spread to India, China, Assyria, and Africa by the first millennium BC. Below is a timeline of human use of the fascinating, many-faceted substance known as cannabis and marijuana (*see* references point out specific encyclopedia entries that provide additional information).

8000 BC
The oldest known use of cannabis by inhabitants of Oki Islands is near Japan where cannabis residue was found near graves.

5000 BC
Evidence of hemp use is found in cultures throughout Southeast Asia from Neolithic Age in Yangshao culture (currently China and Taiwan). Hemp fibers are used in fabrics and shoes. There is evidence that hemp was considered to be one of the "five grains" of China and thus a major food crop.

Scythians used hemp during funeral rites (*see* Hemp).

3200 BC
Ancient Aryans migrate from Indus Valley, bringing cannabis to people of Assyria, Europe, and Africa. Assyrians begin cultivating cannabis.

2737 BC
First written documentation of medical use of cannabis is found in *Pen Ts'ao Ching*, an ancient book of Chinese medicinal practices. Hemp is recommended for treating numerous aliments including gout, malaria, and rheumatism (*see* Hemp; Medical Uses).

2000–800 BC
Sacred texts of Hinduism discuss cannabis as a medicine and a "source of happiness" and "bringer of freedom" (*see* Ancient Religions).

Bhang (a mixture of marijuana, milk, kusha grass, sugar, fruit, and spices) is used in India and South Asia as an anti-phlegmatic and anesthetic.

Cannabis use spreads from Asia to Europe, Middle East, and Africa.

500–200 BC
Cannabis is burned during funeral rites of shaman in China and Siberia. Egyptians use cannabis to treat inflammation and other ailments. Greek and Roman civilizations use cannabis to soothe pain and inflammation.

440 BC
Herodotus writes in *Histories* that cannabis is smoked for spiritual and recreational purposes in Greece, Western Asia, and Northern Africa and that people smoking marijuana "howl with pleasure."

400 BC
Hashish oil is used throughout the Middle East and much of Asia.

70 AD
Roman medical texts list cannabis as a cure for earaches; a means of suppressing sexual desire; and as a useful treatment for gout, arthritis, and general pain.

800–900
Use of cannabis for treating migraines, pain, and syphilis is common throughout Middle East, Eastern Europe, and North Africa.

900–1100
Cannabis use spreads to Western Europe. German philosopher Hildegard Von Bingen describes cannabis as a miracle herb in *Physica* in 1101.

1300–1400
Pipes are used to smoke marijuana in Ethiopia and use of cannabis spreads to central and southern Africa (*see* Africa).

1400–1500
The English document numerous medicinal uses of marijuana, including as treatment for cramps, rheumatism, gout, insomnia, and convulsions.

1545
Cannabis is brought to western hemisphere by Spaniards.

1585
First documented use of marijuana in East Africa (*see* Africa).

1600s
Laws requiring farmers to grow hemp are passed in Massachusetts and Connecticut. Hemp is exchanged as legal tender in Pennsylvania, Virginia, and Maryland.

1619
Virginia Assembly passes legislation requiring farmers to grow hemp.

1700s
Hemp is regularly grown for textiles, sails, and rope.

1700–1800
Marijuana is used by slaves in Caribbean, South America, and the United States.

1765
George Washington, who cultivated hemp on his planation at Mount Vernon, writes about the potential medicinal uses of marijuana in his journals. Thomas Jefferson and James Monroe similarly grow hemp on their plantations. Personal correspondence suggests these American Presidents may have used the drug recreationally (*see* American Presidents).

1809
President James Madison reportedly smokes marijuana (*see* American Presidents).

1829
President Andrew Jackson reportedly smokes marijuana (*see* American Presidents).

1830
Municipal Council of Rio de Janeiro bans all cannabis imports to the city and prohibits the use of cannabis by slaves.

1830s
Sir William Brooke O'Shaughnessy finds cannabis extracts can reduce pain and vomiting in cholera patients.

1840
Marijuana is widely accepted in western mainstream medicine, joining long-standing practices in medicinal practices in Asia and Africa.

1850s
Marijuana is added to the U.S. Pharmacopoeia as treatment for opioid withdrawal, relief of nausea, appetite stimulation, and treatment of mild pain.

Marijuana is introduced to Africa's Congo Basin by merchants from east and southern Africa.

1860s
Hashish candy is widely available in the United States and Europe.

1860s–1900
Domestic production of hemp flourishes until other materials replace hemp for production of rope, sails, and other products.

1880s–1900
Marijuana extracts are common ingredient in numerous medicines sold in pharmacies and by physicians in Europe and the United States.

1890s
Recreational hashish use becomes increasingly common in France and, to a lesser extent, the United States.

1906
Pure Food and Drug Act is passed, requiring drugs meet purity levels established by the United States Pharmacopoeia or National Formulary and that all ingredients be clearly and accurately labeled on a drug's packaging.

1910
Following the Mexican Revolution, immigrants fleeing the violence come to the United States, reintroducing the recreational use of marijuana.

Marijuana becomes associated with immigrants, and anti-marijuana campaigns warn about the "Marijuana Menace" and the alleged violence associated with its use.

1911
Massachusetts requires prescription for sales of hemp.

1914
Harrison Narcotic Tax Act of 1914 is passed requiring licensing of distributors; detailed records of trade and production; and taxation on production, importation, manufacturing, compounding, selling, and distribution of opium or coca and their derivatives. The act serves as the basis for U.S. Federal laws until 1970 and marks the beginning of the criminalization of addiction in American society.

1915–1933
Twenty-nine states pass laws criminalizing marijuana.

1925
Mexico prohibits the exportation of marijuana to the United States following the International Opium Conference.

1930
Federal Bureau of Narcotics is created. Harry J Anslinger is appointed as Commissioner and serves in that role until 1962 (*see* Anslinger, Harry).

1930s
Federal Bureau of Narcotics launches a major anti-marijuana campaign in the popular press (*see* Anti-Marijuana Campaigns in Popular Press).

1934
Due to lack of restrictions in the Harrison Act, the Uniform State Narcotic Drug Act makes laws uniform across states with respect to policing the sale and use of "narcotic drugs." *Cannabis indica* and *Cannabis sativa* are defined as "narcotic drugs" and considered "habit-forming drugs" along with coca and opium (*see Cannabis indica*; *Cannabis sativa*).

1936
Anti-marijuana movie *Refer Madness*, produced by George Hirlman and directed by Louis Gasnier, is released (*see Reefer Madness*)

1937
Marijuana Tax Act of 1937 is passed. Act places a tax on the sale of marijuana (*see* Marihuana Tax Act).

1942
Marijuana is removed from the U.S. Pharmacopoeia. Physicians begin to question and discredit the medicinal use of marijuana.

As part of the "Hemp for Victory" program, the United States Department of Agriculture distributes hemp seeds and offers draft deferments to famers willing to grow hemp, leading to over 375,000 acres of hemp being cultivated by 1943 (*see* Hemp).

1944

The New York Academy of Medicine publishes the La Guardia Report, which states marijuana is a mild intoxicant and does not induce violence, hypersexuality, insanity, or addiction to other drugs.

1951

Boggs Act passes, amending the Narcotic Drugs Import and Export Act and setting mandatory sentences for drug convictions, including 2–10 years imprisonment and up to a $20,000 fine for marijuana possession.

1956

Narcotics Control Act passes, amending the 1956 Internal Revenue Code and the Narcotic Drugs Import and Export Act. The act specifies penalties for the unlawful acquisition and transportation of marijuana, sets mandatory sentences for drug convictions, denies probation and parole for offenders, and allows for the death penalty for those convicted of distributing narcotics to minors.

1950s

Beat subculture promotes drug use, including marijuana use, claiming use promotes creativity (*see* Beat Generation Writers).

1955

Allen Ginsberg's poem "Howl" released. The poem, considered by some as one of the great works of American literature, critiques American society and openly discusses drug use and sex (see "Howl").

1957

520 copies of Allen Ginsberg's "Howl" being shipped from England are seized by custom officials because its discussion of illicit drug use and sexual practices were deemed obscene. Publisher Lawrence Ferlingheti ultimately wins the case, though, as the poem is seen as having redeeming societal importance (*see* Beat Generation Writers; "Howl").

1960

Drug use in general, and marijuana use specifically, gains popularity among youth in the United States and Europe. Marijuana becomes increasingly popular among counterculture of college students, anti-war activists, and hippies (*see* Hippies).

1965

Jerome "Jerry" Garcia forms the acid-rock band The Grateful Dead (*see* Garcia, Jerry).

Reggae legend Bob Marley releases first album, *The Wailing Wailers* (*see* Marley, Bob).

1966

Beatles *Revolver* album released (*see* Beatles, The).

Allen Ginsburg publishes "The Great Marijuana Hoax" (*see* Beat Generation Writers).

Narcotic Addict Rehabilitation Act passes, allowing drug users to seek rehabilitation without receiving a criminal record.

1968

Drug Abuse Control Act (DACA) of 1965 is amended. DACA differentiates between "possession," which was a misdemeanor, and "manufacturing and distributing," which were felonies. The 1968 DACA amendment allows for criminal sentences to be suspended and records to be expunged if no further drug violations occur within one year of conviction.

1969

Marijuana Tax Act is ruled unconstitutional as violating the Fifth Amendment in *Leary v United States*. This ruling helps lead to the drafting of the Controlled Substance Act as Title II in the Comprehensive Drug Abuse Prevention and Control Act of 1970 (*see* Comprehensive Drug Abuse Prevention and Control Act; Marihuana Tax Act).

Woodstock music festival is held from August 15 to 18, 1969, in Bethel, New York. Over 400,000 attend the three-day event in which marijuana and other drugs are commonly and openly used by concertgoers (*see* Woodstock).

Operation Intercept is launched by President Nixon's administration. The initiative is designed to reduce the transnational shipment of marijuana between Mexico and the United States. It runs from September 21 to October 11, 1969, and results in a near shutdown of border crossings from Mexico to the United States.

1970

The Comprehensive Drug Abuse Prevention and Control Act passes and reorients the United States' approach to drug control. Title II, known as the Controlled Substance Act, creates drug schedules that classify drugs into five categories based on the drug's medical utility and potential for abuse. Marijuana is classified as a Schedule I drug along with heroin, LSD, methaqualone, and peyote. Schedule I drugs are drugs considered to have no accepted medical use and a high potential for abuse (*see* Comprehensive Drug Abuse Prevention and Control Act).

National Organization for the Reform of Marijuana Laws (NORML) is founded to lobby for reforming and liberalizing state and federal marijuana laws (*see* National Organization for the Reform of Marijuana Laws).

1971

President Richard Nixon declares drug abuse "public enemy number one" and launches the "War on Drugs" (*see* Nixon Administration "War on Drugs").

Teenage boys in California allegedly use the code name "420" to refer to marijuana for the first time (*see* 420).

1972

National Commission on Marijuana and Drug Abuse, better known as the Shafer Commission, releases "Marijuana: A Signal of Misunderstanding." The report recommends lessening penalties for possession of marijuana.

National Institute on Drug Abuse (NIDA) is formed (*see* National Institute on Drug Abuse).

1973

Drug Enforcement Administration (DEA) is created by the Nixon administration to consolidate and coordinate the government's drug control efforts. The DEA merges Bureau of Narcotics and Dangerous Drugs and Office of Drug Abuse Law Enforcement (*see* Drug Enforcement Administration).

Texas revises law so that possession of four ounces of marijuana or less is a misdemeanor offense.

Oregon becomes first state to decriminalize cannabis. Possession of up to one ounce of marijuana results in a $100 fine (*see* Decriminalization).

1974

High Times, a popular magazine dedicated to marijuana news, culture, and legalization, is founded (*see High Times*).

1975

Monitoring the Future: A Continuing Study of American Youth (MTF) begins collecting data. The nationally representative sample of high school students has been collected annually. The sample was initially limited to high school seniors, but has included eighth and tenth grades since 1991.

Alaska, Maine, Colorado, California, and Ohio decriminalize marijuana (*see* Alaska; California; Colorado; Decriminalization).

1976

Monitoring the Future reports that 44.5 percent of high school seniors had used marijuana in the past year.

Minnesota decriminalizes marijuana.

Coffeeshops open in Amsterdam (*see* Coffeeshops).

Tom Petty and the Heartbreakers release debut album (*see* Petty, Tom).

1977

Mississippi, New York, and North Carolina decriminalize marijuana (*see* Decriminalization).

President Carter delivers "Drug Abuse Message to Congress" (*see* "Drug Abuse Message to Congress").

1978

President Carter creates the Compassionate Investigational New Drug Program to provide cannabis to select patients.

Nebraska decriminalizes marijuana (*see* Decriminalization).

New Mexico passes Controlled Substance Therapeutic Research Act, becoming first state to formally recognize medical utility of marijuana (*see* Medical Marijuana and the Law).

Comedians Cheech and Chong release *Up in Smoke* (*see* Cheech and Chong).

1979

Over 50 percent of high school seniors report using marijuana annually in the Monitoring the Future dataset. This is the highest rate recorded since these data began being collected in 1975.

Virginia allows doctors to recommend cannabis to glaucoma patients and those suffering from side effects of chemotherapy.

1981

Recreational marijuana use peaks in the United States as highest rates since criminalization are recorded.

1982

First Lady Nancy Reagan starts the "Just Say No" campaign (*see* Reagan Administration "War on Drugs").

1983

The Drug Abuse Resistance Education (DARE) program is established (*see* Drug Abuse Resistance Education).

1986

Anti-Drug Abuse Act of 1986 is passed by Congress and enacted by Reagan administration. The act increases penalties for drug possession and establishes mandatory minimum sentences (*see* Anti-Drug Abuse Acts of 1986 and 1988).

1988

Anti-Drug Abuse Act of 1988 is passed by Congress and enacted by Reagan Administration. The law revises mandatory minimum sentences for drug possession and establishes the Office of National Drug Control Policy (*see* Anti-Drug Abuse Acts of 1986 and 1988; Office of National Drug Control Policy).

Hip-hop band Cypress Hill is founded (*see* Cypress Hill).

1989

President George H. W. Bush launches Operation Green Merchant to disrupt businesses selling horticultural equipment used to grow marijuana (*see* Bush [George H.W.] Administration "War on Drugs").

1990

Alaska uses voter initiative to recriminalize possession of marijuana.

1991

U.S. Department of Justice initiates Weed and Seed program to combat drug use, drug trafficking, and violent crime (*see* Weed and Seed Programs).

1992

Rates of marijuana use fall to lowest levels since widespread data collection efforts began in early 1970s. Only 21.9 percent of high school seniors report annual use of marijuana, down from the peak of 50.8 percent recorded in 1979.

First medical marijuana dispensary opens in California (*see* Dispensaries).

1993

President Clinton admits to smoking marijuana recreationally, famously claiming he did not enjoy it and never inhaled (*see* American Presidents; Clinton, Bill).

Movie *Dazed and Confused* is released (*see Dazed and Confused*).

Snoop Dogg's debut studio album, *Doggystyle*, is released, launching the rapper and multimedia superstar's career (*see* Snoop Dogg).

1994

The Violent Crime Control and Law Enforcement Act of 1994 is passed by Congress and adopted by the Clinton administration. While focused primarily on violent crime, the act also made drug testing mandatory for those serving on federal supervised release. Some argue the bill significantly contributed to increasing arrests of drug offenders guilty of minor marijuana offenses, which significantly contributed to mass incarceration (*see* Clinton, Bill; Incarceration Rates).

1995

Marijuana Policy Project is founded (*see* Marijuana Policy Project).

1996

California's Proposition 215, also known as the Compassionate Use Act of 1996, passes, making California the first state to legalize marijuana for medicinal use by people suffering from severe or chronic illnesses (*see* California; Compassionate Use Act; Medical Marijuana and the Law).

1998

Oregon, Alaska, Washington, and Nevada legalize medical marijuana (*see* Alaska; Medical Marijuana and the Law; Washington State).

The Big Lebowski movie is released (*see Big Lebowski, The*).

Television series *That '70s Show* airs and runs for eight seasons (*see That '70s Show*).

1999

Maine legalizes medical marijuana (*see* Medical Marijuana and the Law).

2000

Colorado, Hawaii, and Nevada legalize the use of medical marijuana (*see* Colorado; Medical Marijuana and the Law).

Drug Policy Alliance is formed (*see* Drug Policy Alliance).

2001

President George W. Bush admits to smoking marijuana recreationally (*see* Bush [George W.] Administration "War on Drugs").

2002
U.S. Supreme Court rules in *Conant v. McCaffrey* that physicians can recommend, but not prescribe, cannabis for medicinal purposes (*see Conant v. McCaffrey*; Medical Marijuana and the Law).

Law Enforcement Action Partnership (LEAP) is founded (*see* Law Enforcement Action Partnership).

2004
Montana and Vermont legalize medical marijuana use for patients with specific conditions (*see* Medical Marijuana and the Law).

2005
U.S. Supreme Court rules in *Gonzalez v Raich* that the production and use of homegrown marijuana was illegal under federal law even if state law allowed its use for medicinal purposes (*see Gonzalez v. Raich*).

Television series *Weeds* airs and runs for eight seasons (*see Weeds*).

2007
New Mexico and Rhode Island legalize medical marijuana, and Vermont expands the use of medical marijuana to permit use for additional medical conditions (*see* Medical Marijuana and the Law).

2008
Michigan legalizes medical marijuana (*see* Medical Marijuana and the Law).

2009
Obama administration releases memo encouraging federal prosecutors to not prosecute people distributing medical marijuana, provided they are in compliance with state and local laws (*see* Obama, Barack).

President Obama admits to using marijuana recreationally, famously saying, "I inhaled. That was the point" (*see* American Presidents; Obama, Barack).

New Jersey legalizes medical marijuana (*see* Medical Marijuana and the Law).

2010
Arizona and District of Columbia legalizes medical marijuana (*see* Medical Marijuana and the Law).

2011
Delaware and Montana legalize medical marijuana (*see* Medical Marijuana and the Law).

2012
Colorado and Washington becomes first states to legalize the recreational use of marijuana (*see* Colorado; Recreational Marijuana Laws; Washington State).

2013
New Hampshire legalizes medical marijuana, and Illinois allows the compassionate use of medical marijuana (*see* Medical Marijuana and the Law).

2014

Alaska, Oregon, and District of Columbia legalize recreational marijuana (*see* Alaska; Oregon; Recreational Marijuana Laws; Washington D.C.).

Minnesota and New York legalize medical marijuana (*see* Medical Marijuana and the Law).

2016

California, Massachusetts, and Nevada legalize recreational marijuana (*see* California; Recreational Marijuana Laws).

Arkansas, Florida, North Dakota, Ohio, and Pennsylvania legalize medical marijuana (*see* Medical Marijuana and the Law).

2017

West Virginia legalizes medical marijuana (*see* Medical Marijuana and the Law).

2018

Trump administration reverses Obama administration's policy related to enforcing federal marijuana laws in states and localities that have legalized marijuana (*see* Trump, Donald).

Vermont legalizes recreational marijuana use (*see* Recreational Marijuana Laws).

Oklahoma legalizes medical marijuana (*see* Medical Marijuana and the Law).

2019

U.S. House of Representatives approves Marijuana Opportunity Reinvestment and Expungement Act (MORE) of 2019 that calls for marijuana to be decriminalized at the federal level and removed from Schedule I of the Controlled Substance Act (*see* Marijuana Opportunity Reinvestment and Expungement Act of 2019).

Alaska becomes first state to allow on-site consumption of marijuana at sale location (*see* Alaska).

2020

New Jersey, Vermont, Arizona, and Montana legalize recreational marijuana. South Dakota legalizes both medical and recreational marijuana (*see* Recreational Marijuana Laws).

A

Africa

Although marijuana is not indigenous to Africa, it is one of the most commonly and widely consumed drugs on the continent; it is both cultivated and grows in the wild. An estimated 38,000 tons of cannabis is produced in Africa each year, making the continent a prime hub for trafficking.

ORIGINS OF CANNABIS IN AFRICA

Cannabis was originally introduced to the continent from southern Asia. Evidence suggests that cannabis existed on the continent in the fifteenth century, with rapid dispersal throughout the rest of Africa occurring in the 1500s. Some scholars suggest that the cultivation of cannabis was introduced to Africa from India by Islamic Sufi mystics. Other scholars suggest that it was introduced by Arab or Chinese merchants and travelers and that knowledge of its uses spread around the world—including Africa—along more than one path. Evidence suggests that cannabis arrived in East Africa from travelers as well as in North Africa through the Mediterranean Sea about 1,000 years ago (Duvall 2019).

Archaeobotanical research suggests that the earliest cultivation of marijuana in Africa may have been in Egypt (which included present-day South Sudan). The earliest evidence of African cannabis use outside of Egypt comes from fourteenth-century Ethiopia, where water pipes with traces of marijuana were found by archaeologists (Van Der Merwe 1975). This suggests that the rapid adaptation of marijuana in the rest of the continent may have been through Ethiopia. The plant then dispersed widely throughout the sub-Saharan region by the 1500s. Prior to this, there is no known evidence of widespread use of marijuana in Africa as a medium in religious rituals, for mystical purposes, or in ceremonies as indigenous practices prior to its introduction from Asia. In West Africa, for example, there is no known indigenous name for marijuana. The earliest known documentation of cannabis use in the sub-Saharan region came from European travelers. They first documented its use in East Africa around 1585, in Southern Africa in 1713, and in western Africa in 1803 (Duvall 2014). There is documentation of marijuana presence in Gambia, Liberia, Nigeria, Niger, Senegal, and Sierra Leone by the nineteenth century. However, its presence in Africa predated observations from European travelers.

The introduction of marijuana had a significant impact in Africa. Cultural traditions of marijuana use for religious, medical, and recreational purposes developed throughout the continent. The plant was used widely as a remedy for asthma symptoms. It was also used as a remedy for anthrax, malaria, black fever, dysentery, and other ailments in Zimbabwe and as a cure for snake bites by the Khoikhoi.

Prior to its introduction into Africa, cannabis had largely been taken orally in Asia. Cannabis use merged with an existing smoking tradition in Africa to initiate the practice of smoking marijuana—a method of consumption that spread quickly. Smoking marijuana meant that the pharmacological effects were felt in the body much more quickly and the dosage could be controlled. Therefore, this practice spread quickly between ethnic groups throughout the continent. Smoking marijuana led to the creation of new paraphernalia, such as water pipes, bowls, and other pipe forms. These were made of materials like wood, coconut, stone, bone, bamboo stalks, or pottery.

Smoking transformed a number of cultures in southern Africa by turning the use of marijuana from an individual practice into a communal one. It also encouraged creation of new smoking-related games and religious rituals. In the case of the politico-religious movement Bena Diamba (*diamba* meaning "marijuana" in Central Africa), or "Marijuana Brotherhood," it's also said to have helped the Bashilenge, an ethnic group in Equatorial Guinea that was previously belligerent, convert into a peace-loving one. Smoking and other African marijuana practices eventually became global, spreading worldwide through interactions between enslaved Africans, nomadic groups, traders, and other non-African travelers.

RACISM-TINGED MYTHS

Many of the early accounts about the impact and usage of marijuana in Africa have been faulted for being inaccurate. The narratives are heavily drawn from European observers who have been criticized by scholars for trafficking in common myths and stereotypes of that period about race and class (Duvall 2019). In reality, these accounts of cannabis use in Africa were oftentimes fictionalized, exaggerated, and rife with racist sentiments. As an example, American explorer and journalist Henry Morton Stanley asserted that marijuana had rendered many Africans useless. His counterpart, British missionary David Livingstone, wrote that watching members of the Bakota ethnic group smoke marijuana left a "feeling of disgust in the spectator" (Clarke and Merlin 2013, 236). European travelers often depicted drug use as racially determined behavior and Africans as inherently inclined to drug use. They also depicted drug use by Africans as "backward," especially in comparison to tobacco use, a common habit of white Europeans that was portrayed as sophisticated and indicative of more refined taste. Their accounts propagated widespread myths about African usage of the plant, which was based on ignorance about motivations for cannabis use in Africa.

ANTI-MARIJUANA LAWS

European colonial governments throughout the continent began to outlaw the use of marijuana in the 1920s, citing negative effects on the productivity of African laborers. Prohibition was met with resistance, though, because marijuana use was embedded into African cultures by that point.

The roots of global prohibition of the drug originated in Africa led by international concerns. Myths about marijuana usage and its perceived effects on Africans led to increased efforts to control it by colonial governments. This was informed by racialized ideas aimed at controlling enslaved Africans, poor whites, Asians, or other laborers who were the drug's primary users. However, cannabis prohibition first appeared at the international level at the 1925 International Opium Convention, where an agreement for cannabis control was signed in Geneva at the insistence of South Africa and Egypt, which had already outlawed marijuana use at home by the 1870s. All colonial governments started prohibiting the drug's use, possession, sale, and cultivation by the 1920s (Abel 1980; Duvall 2017). However, Africans resisted prohibition throughout the continent, and its production continued. For example, evidence suggests that soldiers returning from the World War II were responsible for the resurgence of marijuana use in countries such as Nigeria.

Cannabis cultivation and consumption continued in spite of it being outlawed even after the colonial era ended, as African governments continued to criminalize its use for decades after independence. Even so, the 1970s saw an increase in marijuana tourism in African countries such as Malawi. Marijuana thus remained socially and economically significant in many parts of the continent despite its continued criminalization.

Marijuana is currently criminalized in most African countries. Nonetheless, the continent produces an estimated 38,000 tons of marijuana annually. The World Health Organization estimates South Africa to be the third largest producer of cannabis in the world. However, due to criminalization most marijuana production in Africa is grown illegally (United Nations Office on Drugs and Crime 2018). Countries such as Ghana, Nigeria, Mozambique, and Eswatini are prime distribution points for marijuana. Most production is consumed within the region, with South Africa being a prime destination. Marijuana from countries such as Nigeria, Ghana, South Africa, and Zambia is also exported to Europe. Encouraged by increasing global demand, potential for huge profits, medical usage, Rastafarianism, and marijuana tourism, many African countries are reviewing their marijuana laws (Prohibition Partners 2019). This has already prompted Uganda, Zimbabwe, and Malawi to decriminalize its production for medicinal and industrial use. It is legal and regulated in South African and Lesotho.

Sitinga Kachipande

See also: Religion; Trafficking.

Further Reading

Abel, E. L. *Marijuana the First Twelve Thousand Years Plenum Press.* New York: Plenum Press, 1980.

Asuni, T., and O. A. Pela. "Drug Abuse in Africa." *Bulletin on Narcotics* 38, no. 1 (1986): 55–56.

Clarke, Robert C., and Mark D. Merlin. *Cannabis: Evolution and Ethnobotany.* Los Angeles: University of California Press, 2013.

Duvall, Chirs S. *The African Roots of Marijuana.* Durham, NC: Duke University Press, 2019.

Duvall, Chris S. *Cannabis.* London, UK: Reaktion Books, 2014.

Duvall, Chirs S. "Cannabis and Tobacco in Precolonial and Colonial Africa." In *Oxford Research Encyclopedia of African History.* Oxford, UK: Oxford University Press, 2017.

Hawdon, James. *Drug and Alcohol Consumption as Functions of Social Structures: A Cross-cultural Sociology.* No. 47. Lewistown, NY: Edwin Mellen Press, 2005.

Klantschnig, Gernot, Neil Carrier, and Charles Ambler, eds. *Drugs in Africa: Histories and Ethnographies of Use, Trade, and Control*. New York: Springer, 2014.

Prohibition Partners. *The African Cannabi Report*. London, UK: Prohibition Partners, 2019.

United Nations Office on Drugs and Crime. *World Drug Report: Analysis on Drug Markets: Opiates, Cocaine, Cannabis, Synthetic Drugs*. Vienna, Austria: Division for Policy Analysis and Public Affairs, 2018.

Van der Merwe, Nikolaas J. "Cannabis Smoking in 13th–14th Century Ethiopia: Chemical Evidence." *World Anthropology: Cannabis and Culture* 1 (1975): 77–80.

Age

Medical and recreational marijuana use has become widespread and likely increased the availability of marijuana products (Scheier and Griffin 2020). Substance use is a relatively normative part of the human life course (Patrick et al. 2011), and experimenting with or using marijuana is popular among many age groups (Johnston et al. 2019; National Academies of Sciences, Engineering, and Medicine 2017). Research on marijuana use in the United States provides comprehensive information on national estimates for use, usage patterns, and correlation. According to a 2018 report of the National Institute on Drug Abuse (NIDA), marijuana remains the most commonly used illegal substance in the United States. Marijuana usage rates have grown notably among various adult age groups, especially among young populations (Substance Abuse and Mental Health Services Administration 2019). Especially past month marijuana vaping has increased in popularity among 10th and 12th graders, outpacing daily cigarette use (NIDA 2018).

When it comes to marijuana use, the age of onset (first use of marijuana) is crucial. Survey data on the national and state level estimate that for individuals between 12 and 17 years old, the average age of marijuana initiation is somewhere around 15, and for the overall population, it is less than 19 (Azofeifa et al. 2016). When first use occurs prior to the age of 18, the likelihood of developing marijuana addiction increases notably (Substance Abuse and Mental Health Services Administration 2019). Research shows that early marijuana use is related to more frequent and longer duration of marijuana use throughout life. Early-onset individuals also report using higher amounts of marijuana per week when compared to late onset individuals (Gruber et al. 2012). Research following marijuana use trends among youth has found that those youths who initiated marijuana use in high school or during young adulthood had the highest rates of problematic use in their early twenties (Nelson, Van Ryzin, and Dishion 2015).

The Centers for Disease Control (CDC) reports that individuals age 12 and older perceive marijuana as fairly easy or very easy to obtain (Azofeifa et al. 2016). Changes have also occurred in overall marijuana perception, as an increasing number of young people consider regular marijuana use as a nonrisky behavior (NIDA 2018). These trends are further reflected on user statistics, indicating that a decline in perceived risk is accompanied by an increase in marijuana use rates among adolescents (Johnston et al. 2019). Similar changes in marijuana perception have been observed among other age cohorts: Among women of reproductive age (18–44), about 70 percent believe that there is slim to no risk of harm in using marijuana once or twice a week, whether pregnant or not during the use (Ko et al. 2015). However, marijuana use by women of reproductive age can cause health problems in the user and has risks to the infant (CDC 2018).

Marijuana is most typically used by smoking in hand-rolled cigarettes (i.e., joints) or in pipes. However, marijuana can be also consumed as edibles when mixed in food, such as cookies, brownies, or candies (Cao et al. 2016; NIDA 2018). According to reports to U.S. poison centers, intentional exposure to edible marijuana products is most common among 6- to 19-year-old individuals, with 47 percent of exposures pertaining to this age group. Unintentional exposure to edible marijuana products, on the other hand, is more common among children five years of age or younger, with a rate of 0.15 calls to poison centers per 100,000 population per year, and among teens between 13 and 19 years old, with 0.09 calls to poison centers per 100,000 population per year (Cao et al. 2016). Edible marijuana products might be indistinguishable from their nonmarijuana counterparts, making them appealing and appetizing to small children and young individuals (Cao et al. 2016).

Marijuana use is predominantly common among young individuals between 18 and 25 years of age in the United States (NIDA 2018; Azofeifa et al. 2016). Decreased perception of risk, fewer legal penalties, and increased availability are likely factors when explaining the prevailing marijuana trends and popularity of the product among Americans across age groups (Azofeifa, et al. 2016). However, reasons to initiate and continue marijuana use change with age. While younger individuals more typically associate marijuana use with experimentation, having a good time with friends, or fitting in with a group, older individuals associate marijuana use as a way to get high, to relax, and to decrease the effects of other drugs (Patrick et al. 2011). Marijuana is also used for medical purposes, the most common use for medical marijuana being pain control (Park and Wu 2017). According to a study using a national sample, individuals in the 18–25 age group and those 50 years and older had higher rates of medical marijuana use when compared to adults in the 26–34 and 35–49 age groups (Lin et al. 2016). Another study found a decisive majority (81 percent) of U.S. adults believe that marijuana use has at least one benefit, and in line with medical marijuana use, the most important benefit reported by adults is pain management. Marijuana use is also reported to relieve anxiety, depression, and stress (Keyhani et al. 2018). However, it should be noted that marijuana users are more likely than nonusers to agree with statements indicating that marijuana use has no risks and that marijuana use has benefits (Keyhani et al. 2018).

Marijuana use can have serious short- and long-term effects that manifest in many ways in different individuals. These effects are typically heightened among young users. When initiated during adolescence, marijuana use may impair brain development, learning, and memory functions, reflecting through adult years (NIDA 2018). Among older individuals, marijuana use may increase a variety of mental and physical health problems, including the chance of heart attack. Though much is known about the age-related use of marijuana and its consequences, research on these correlates is continuing, to better understand their complex interactions and effects.

Iina Savolainen

See also: Gender; Race.

Further Reading

Azofeifa, Alejandro, et al. "National Estimates of Marijuana Use and Related Indicators—National Survey on Drug Use and Health, United States, 2002–2014." *Morbidity and Mortality Weekly Report: Surveillance Summaries* 65, no. 11 (2016): 1–25.

Cao, Dazhe, Sahaphume Srisuma, Alvin C. Bronstein, and Christopher O. Hoyte. "Characterization of Edible Marijuana Product Exposures Reported to United States Poison Centers." *Clinical Toxicology* 54, no. 9 (2016): 840–846.

Centers for Disease Control and Prevention (CDC). "What You Need to Know about Marijuana Use and Pregnancy." 2018. https://www.cdc.gov/marijuana/factsheets/pregnancy.htm

Goncy, Elizabeth A., and Sylvie Mrug. "Where and When Adolescents Use Tobacco, Alcohol, and Marijuana: Comparisons by Age, Gender, and Race." *Journal of Studies on Alcohol and Drugs* 74, no. 2 (2013): 288–300.

Gruber, Staci A., et al. "Age of Onset of Marijuana Use and Executive Function." *Psychology of Addictive Behaviors* 26, no. 3 (2012): 496–506.

Johnston, L. D., et al. *Monitoring the Future: National Survey Results on Drug Use 1975–2018: Overview, Key Findings on Adolescent Drug Use.* Ann Arbor: University of Michigan Institute for Social Research, 2019.

Keyhani, Salomeh, et al. "Risks and Benefits of Marijuana Use: A National Survey of U.S. Adults." *Annals of Internal Medicine* 169, no. 5 (2018): 282–290. doi:10.7326/M18-0810

Ko, Jean Y., et al. "Prevalence and Patterns of Marijuana Use among Pregnant and Nonpregnant Women of Reproductive Age." *American Journal of Obstetrics and Gynecology* 213, no. 2 (2015): 201.e1–201.e10.

Lin, L. A., et al. "Comparing Adults Who Use Cannabis Medically with Those Who Use Recreationally." *Addictive Behaviors* no. 61 (2016): 99–103. doi:10.1016/j.addbeh.2016.05.015

National Academies of Sciences, Engineering, and Medicine. *The Health Effects of Cannabis and Cannabinoids.* Washington, DC: The National Academies Press, 2017. doi:10.17226/24625

National Institute on Drug Abuse (NIDA). *Marijuana.* 2018. https://www.drugabuse.gov/publications/drugfacts/marijuana

Nelson, Sarah E., Mark J. Van Ryzin, and Thomas J. Dishion. "Alcohol, Marijuana, and Tobacco Use Trajectories from Age 12 to 24 Years: Demographic Correlates and Young Adult Substance Use Problems." *Development and Psychopathology* 27, no. 1 (2015): 253–277.

Park, Ji-Yeun, and Li-Tzy Wu. "Prevalence, Reasons, Perceived Effects, and Correlates of Medical Marijuana Use: A Review." *Drug and Alcohol Dependence* 177 (2017): 1–13. doi:10.1016/j.drugalcdep.2017.03.009

Patrick, Megan E., et al. "Age-related Changes in Reasons for Using Alcohol and Marijuana from Ages 18 to 30 in a National Sample." *Psychology of Addictive Behaviors* 25, no. 2 (2011): 330.

Scheier, Lawrence M., and Kenneth W. Griffin. "Youth Marijuana Use: A Review of Causes and Consequences." *Current Opinion in Psychology* (2020): 11–18. doi.org/10.1016/j.copsyc.2020.06.007

Substance Abuse and Mental Health Services Administration (SAMHSA). *Know the Risks of Marijuana.* 2019. https://www.samhsa.gov/marijuana

Alaska

Alaska was the second state in the United States to decriminalize cannabis (marijuana) use. A $100 fine for possession of small amounts of cannabis was imposed in 1975, effectively decriminalizing the use of marijuana. That same year, the Alaskan Supreme Court ruled adults had the right to possess and consume small amounts of cannabis. Years later in 1982, the monetary fine for possessing cannabis was removed, and the Alaskan state legislature decriminalized the possession of up to four ounces of cannabis within the home and one ounce outside the home. However, cannabis was not yet legalized in the state (Weedmaps n.d.).

While Alaska was a pioneer in the decriminalization of cannabis, legislators were pressured to take a firmer approach to the use of cannabis following several high-profile incidents of individuals involved in automobile accidents while intoxicated on cannabis. Indeed, in 1990 a law was passed that reversed prior rulings and recriminalized the possession of small amounts of marijuana. However, in 1998, the pendulum once again swung, and Alaska legalized the medical use of cannabis with the passage of the Alaska Medical Marijuana Initiative, which was supported by 58 percent of Alaska voters. More than a decade later, in November 2014, Alaska became the third state in the United States to legalize the production, sale, and use of recreational cannabis by adults 21 years of age or older. The law permitted Alaskan adults to possess up to one ounce of cannabis and up to six marijuana plants, as long as three or fewer were mature and flowering. Cultivation of cannabis is legal in Alaska as long as individuals cultivate the plant for noncommercial purposes. However, the cultivation must be outside public view, and cultivators are responsible for securing their marijuana plants to maintain public safety (Potguide.com n.d.).

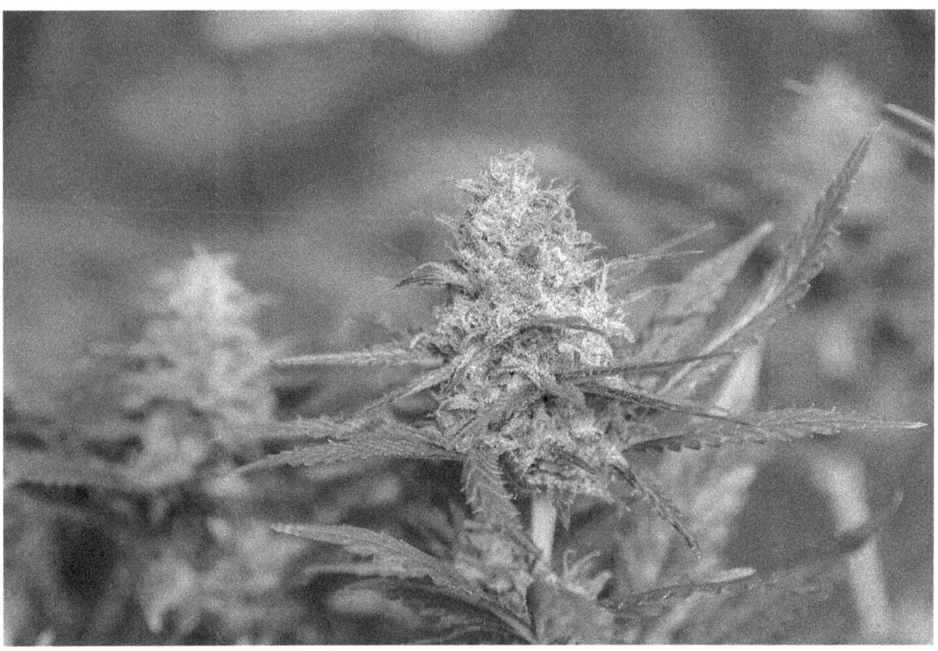

Alaskan purple variety of marijuana. Alaska legalized recreational cannabis use in 2014. (Michael Nosek/Dreamstime.com)

Punishments for violating Alaskan cannabis laws vary in severity. If an individual possesses between one and four ounces of marijuana, they may be punished by up to one year imprisonment and/or a fine up to $10,000. Possession of between one and four ounces of cannabis, including possession with the intent to distribute, is considered a Class A misdemeanor. Possession, as well as possession with the intent to distribute, of more than four ounces of marijuana constitutes a Class C felony, and the possible punishments include up to five years imprisonment and/or a $50,000 fine. Likewise, possession of more than four ounces of marijuana near school grounds or youth centers constitutes a Class C felony (NORML n.d.).

Continuing to blaze a trail in legal cannabis use, in 2019 Alaska became the first state in which consumers of marijuana can buy and consume their cannabis at the same location. While numerous states previously allowed licensed storefront dispensaries to regulate the sale of cannabis, Alaska was the first to issue permits for on-site consumption. Cannabis consumption areas must remain physically apart from retail areas under the newly passed legislation, and adequate ventilation is required for businesses that allow on-site smoking. Local governments, however, retain the power to prohibit on-site consumption or impose specific regulations. Outdoor smoking of marijuana remains illegal in Alaska (Roberts 2019).

Matthew Costello

See also: California; Colorado; Decriminalization; Taxation; Vermont; Washington D.C.; Washington State.

Further Reading

National Organization for the Reform of Marijuana Laws (NORML). "Alaska Laws and Penalties." n.d. Accessed August 20, 2021. https://norml.org/laws/item/alaska-penalties

Potguide.com. "Alaska Marijuana Laws." n.d. Accessed August 20, 2021. https://potguide.com/alaska/marijuana-laws/

Roberts, Chris. "Alaska Is Officially the First State to License On-Site Marijuana Consumption at Cannabis Stores." *Marijuana Moment*, March 13, 2019. https://www.marijuanamoment.net/alaska-is-officially-the-first-state-to-legalize-on-site-marijuana-consumption/

Weedmaps. "Learn Laws and Regulations: Alaska." n.d. Accessed August 20, 2021. https://weedmaps.com/learn/laws-and-regulations/alaska/

American Presidents

At least 11 U.S. presidents used marijuana medicinally or recreationally. In early America, George Washington (1732–1799) grew hemp and cultivated marijuana for its medicinal purposes. Thomas Jefferson (1743–1826) also grew hemp and smoked it to treat his migraine headaches. James Madison (1751–1836), James Monroe (1758–1831), Andrew Jackson (1767–1845), Zachary Taylor (1784–1850), Franklin Pierce (1804–1869), and Abraham Lincoln (1809–1865) also reportedly smoked marijuana. In more recent years, Bill Clinton (1946–), George W. Bush (1946–), and Barack Obama (1961–) admitted to smoking marijuana recreationally. Today, the stance on marijuana legalization is often a part of presidential candidates' platforms.

In his diary, George Washington wrote that he intentionally grew marijuana with a high tetrahydrocannabinol (THC) content to be used medicinally. Scholars believe that Washington used marijuana for his toothaches. Washington also gifted "smoking blends" of marijuana to Thomas Jefferson. Jefferson, who also used marijuana medicinally, reciprocated by sending his own special marijuana blends to Washington. Andrew Jackson, Zachary Taylor, and Franklin Pierce reportedly enjoyed smoking marijuana with their troops. Abraham Lincoln grew up smoking marijuana rather than tobacco because the latter was more expensive. He reportedly said that "he liked nothing better than sitting on his front porch smoking from his hemp pipe" (Deitch 2003).

In 1992, presidential candidate Bill Clinton admitted that he tried, but "didn't inhale," marijuana in his youth. Clinton's successor, George W. Bush, also admitted to experimenting with marijuana (and to inhaling). By this time, however, smoking marijuana had become less of a taboo to the American public. Before he was officially a presidential candidate, Barack Obama was asked if he inhaled when he smoked marijuana as a youth. He responded, "When I was a kid, I inhaled. That was the point." Obama's admission received even less negative attention than Bush's.

Despite its use by several early and more recent presidents, many presidents took official stances opposing the use of marijuana and pursued policies that criminalized it at the federal level. For example, Franklin Roosevelt (1882–1945) adopted the Uniform State Narcotic Act in 1932. This law encouraged states to criminalize and regulate marijuana use. He also signed the Marijuana Tax Act of 1937 into law. Similarly, Harry S. Truman (1884–1972) signed the Boggs Act into law in 1952, and Dwight D. Eisenhower (1890–1969) signed the Narcotics Control Act of 1956. These acts set mandatory sentences for drug-related offenses, including marijuana offenses, for which a first offense for possession could result in a minimum sentence of 2–10 years and a fine of up to $20,000.

In 1971, President Richard Nixon (1913–1994) declared a "War on Drugs." This led to increased penalties for marijuana charges, including longer mandatory minimum sentences and the "three strikes rule." During his presidency, marijuana was labeled a Schedule I narcotic along with drugs like heroin. Nixon was vehemently against marijuana use and used it to disparage anti-Vietnam War protestors, who he claimed were "all on drugs" (Lee 2012). In 1980, presidential candidate Ronald Reagan (1911–2004) claimed that marijuana was "probably the most dangerous drug in America" (Gerber 2004). Once in office, his wife, Nancy Reagan (1921–2016), began the "Just Say No" campaign, which aimed to discourage children from using drugs, particularly marijuana. Reagan's successor, George H. W. Bush, continued the crusade against marijuana by reinvigorating the War on Drugs. The Obama administration, however, adopted the policy of not interfering with the distribution of medical or recreational marijuana in states that had legalized its use at the state level, despite the drug remaining a Schedule I drug at the federal level. President Donald Trump (1946–), the first president since George H. W. Bush to deny ever smoking marijuana, has taken a more laissez-faire approach to the legalization debate than most of his fellow Republicans. He argues that marijuana legalization should be left up to the states.

Amanda M. Burroughs

See also: Colonial America; Reagan Administration "War on Drugs."

Further Reading

Deitch, Robert. *Hemp—American History Revisited: The Plant with a Divided History*. New York: Algora Publishing, 2003.

Gerber, Rudolph Joseph. *Legalizing Marijuana: Drug Policy Reform and Prohibition Politics*. Westport, CT: Greenwood Publishing Group, 2004.

Gonzalez, Jay, and Mickey P. McGee, eds. *Legal Marijuana: Perspectives on Public Benefits, Risks and Policy Approaches*. Jefferson, NC: McFarland, 2019.

Hudak, John. *Marijuana—A Short History*. Washington, DC: Brookings Institution Press, 2016.

Lee, Martin A. *Smoke Signals: A Social History of Marijuana—Medical, Recreational and Scientific*. New York: Simon and Schuster, 2012.

Ancient Religions

Cannabis was a staple of the ancient Eurasian world. This ancient world, much like today, had a fixation on death and gods and how to communicate with these entities. Cannabis became an important tool in these efforts for some ancient civilizations.

Cannabis was first cultivated in the Neolithic period (4500–2000 BCE) but was not used religiously until 2000 BCE, when it was used by Chinese shamans to talk to the dead and help them cross over to the afterlife. It was later used in China as both a medicine and religious tool.

Ancient cannabis has also been found in northern Europe, where the Vikings and Germanic tribes used it in ceremonies to contact the dead. Northern Europeans also used cannabis for love charms and to gain the favor of gods.

The use of mind-altering substances is not a modern idea; it is an ancient one. Mind-altering substances have been used in religious ceremonies, rites of passages, love charms, and even rituals of war. Cannabis is the most common of these mind-altering substances in the Eurasian world. Cannabis has been used as a fiber, medicine, magic, and a religious substance across Europe and Asia since the beginning of agriculture. The cultivation of cannabis dates back to the Neolithic period in northern China (McClain 2016), where it was so commonplace that the region was commonly referred to as the "land of mulberry and hemp" (McClain 2016). Cannabis was first used as a fiber and was later ritualistically used in funeral attire. The first recorded use of cannabis as an internal medicine dates to around 4000 BCE; however, it was not until 2000 BCE that shamans in China began ingesting cannabis ritualistically (McClain 2016). According to ancient Chinese (pre-Shang dynasty) manuscripts, these shamans drank a cannabis-infused beverage to help souls of the dead cross over to the afterlife.

Throughout history, cannabis also has been associated with death and death cults. One example of this phenomenon comes from the Scythians (Eurasian nomads who existed as early as the ninth century BCE until the second century CE) and their cult of the dead. After a Scythian leader died, the body was taken on a tour of the region and was buried. When the burial was completed, tepee-like structures were built to allow mourners to gather inside and stoke fires, where hemp seeds were thrown on the coals or cooked in vessels. The mourners inhaled the vapors from these seeds in the belief that the ensuing out-of-body experiences would help cleanse their souls and minds. This activity was recorded in the Histories of Herodotus (verses 73–75), but for many years was discounted as an exaggeration until excavations of Scythian sites took place in 2013 at Sengileevskoe (a Russian city). Archeologists found a black sticky substance in vessels—a substance that was later found to be a mixture of cannabis and opium (Graham 2015).

The mixing of drugs (e.g., cannabis and opium) in the ancient world was not exclusive to the Scythians. The Hindus, both modern and ancient, partook of a drink called bhang (McClain 2016). Bhang is primarily made of cannabis but also contains poppy seeds, cloves, cinnamon, and milk. Bhang was drunk during the Festival of Holi and on the Night of Shivratri, which is celebrated in honor of Lord Shiva who is the Lord of Bhang (McClain 2016). Bhang was ingested in other regions outside of India including Persia (within modern-day Iran). The Sufi order, located in Persia, was a mystic sect of Islam that used cannabis to make hashish. Hashish is a smokable paste made from the resin found in the flowers of the cannabis plant. Hashish contains up to four times as much THC (the principal psychoactive compound in marijuana) as marijuana and thus is a more potent compound. Subsects of the Sufi order called themselves the Hashishin, which comes from the root word hashish. The Hashishin were a notorious assembly of assassins (1090–1275 CE). These assassins were so prolific that the English word "assassin" is believed to have originated from the word "Hashishin." The use of hashish by the assassins, it was believed, allowed the user to enter a mystic trance, which would give the user enhanced abilities (McClain 2016).

In ancient China, medicine and rituals were tightly bound. The Dunhuang Medical Manuscripts (a collection of medieval Chinese manuscripts describing medical and spiritual practices dating from around the fourth century CE) describe both medical and spiritual uses of cannabis. One text of this collection that details the Daoist religion describes a miraculous fragrant pill called miaoziang wan (Lo 2004). These pills are widely believed to be cannabis, used to heal both the body and the spirit. Several ancient manuscripts blur the lines between medicinal and religious uses. Ts'ao Ching (451–536 CE) wrote a work detailing herb use, which describes how the seeds of the plant were used in stories of necromancy and when trying to speak to the dead. Speaking with the dead in this way was a recurring theme in early Chinese culture. Ching wrote, "To take too much makes people see daemons and throw themselves about like maniacs, but if one takes it over a long period of time, one can communicate with the spirits" (Ts'ao Ching, as cited in McClain 2016). Cannabis became sacred in some religions, including Daoism. Daoism is a Chinese religious philosophy of living in harmony with the "way" or "path." One of Daoism's principle deities, Ma Gu, was considered the "hemp maiden" (Ferrara 2016). Another ancient eastern religion, Buddhism, also considered cannabis sacred. According to Tantric Buddhism, Siddhartha Gautama (the primary figure in Buddhism) ate one hemp seed per day in order to achieve enlightenment.

Cannabis use in ritualistic and religious practices is not confined to the East. In the Viking and Germanic world of Northern Europe, cannabis had a similar role, if not an even more mystical one. In this ancient Germanic world, a group of people called the Völur (793–1066 CE) consumed cannabis and other drugs in order to travel between the worlds of the living and the dead. The word "Völur" means wand-carrier or staff bearer (Rysdyk 2016). These wand-carriers were mostly high-status women (with a few men added to their ranks) who were believed to have mystical powers. It was believed, for example, that they could travel into the realm of the spirits by consuming cannabis seeds and henbane, a plant that can cause hallucinations (Rysdyk 2016). Excavations have found these women and men buried with small bags of cannabis and henbane, which were believed to aid in their journeys after death (Brink and Price 2012). Hemps seeds were not just for the dead in the north of Europe, though. The sowing of hemp seeds in these Germanic areas was considered a love charm performed by men, and hemp blossoms were even eaten on Fridays by barren women to gain favor with Feira, the goddess of fertility (Rätsch and Müller-Ebeling 2006).

There are even some residual traditions from these ancient religions that are observed today. One such tradition is the cooking of a traditional Silesian soup with hemp seeds called siemieniotka (Rätsch and Müller-Ebeling 2006). This soup is offered to the family's ancestors on Christmas night. This practice remains today, along with several other cannabis-laced traditions. Bhang, cannabis-infused drink, is still consumed during Hindu religious festivals, and while religion is not at the forefront of many aspects of modern medicine, cannabis is increasingly touted as a plant with pain management benefits and other therapeutic advantages by its proponents.

Ben Stickle and Virginia Benefield

See also: Cannabis Drinks; China and Southeast Asia; Europe; Hashish; Religion.

Further Reading

Brink, Stafan, and Neil Price. "Gods and Humans." In *The Viking World,* edited by Stafan Brink and Neil Price. London: Routledge, 2012, 245–260.

Ferrara, Mark S. 1890 *Sacred Bliss: A Spiritual History of Cannabis*. Lanham, MD: Rowman & Littlefield, 2016.

Graham, Karl. "Ancient Scythians Spread the Use of Cannabis in Death Rituals." *Digital Journal*, May 25, 2015. http://www.digitaljournal.com/science/gold-artifacts-of-ancient-scythians-reveals-bastard-war-and-drugs/article/434123

Hawdon, James. *Drug and Alcohol Consumption as Functions of Social Structures: A Cross-cultural Sociology*. No. 47. Lewistown, NY: Edwin Mellen Press, 2005.

Herodotus. *The History of Herodotus*. Translated by G. C. Macaulay. Whitefish, MT: Kessinger Publishing.

Lo, Vivienne, and Christopher Cullen. *Medieval Chinese Medicine: The Dunhuang Medical Manuscripts*. London: Routledge, 2004, 278–290.

McClain, Matthew Sean. *Herb & Shaman: Recreating the Cannabismythos*. Carpinteria, CA: Pacifica Graduate Institute, 2016.

Rätsch, Christian, and Claudia Müller-Ebeling. *Pagan Christmas: The Plants, Spirits, and Rituals at the Origins of Yuletide*. New York: Simon and Schuster, 2006.

Rysdyk, Evelyn C. *The Norse Shaman: Ancient Spiritual Practices of the Northern Tradition*. New York: Simon and Schuster, 2016.

Anslinger, Harry (1892–1975)

Harry Jacob Anslinger (1892–1975) was the first commissioner of the Federal Bureau of Narcotics (FBN) and was influential in shaping public opinion about marijuana in the 1930s.

Anslinger was born on May 20, 1892 in Altoona, Pennsylvania, to Robert John and Christina Fladtt Anslinger, both immigrants from Switzerland. Harry Anslinger grew up with glimpses of drug addiction. For example, when he was twelve years old, he was told to go buy morphine to save his neighbor's life. At the time he did not know what morphine was and was unaware of the concept of addiction, but he recognized that the woman was screaming in pain until she received her morphine (Carroll 2004).

Anslinger attended Pennsylvania State College (now Pennsylvania State University) from 1913 to 1915 and also obtained an LLB from American University in 1930. After graduating from Pennsylvania State, Anslinger held many different jobs requiring sensitivity and diplomacy with the U.S. government from 1918 until his retirement in 1963. These positions included consular posts (1918–1926), Chief of the Division of Foreign Control for the Treasury Department (1926–1929), assistant commissioner of prohibition (1929–1930), and Commissioner of the Bureau of Narcotics (1930–1963).

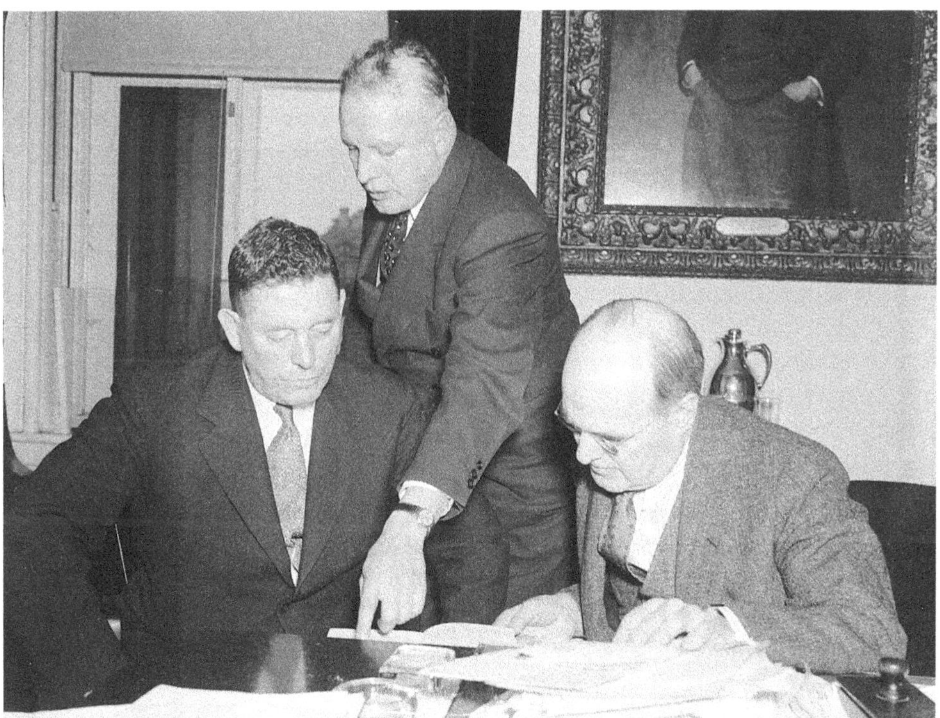

Harry Anslinger was the first Commissioner of the Federal Bureau of Narcotics. He is known for his anti-marijuana campaign of the 1930s that resulted in the Marihuana Tax Act. He served as Commissioner from 1930 to 1962. (Library of Congress)

Anslinger remains best known for his tenure as Commissioner of the Bureau of Narcotics, which made him the chief American law enforcement officer on drugs. The Federal Narcotics Bureau had been created in 1930, when only 16 states had laws outlawing marijuana—and none of them were doing much to enforce those laws (Armstrong and Parascandola 1972). Prior to the creation of the Federal Narcotics Bureau, marijuana was not considered an issue even worth mentioning, let alone pouring resources into. In fact, prior to 1936 Anslinger and the FBN thought of it mainly as a "nuisance drug" and regarded heroin as the most dangerous drug of all (Carroll 2004, 68).

Anslinger and the FBN drastically changed their stances on marijuana in early 1936, however. In January 1936, a bill known as the Secret Service Reorganization Act was introduced that would have forced Anslinger out of his position and dissolved the FBN (Carroll 2004). This political pressure led Anslinger to launch a campaign to save the bureau and his position, and one of his main tactics in this regard was to fabricate or exaggerate horror stories connecting marijuana use and crime (Carroll 2004). Anslinger was also associated with the creation of several educational films and articles about marijuana such as *Assassin of Youth*, *Marihuana, the Weed with Roots in Hell*, and *Tell your Children* (also known as *Reefer Madness*) (Boyd 2009; Becker 1963). These works depicted marijuana as an assassin of youthful innocence and health, and they breathlessly recounted examples of heinous crimes that had supposedly been committed by people under the influence of marijuana (Armstrong and Parascandola 1972). According to this propaganda, marijuana use could cause people to go insane, hallucinate, and even kill other people. The most famous article is one of a young man in Florida who killed his whole family with an ax after smoking marijuana (Cooper and Anslinger 1937). Popular journals, including medical journals, responded to this surge of stories about marijuana by dramatically increasing their coverage of marijuana as well (Armstrong and Parascandola 1972; Becker 1963).

Anslinger's campaign saved the bureau and his own career, became a springboard for new laws designed to stamp out marijuana use, and did much to establish pot as a dark and threatening drug in American popular opinion (Armstrong and Parascandola 1972; Nicholas and Churchill 2012). Despite the lack of scientific or medical evidence to support the claims, these horror stories were presented to Congress, and they directly contributed to the passage of a variety of antidrug laws, including the Marihuana Tax Act of 1937, the Boggs Act of 1951, and the Narcotics Control Act of 1956.

Alexandria Goldstein and Richard Stringer

See also: Anti-Marijuana Campaigns in Popular Press; Drug Abuse Resistance Education (DARE); Drug Policy Alliance (DPA); Moral Panics; *Reefer Madness*.

Further Reading

Armstrong, William D., and John Parascandola. "American Concern over Marihuana in the 1930's." *Pharmacy in History* 14, no. 1 (1972): 25–35.

Becker, Howard S. *Outsiders: Studies in the Sociology of Deviance*. New York: Free Press of Glencoe, 1963.

Boyd, Susan C. *Hooked: Drug War Films in Britain, Canada, and the United States*. Toronto: University of Toronto Press, 2009.

Carroll, Rebecca. "Under the Influence: Harry Anslinger's Role in Shaping America's Drug Policy." In *Federal Drug Control: The Evolution of Policy and Practice*, edited by Jonathon Erlen and Joseph Spillane. Binghamton, NY: Pharmaceutical Products Press, 2004, 61–99.

Cooper, Courtney Ryley, and H. J. Anslinger. "Marihuana, Assassin of Youth." *American Magazine* 124 (1937): 18–19.

Nicholas, Phil, and Andrew Churchill. "The Federal Bureau of Narcotics, the States, and the Origins of Modern Drug Enforcement in the United States, 1950–1962." *Contemporary Drug Problems* 39, no. 4 (2012): 595–640.

Anti-Drug Abuse Acts of 1986 and 1988

The Anti-Drug Abuse Acts of 1986 and 1988 were two distinct antidrug bills that were signed into law by President Ronald Reagan (1911–2004). In essence, these laws created mandatory minimum sentences for conspiracy to sell, attempts to sell, or sale of a number of illegal drugs, including marijuana. These acts were seen as critical parts of the Reagan administration's so-called "War on Drugs," an effort to use law enforcement, education, and public health resources of the federal government to reduce drug use in the United States, especially among young people. These laws, however, also contributed to the rapid increase in incarceration rates experienced in the United States beginning in the 1980s, especially among African American citizens. In fact, they resulted in "historically unprecedented rates of imprisonment for drug use and possession" (Travis, Western, and Redburn 2014, 120).

ANTI-DRUG ABUSE ACT OF 1986

The Anti-Drug Abuse Act of 1986 was fueled by a rise in the use of crack cocaine in America's inner cities. The bill was also a response to the drug and alcohol overdose death in June of that year of University of Maryland basketball star Len Bias (1963–1986), who had just been drafted by the Boston Celtics. Although it was later determined that Bias died of a powder cocaine overdose, most people believed he had used crack cocaine. This mistaken belief made crack cocaine a leading focus of the sentencing guidelines established in this act.

The law reflected a widespread belief, both in Congress and among the American public, that crack cocaine was more addictive and caused more harm to people than powder cocaine. But critics asserted that there was a racial component to the law as well, since crack cocaine was more popular with African Americans than powder cocaine, which was more often used by white Americans.

The act included harsher punishments for individuals convicted of crack-related offenses than those who were caught selling, possessing, or using the powder form of the drug. Specifically, possession of 5 grams of crack cocaine (the weight of 2 pennies) and 500 grams of powder cocaine each resulted in a minimum of 5 years in prison regardless of mitigating factors. Similarly, possession of 50 grams of crack cocaine (the weight of a candy bar) and 5,000 grams of powder cocaine each resulted in a minimum of at least 10 years in prison. These standards became known as the 100 to 1 rule. The Fair Sentencing Act of 2010 reduced this disparity to 18:1.

In addition to the minimum sentences associated with cocaine offenses, the 1986 law required a minimum sentence of 5 years for offenses involving 1 kilogram of heroin, 40 grams of any substance with a detectable amount of fentanyl, or 5 grams of methamphetamine. A minimum sentence of 10 years imprisonment resulted from drug offenses involving 1 kilogram of heroin, 400 grams of a substance with a detectable amount of fentanyl, and 50 grams of methamphetamine. With respect to marijuana, a 5-year minimum sentence was set for offenses involving 100 kilograms of a mixture of substance containing a detectable amount of marijuana or 100 plants of marijuana regardless of weight and a sentence of at least 10 years for offenses involving 1,000 kilograms or more of a mixture of substance containing a detectable amount of marijuana or 1,000 plants of marijuana regardless of weight.

ANTI-DRUG ABUSE ACT OF 1988

The Anti-Drug Abuse Act of 1986 was amended by the Anti-Drug Abuse Act of 1998. The act contained numerous changes, including enhanced penalties and funding for the War on Drugs. While still focusing on drug selling, it broadened the efforts of the federal government to stamp out drugs by establishing more severe punishments for drug use. The increased penalties for drug offenses included the death penalty for those actively involved in a criminal enterprises such as drug sales or distribution or those who commit federal felonies, such as murder, while committing a drug-related offense. The law also closed a loophole in the Anti-Drug Abuse Act 1986 by allowing authorities to hold anyone involved in the criminal enterprise of selling or distributing drugs liable for the criminal enterprise. For example, a smalltime dealer caught selling drugs could receive enhanced penalties if the case could be made that he or she was connected to a larger enterprise or distribution network. The Anti-Drug Abuse Act of 1988 also created the Office of National Drug Control Policy, or ONDCP.

Similar to the earlier bill, the focus of this bill was disproportionally on crack cocaine rather than powder cocaine, again meting out harsher sentences for crack versus powder users. Specifically, the act established a 5-year mandatory minimum and 20-year maximum for simple possession of 5 grams (the weight of 2 pennies) of crack cocaine and a maximum of no more than 1 year for simple possession of powder cocaine or any other drug. The act also amended the 1986 act to make crack cocaine the only drug with a mandatory minimum penalty for a first offense of simple possession. In addition, the act also established a 5-year minimum penalty for lower possession amounts if the person had a previous drug conviction. In addition to updating the mandatory minimum sentences, the 1988 act also established the Office of National Drug Control Policy and created a policy goal of a drug-free America.

IMPACT OF THE ACTS

The acts contributed to massive growth in rates of incarceration in the United States. While the incarceration rate hovered around 100 per 100,000 population from the early part of the twentieth century until the early 1970s, it began increasing in 1972, and the rate of increase accelerated appreciably after the antidrug abuse acts of the 1980s. In 1984, the incarceration rate in jails and prisons was approximately 300 per 100,000 population, and this rate increased to over 700 per 100,000 population by 1994 (Travis, Western, and Redburn 2014). These laws also contributed to a significant jump in sentencing disparities between Black and white citizens. Before the passage of the 1986 law, sentences for Black Americans were 11 percent higher than white Americans. After the law's passage, that disparity rose to 49 percent (Vagins and McCurdy 2006).

Katherine Ayers

See also: Comprehensive Drug Abuse Prevention and Control Act (1970); Marihuana Tax Act (1937); Office of National Drug Control Policy; Racial Inequalities in Sentencing; Reagan Administration "War on Drugs."

Further Reading

Travis, Jeremy, Bruce Western, and F. Stevens Redburn. *The Growth of Incarceration in the United States: Exploring Causes and Consequences.* Washington, DC: National Research Council, 2014.

Vagins, Deborah J., and Jesselyn McCurdy. *Cracks in the System: Twenty Years of the Unjust Federal Crack Cocaine Law.* Washington, DC: American Civil Liberties Union, 2006.

Anti-Marijuana Campaigns in Popular Press

While anti-marijuana propaganda campaigns in the United States date to the mid-nineteenth century, one of the most orchestrated campaigns appeared in the wake of the formation of the Federal Bureau of Narcotics (FBN) in 1930. Even though marijuana had already been prohibited in several states—mainly in Southwestern states such as California and Texas—there were few campaigns against its use in the popular press. Within his first two years as the first commissioner of the FBN, however, Harry J. Anslinger (1892–1975) launched a major anti-marijuana campaign. Anslinger orchestrated the publication of anti-marijuana articles in numerous national and local newspapers. These articles sought to frighten readers about the alleged hazards of marijuana use, often by highlighting an alleged relationship between marijuana use and violent crimes.

Following the passage of the Marijuana Tax Act of 1937, Commissioner Anslinger intensified the ongoing anti-marijuana campaign in the American press. He published a highly sensationalized article, "Marijuana: Assassin of Youth," in *The American Magazine*'s July 1937 issue. The article begins:

> Not long ago the body of a young girl lay crushed on the sidewalk after a plunge from a Chicago apartment window. Everyone called it suicide, but actually it was murder. The killer was a narcotic known to America as marijuana, and to history as hashish. Used in the form of cigarettes, it is comparatively new to the United States and as dangerous as a coiled rattlesnake.

The story, which was republished in numerous other outlets, describes murders, suicides, robberies, and other "maniacal deeds" committed by marijuana "addicts." The effect of this story was powerful, in spite of the objections of different scientific organizations such as the American Medical Association (AMA) whose research suggested possible medicinal uses of cannabis. Over time, the campaign's tactics included visual ads in newspapers, pamphlets, comics, and even movies like *Reefer Madness* (1936). During this time Anlinsger relied heavily on what was known as his "gore file"—stories of alleged crimes committed by people under the influence of marijuana. These stories were reported in influential newspapers, including the *New York Times*. This sustained, negative messaging was effective in turning public sentiment firmly against marijuana, which came to be increasingly associated with crime, violence, immoral behavior, death, suicide, and the devil. These campaigns reinforced Commissioner Anslinger's anti-marijuana agenda and legitimized the ongoing FBN initiatives.

During the following decades, anti-marijuana campaigns continued to be presented in the popular press, often as Public Service Announcements or PSAs. In the 1950s, the fundamental argument was that marijuana was a "gateway drug" that would inevitably lead to heroin addiction. By the 1960s, the message was tempered somewhat, but federal authorities still argued that marijuana use was a life-ruining experience.

As drug use continued to increase in the 1970s despite these anti-marijuana campaigns, the Nixon administration launched a "war on drugs" in 1971 and called drug abuse "public enemy number one." These anti-marijuana campaigns frequently returned to the old messages that marijuana was a gateway drug that would lead to even worse forms of drug addiction, higher rates of crime, and psychosis and other forms of mental deterioration. In the 1980s, the Reagan administration launched a new "War on Drugs" that placed a greater focus on combating crack cocaine, but anti-marijuana campaigns continued to promote the idea that marijuana use would lead to addiction and ruin.

Since the 1990s, and especially since 2012 when the states of Colorado (Amendment 64) and Washington (Initiative 502) legalized the recreational use of marijuana, anti-marijuana campaigns in the American press have decreased substantially. Nonetheless, there is still an important number of organizations and activists, as well as governmental agents, who promote and support anti-marijuana campaigns on digital platforms.

Antonio Paniagua Guzmán

See also: Alaska; Anslinger, Harry (1892–1975); California; Colorado; Marihuana Tax Act (1937); Medical Marijuana and the Law; *Reefer Madness*; Vermont; Washington D.C.; Washington State.

Further Reading

Booth, Martin. *Cannabis: A History*. London, UK: Doubleday, 2003.

Chasin, Alexandra. *Assassin of Youth: A Kaleidoscopic History of Harry J. Anslinger's War on Drugs*. Chicago: The University of Chicago Press, 2016.

Chasteen, John C. *Getting High: Marijuana through the Ages*. Lanham, MD: Rowman & Littlefield, 2016.

Lee, Martin A. *Smoke Signals: A Social History of Marijuana—Medical, Recreational, and Scientific*. New York: Scribner, 2012.

McWilliams, John C. *The Protectors: Harry J. Anslinger and the Federal Bureau of Narcotics, 1930–1962*. Newark: University of Delaware Press, 1990.

Anxiety

Medical marijuana as a treatment for anxiety disorder is controversial. In anxiety disorders, an excessive fear and/or anxiety about a perceived threat results in potential negative impacts on behavior. Some examples of anxiety disorders include generalized anxiety disorder, panic disorder, social anxiety disorder, phobias, and post-traumatic stress disorder (PTSD). Approximately 18 percent of Americans suffer from anxiety disorders in a year.

Most states that have legalized the use of medical marijuana have approved it for the treatment of PTSD, but as of early 2020, few of these states allow medical marijuana for treating other types of anxiety disorders. Two exceptions are New Jersey for anxiety disorder and West Virginia for refractory generalized anxiety disorder. Despite the scarcity of states approving medical marijuana for anxiety disorders, relief from anxiety appears to be a major reason that people seek medical marijuana. For example, physicians in nine California assessment clinics indicated that, after pain and insomnia, the third most common condition for prescribing medical marijuana was anxiety (Reinarman et al. 2011).

Medical marijuana users are more likely to report being diagnosed with anxiety disorders (Compton et al. 2017). When combined use is considered, marijuana users who reported both medical and nonmedical use have higher rates of anxiety disorders. The association between medical marijuana and anxiety disorders could simply indicate that medical marijuana users are using marijuana to cope with anxiety. Indeed, young adult medical marijuana patients are more likely to report using marijuana to relieve feelings of anxiety compared to non-patient marijuana users (Lankenau et al. 2018).

Medical marijuana appears to relieve various symptoms of anxiety (Park and Wu 2017). Cannabidiol (CBD), an essential component of medical marijuana, is considered to have properties similar to other drugs used to treat symptoms of anxiety that result in decreased subjective anxiety and increased mental sedation (Crippa et al. 2004). CBD's anxiolytic properties appear to operate by affecting cerebral blood flow, especially to the limbic and paralimbic areas of the brain (Crippa et al. 2004). CBD has been shown to be effective in addressing a wide range of anxiety disorders including generalized anxiety disorder, panic disorder, social anxiety disorder, obsessive compulsive disorder, and PTSD (Blessing et al. 2015). However, a separate review of the research literature concluded that CBD is a promising but insufficiently proven treatment for anxiety (Rong et al. 2017). Medical marijuana can also be useful for treating the physical symptoms of anxiety. For example, medical marijuana may be beneficial for sleep problems, although research on this issue is not definitive due to methodological concerns.

Although medical marijuana is considered a potential treatment for anxiety disorders, marijuana use has been shown to be associated with an increased risk of anxiety (Volkow et al. 2014), particularly for chronic cannabis users (Crippa et al. 2009). Despite the co-occurrence between marijuana use and anxiety disorder, it is unclear whether marijuana use actually causes anxiety or whether those who are more prone to anxiety simply are more likely to use marijuana (possibly as a form of self-medication). Research supports the latter, since anxiety sensitivity—that is, fear and concern about the negative consequences of anxiety symptoms—is associated with using marijuana as coping (Bonn-Miller, Zvolensky, and Bernstein 2007). Even though marijuana use might not be a causal factor triggering anxiety disorders, it should be noted that anxiety is a potential symptom of cannabis withdrawal (Volkow et al. 2014).

Anastasia S. Vogt Yuan

See also: Medical Marijuana and the Law; Medical Uses; Mental Illness.

Further Reading

Blessing, Esther M., et al. "Cannabidiol as a Potential Treatment for Anxiety Disorders." *Neurotherapeutics* 12, no. 4 (2015): 825–836.

Bonn-Miller, Marcel O., Michael J. Zvolensky, and Amit Bernstein. "Marijuana Use Motives: Concurrent Relations to Frequency of Past 30-day Use and Anxiety Sensitivity among Young Adult Marijuana Smokers." *Addictive Behaviors* 32, no. 1 (2007): 49–62.

Compton, Wilson M., Beth Han, Arthur Hughes, Christopher M. Jones, and Carlos Blanco. "Use of Marijuana for Medical Purposes among Adults in the United States." *JAMA* 317, no. 2 (2017): 209–211.

Crippa, José Alexandre, et al. "Cannabis and Anxiety: A Critical Review of the Evidence." *Human Psychopharmacology: Clinical and Experimental* 24, no. 7 (2009): 515–523.

Crippa, José Alexandre de Souza, et al. "Effects of Cannabidiol (CBD) on Regional Cerebral Blood Flow." *Neuropsychopharmacology* 29, no. 2 (2004): 417.

Lankenau, Stephen E., et al. "Health Conditions and Motivations for Marijuana Use among Young Adult Medical Marijuana Patients and Non-patient Marijuana Users." *Drug and Alcohol Review* 37, no. 2 (2018): 237–246.

Park, Ji-Yeun, and Li-Tzy Wu. "Prevalence, Reasons, Perceived Effects, and Correlates of Medical Marijuana Use: A Review." *Drug and Alcohol Dependence* 177 no. 1 (2017): 1–13.

Reinarman, Craig, Helen Nunberg, Fran Lanthier, and Tom Heddleston. "Who Are Medical Marijuana Patients? Population Characteristics from Nine California Assessment Clinics." *Journal of Psychoactive Drugs* 43, no. 2 (2011): 128–135.

Rong, Carola, et al. "Cannabidiol in Medical Marijuana: Research Vistas and Potential Opportunities." *Pharmacological Research* 121 (2017): 213–218.

Volkow, Nora D., Ruben D. Baler, Wilson M. Compton, and Susan R. B. Weiss. "Adverse Health Effects of Marijuana Use." *New England Journal of Medicine* 370, no. 23 (2014): 2219–2227.

B

Beat Generation Writers

The Beat Generation is an American social, cultural, and literary movement that came of age post-World War II. It was led by writers and artists "disenchanted with . . . an excessively repressive, materialistic, and conformist society" (Petrus 1997, 3). Beat writers are known for their individualistic, romantic, and even idealistic pursuits. They were the first wave of American writers to be both highly influenced by marijuana and forthcoming about their enthusiasm for the drug (Glass 2015). Because marijuana significantly impacted their lifestyle and aesthetic sense, it necessarily also impacted their writing, including the experiences they impart to the reader, their methods of composition, and the unique styles of prose and poetry they explored (Glass 2015).

In order to understand the relationship between marijuana and members of the Beat Generation, it is instructive to hear from two of its principals, namely William Burroughs, author of the seminal Beat texts *Naked Lunch* and *Junky*, and poet Allen Ginsberg, who wrote an entire essay on what he termed "The Great Marijuana Hoax."

In Burroughs' prologue to *Junky* (1953), which concerns heroin addiction, he takes pains to contrast that hard drug with marijuana, which he describes simply as a "means to increased enjoyment of life." In *Naked Lunch* (1959), meanwhile, Burroughs wrote that:

> When I speak of drug addiction I do not refer to keif, marijuana or any preparation of hashish, mescaline, Bannisteria Caapi, LSD6, Sacred Mushrooms or any other drug of the hallucinogen group . . . . There is no evidence that the use of any hallucinogen results in physical dependence. The action of these drugs is physiologically the opposite to the action of junk [heroin]. A lamentable confusion between the two classes of drugs has arisen owing to the zeal of the U.S. and other narcotic departments. (Charters 1992)

Keeping with this theme, Allen Ginsberg, in his essay "The Great Marijuana Hoax," published in *The Atlantic Monthly* in November 1966, writes specifically for those who are not familiar with marijuana and whose attitudes toward it may have been negatively influenced by government bureaucrats, the police, and society. Evoking Howard Becker's (1966) theory of deviance, Ginsberg argues that the criminalization and corresponding persecution of marijuana use is not a function of any inherently deviant characteristics of the substance itself, but is instead a function of bureaucracy, namely, the U.S. Treasury Narcotics Bureau, in its mission to keep its staff busy and thus employed. Ginsberg notes "that a bureaucracy will attempt to find work for itself . . . the agents of this Bureau have a business interest in perpetuating the ideas of a

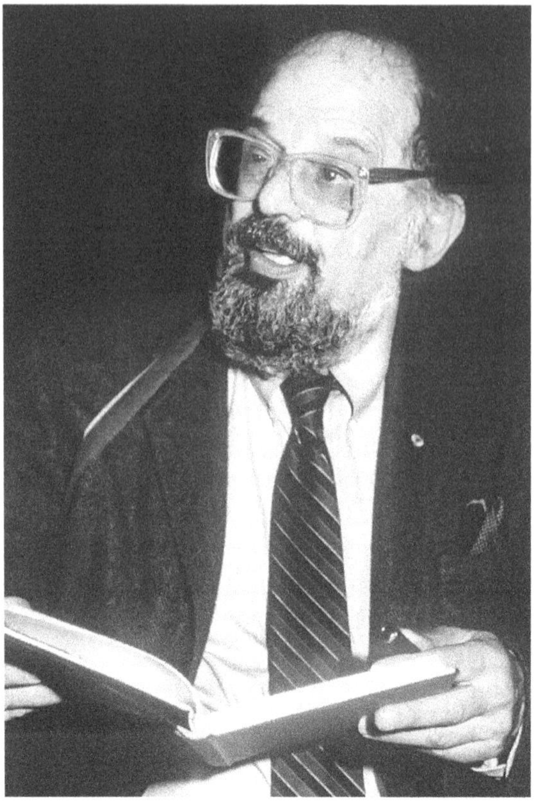

Allen Ginsberg (1926–1997) was a leading Beat Generation poet and writer. He is best known for his poem "Howl" that embraced the drug counterculture of the 1950s. (Laurence Agron/ Dreamstime.com)

marijuana 'menace' lest they lose their employment" (2). Ginsberg also notes, "I have termed [marijuana] an herb—which it is—a leaf or blossom—in order to switch from negative terminology and inaccurate language," and he characterizes former Bureau chief Harry J. Anslinger as "planting the seed of the marijuana 'menace' in the public mind and carefully nurturing its growth over the last few decades until the unsuspecting public was forced to accept an outright lie."

Ginsberg argued that for decades under Anslinger's direction, the Bureau was able to portray marijuana in a negative light and define any user of pot as a "Dope Fiend." The Bureau's mission was largely successful, wrote Ginsberg, until enough people had firsthand experience with marijuana to recognize that the dark warnings about marijuana's perils were "palpable poppycock." This represented a necessary shift in anti-marijuana messaging. Finally, Ginsberg ridiculed the notion that marijuana was a "gateway drug" that would ultimately push users down the path to an even greater evil—heroin. "A greater percent of opiate users started with bananas, cigarettes and alcohol than started with marijuana," declared Ginsberg.

Daisy Ball

See also: Hippies; "Howl"; Marihuana Tax Act (1937); Moral Panics.

Further Reading

Becker, Howard. *Outsiders*. New York: The Free Press, 2008.

Burroughs, William. *Junky*. New York: Penguin, 1953.

Burroughs, William. *Naked Lunch*. New York: Grove Press, 1959.

Charters, Ann, ed. *The Portable Beat Reader*. New York: Viking, 1992.

Drury, Adam. "The Marihuana Tax Act of 1937." *High Times*, July 13, 2018.

Ginsberg, Allen. "The Great Marijuana Hoax: First Manifesto to End the Bringdown." *The Atlantic Monthly*, November 1966.

Glass, Loren. "The Mighty Mezz, Marijuana, and the Beat Generation." *Los Angeles Review of Books*, May 7, 2015.

Hawdon, James. *Drug and Alcohol Consumption as Functions of Social Structures: A Cross-Cultural Sociology*. No. 47. Lewistown, NY: Edwin Mellen Press, 2005.

Petrus, Stephen. "Rumblings of Discontent: American Popular Culture and Its Response to the Beat Generation, 1957–1960." *Studies in Popular Culture* 20, no. 1 (1997): 1–17.

Beatles, The

The Beatles were a rock band formed in 1960 in Liverpool, England, which rose to become one of the most influential and successful popular music acts ever. The members of the Beatles were John Lennon, Paul McCartney, George Harrison, and Ringo Starr.

The Beatles' rapid ascent to the top of the music world in the 1960s included live concert tours around the globe as well as months' long stints in music studios to record albums. The demands of this arduous schedule led members of The Beatles to use purple heart, a street drug that included a mixture of amphetamines and barbiturate, resulting in a rigorous boost in energy. It was not until 1964, however, during a tour in the United States at the height of "Beatlemania," that the band was introduced to marijuana by another rock and roll icon, American singer-songwriter Bob Dylan. A regular user of marijuana, Dylan had misinterpreted several lines from The Beatles' music that had given him the mistaken impression that they were accustomed to marijuana and the use of the drug. In reality, this was the group's first experience with cannabis. After smoking a joint with Dylan, members of The Beatles began to regularly use marijuana.

The recreational use of marijuana became highly influential in their music. In 1965, *Rubber Soul* was released to critical acclaim and blockbuster sales. In a 1983 biography of The Beatles, authors Peter Brown and Steve Gaines noted that the difference between *Rubber Soul* and The Beatles' previous releases was inspired by their use of marijuana.

While many of their subsequent albums and songs referenced drug use, specifically cannabis, "Got To Get You Into My Life," from the 1966 album *Revolver*, was one of The Beatles' most notorious songs about using marijuana. In 1997, McCartney reported to Barry Miles that "Got To Get You Into My Life" was frequently assumed to be about a woman, when in actuality McCartney wrote it shortly after being introduced to marijuana, outlining his plan to continue to use the drug. McCartney acknowledged that *Revolver* focused heavily on the use of marijuana. *Sgt. Pepper's Lonely Hearts Club Band* also referenced drug use throughout the 1967 album. One of the album's songs, "Lucy in the Sky with Diamonds," was even banned from being played on the BBC on the grounds that the song openly promoted the use of lysergic acid diethylamide (LSD), an illicit drug.

In 1967, The Beatles moved beyond recording and performing songs with pro-marijuana lyrics. That year, the band joined forces with more than 60 other people of influence throughout the United Kingdom in signing an advertisement critiquing British law surrounding marijuana. This advertisement, which was published in the *London Times*, called for the removal of cannabis from the list of dangerous

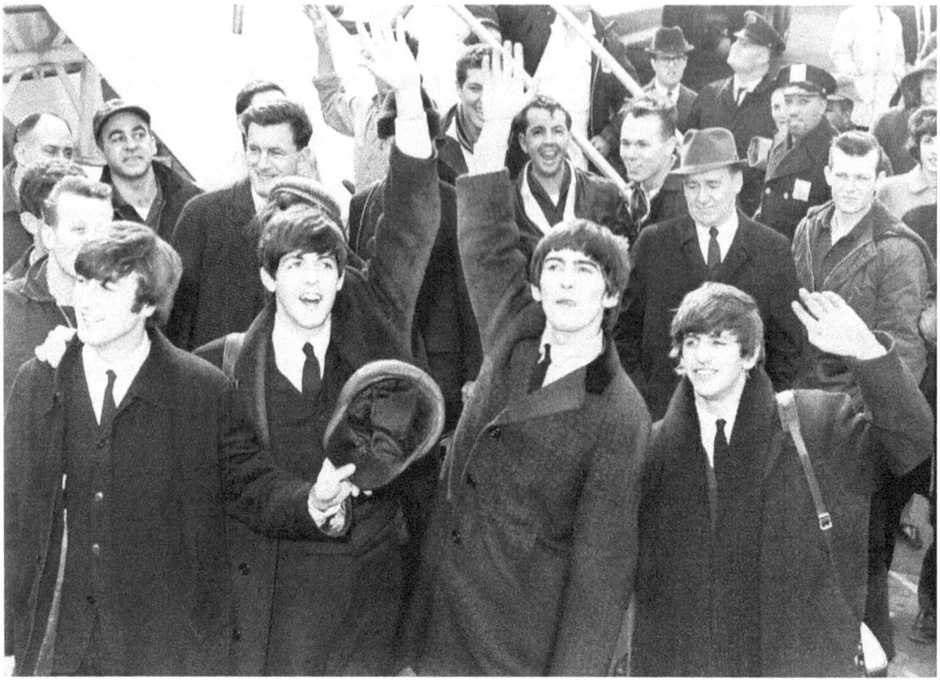

The Beatles arriving in New York, 1964. The English rock band from Liverpool led the British Invasion that revolutionized rock music and ushered in drug-glorifying music of the counterculture. (Library of Congress)

drugs designated by law, release of those imprisoned for possession of marijuana, and approval of cannabis use in privacy. In 1968, the Wootton Report was released by the British Parliament's Advisory Committee on Drug Dependence stating that regular use of marijuana is not detrimental and the laws surrounding the drug are socially harmful. James Callaghan, the Home Secretary in the late 1960s, originally said he would reject the report. Within the next year, Callaghan introduced legislation that paralleled the effects proposed in the Wootton Report.

Anne McNutt Patrick

See also: Garcia, Jerry (1942–1995); Marley, Bob (1945–1981); Monkees, The; Nelson, Willie (1933–).

Further Reading

Bienstock, Richard. "Pot Sounds: The 20 Greatest Weed-Themed Songs of All Time." *Rolling Stone*, August 29, 2019.

Brown, Peter, and Steven S. Gaines. *The Love You Make: An Insider's Story of The Beatles*. New York: New American Library, 1983.

Harry, Bill. *The Beatles Encyclopedia*. London, UK: Virgin Pub, 2000.

Lee, Martin A. *Smoke Signals: A Social History of Marijuana—Medical, Recreational and Scientific*. New York: Scribner, 2012.

Lee, Martin A. "When Bob Dylan Turned the Beatles on to Marijuana." *Project CBD*, August 25, 2016 (updated August 28, 2019). https://www.projectcbd.org/culture/when-bob-dylan-turned-beatles-marijuana

Miles, Barry. *Paul McCartney: Many Years from Now*. London, UK: Harvill Secker, 1997.

Sawyer, June Skinner. *Read the Beatles: Classics and New Writings on the Beatles, Their Legacy, and Why They Still Matter.* Paradise, CA: Paw Prints, 2008.

Sznitman, Sharon Rödner. *A Cannabis Reader: Global Issues and Local Experiences: Perspectives on Cannabis Controversies, Treatment and Regulation in Europe.* Lisbon, Portugal: European Monitoring Centre for Drugs and Drug Addiction, 2008.

Big Lebowski, The

Produced and directed by the Coen Brothers, the 1998 crime comedy *The Big Lebowski* follows Jeff "The Dude" Lebowski (played by Jeff Bridges), an unemployed avid bowler with an affection for white Russians and marijuana who becomes the victim of a case of mistaken identity with a millionaire also named Lebowski (David Huddleston). The movie *The Big Lebowski* showcased the role and acceptance of substance use, both marijuana and alcohol, in popular culture. Portrayal of marijuana use in early 1990s California throughout the movie is underscored as a normative activity that no one even notices. Moreover, the general demeanor and attitude of the main character, The Dude, reflects what has become an almost stereotypical example of a stoner embracing a laidback and carefree lifestyle. The film's relatively benign depiction of marijuana use has been cited as one of many representations in popular culture that increased public acceptance of marijuana and drove support for legalization efforts for both medicinal and recreational use.

While the original release of *The Big Lebowski* received generally average reviews and had a mediocre draw at the box office, over time it has garnered a cult following, and it was chosen to be preserved in the National Film Registry in 2014 (Library of Congress 2014).

The movie starts with The Dude having his rug urinated on by associates of a loan shark and pornographer named Jackie Treehorn (Ben Gazzara), who mistakenly believes that The Dude is a millionaire known as "the Big Lebowski." The associates are actually searching for the Big Lebowski's wife, Bunny Lebowski (Tara Reid), who owes Treehorn a considerable sum of money. The Dude meets with the Big Lebowski in hopes of obtaining some compensation for having his rug soiled. After his request is denied, he steals a replacement rug from the millionaire's home. Eventually, The Dude is contacted by Brandt (Philip Seymour Hoffman), an associate of the Big Lebowski, in hopes of having him deliver a ransom to have his wife Bunny, who had recently been kidnapped, returned unharmed. The Dude agrees. However, things end up going awry when his high-strung friend Walter Sobchak (John Goodman) decides to keep the money rather than pay the ransom. Walter throws a bag full of his underwear, instead of the ransom money, out the window for the kidnappers. Soon after The Dude ends up having his car stolen as well as the rug he took from The Big Lebowski. Eventually, the daughter of the Big Lebowski, Maude (Julianne Moore), calls The Dude to let him know that she took the rug because it had sentimental value. She also later reveals that her father is not actually rich and that he took money from the family foundation to pay the ransom. Bunny eventually returns home unharmed, and it is revealed that the millionaire never actually put money in the briefcase to pay the kidnappers—who were actually friends of Bunny and were in on the plot with her—but rather kept it for himself because he hated his wife.

One of the most common themes throughout the movie is substance use. During the course of the movie, The Dude drinks nine glasses of his signature drink, the white Russian, and also partakes of beer while he bowls with Walter and his sidekick, Donny (Steve Buscemi). Drinking is portrayed as both a social activity and one that The Dude partakes in simply by himself. Neither is framed as particularly controversial or problematic.

Marijuana use is also present within the movie, albeit to a significantly lesser extent than alcohol use. As a whole, there are four instances where The Dude uses marijuana. The first instance of The Dude smoking marijuana is when he sits down with The Big Lebowski after being told that Bunny was kidnapped. While the Big Lebowski is discussing his feelings about the matter, The Dude asks, "Mind if I do a J?"—at which point he pulls out a joint, lights it up, and takes a long hit. The second example is when The Dude is smoking while taking a bath, only to be interrupted by the kidnappers. The third example, which is the only one showcasing simultaneous alcohol and marijuana use, is a scene in which he crashes his car after he drops the last bit of a lit joint (known as "a roach") into his lap. The final example involves the one instance when he smokes with another individual, specifically sharing a roach with Maude right after they have sex.

Aside from marijuana use, there are some more subtle references to marijuana. One involves The Dude visiting the Big Lebowski for the first time, and as he is looking over the awards that the other Lebowski has won, Brandt asks The Dude about never going to college, to which he responds, "Well, yeah I did, but I spent most of my time occupying various, um, administration buildings, smoking Thai-stick, breaking into the ROTC, and bowling . . . ," with the specific reference here being the Thai-stick, marijuana that is tightly packed in a cylindrical form around sticks (IMSDB, n.d). An even subtler reference appears when two cops come to talk to The Dude at his home about his car being stolen and rug being taken. The scene shows two cops sitting on his couch, with the older of the two picking up a bowling pin shaped pipe, looking at it and around a tray of what appears to be discarded roaches, and finally putting the pipe down and saying nothing about it.

Throughout the film, marijuana and marijuana use is portrayed as generally unremarkable. As a whole, substance use in The Big Lebowski, especially for marijuana, is not controversial but rather normative in the sense that little attention is placed on it in a negative manner (or positive even) and generally glossed over.

Jonathan A. Grubb

See also: California; *Dazed and Confused*; *Reefer Madness*; Stoner Films.

Further Reading

Klinger, Barbara. "Becoming Cult: The Big Lebowski, Replay Culture and Male Fans." *Screen* 51, no. 1 (2010): 1–20.

Library of Congress. *Cinematic Treasures Named to National Film Registry "Saving Private Ryan," "Luxo Jr." and "Rosemary's Baby" among Film Additions*. Last modified 2014. https://www.loc.gov/item/prn-14-210/

Robertson, William Preston, et al. *The Big Lebowski: The Making of a Coen Brothers Film.* New York: Norton, 1998.
Rohrer, Finlo. "Is The Big Lebowski a Cultural Milestone?" *BBC News Magazine,* October 10, 2008. http://news.bbc.co.uk/2/hi/uk_news/magazine/7662943.stm

Biosocial Theories

Marijuana is the most commonly used drug in the United States. Even though it is considered mild compared to other drugs, there are still detrimental effects associated with chronic use including low academic achievement, truancy, addiction, and respiratory problems (isolated instances of hallucinations have even been reported in some extreme cases). Several studies find that some of the primary correlates associated with marijuana use are biological/genetic risk factors (i.e., self-control, cognitive abilities, and other significant markers of brain development) and social predictors (i.e., delinquent peer groups, coping mechanisms, parental substance use, and socioeconomic status). The integration of a biosocial perspective provides a theoretical lens to better understand the linkages between biological and environmental factors on marijuana use.

Biosocial theories place emphasis on both biological/genetic and environmental/social factors regarding antisocial behavior and criminality. The emphasis is not solely based on nature or nurture but on the interaction of both components. Biological theories were first established with the ideas of Cesare Lombroso in the late 1800s, which focused on criminal traits. Certain anatomical features of the human body were thought to determine which individuals would become criminal and noncriminal. As time progressed and more sophisticated research methods were applied, studies revealed that aggressive and antisocial behavior could be attributed to biological, neurological, genetic, and physiological factors (i.e., brain chemistry, hormones, and genes) compared to anatomical traits. In addition, environmental factors (i.e., poverty, malnourishment, stress, etc.) have shown to affect—and possibly alter—certain genes, which can increase the likelihood of aggressive and antisocial behavior. Current research suggests that these behaviors are estimated to be over 50 percent inherited, with some estimates showing that such behaviors might be as high as 85 percent inherited.

Studies indicate that there are numerous genetic and biological risk factors associated with increased exposure and/or use of marijuana and related illicit behavior (Bava and Tapert 2010; Beaver et al. 2009; Brook, Zhang, and Brook 2011). The predictors are primarily formed during childhood and adolescence. These studies include research on adolescent brain development as it relates to cognitive/social development (Bava and Tapert 2010; Brook et al. 2011) and genetic risk based on twin association and co-twin delinquency involvement (Beaver et al. 2009). While this research has found reliable results, many of these studies also find that those outcomes leave adolescents *even more* susceptible to substance use when combined with additional social predictors.

During adolescence, there are many changes in brain development, which include sophisticated cognitive functioning, emotional processing, and self-control. While the brain develops during adolescence, brain activity increases so that individuals can mature and cope with complex social and psychological environments. Research suggests this increase of brain activity leaves other areas of adolescent processing more vulnerable to unhealthy environmental influences (Bava and Tapert 2010). Certain delays in social and emotional processing leave an individual more likely to engage in substance abuse and other unhealthy behavior. These specific brain developments (i.e., low self-control and reward-seeking behavior) on their own have been linked to substance use; however, when it is combined with social-environmental influences (i.e., delinquent peers and normalized substance use) adolescents are at an increased risk of using marijuana.

Additional studies also show significant correlations between social problems and substance abuse. For instance, coping strategies are considered one of the most critical components that influence marijuana use (Patrick et al. 2019), which can stem from social/environmental factors such as neglect, poor social and parental relationships, and low academic achievement. Research reveals that coping skills are consistently found among chronic marijuana users throughout the lifetime. This reasoning is rational as many individuals who frequently partake in marijuana use and other drugs do so to relieve stress. The social factors that lead to poor coping skills are equally important to discuss, however.

Longitudinal studies measuring individual marijuana use from early adolescence to early adulthood indicate that parent/child relationships, delinquent peer association, and the social environment are some of the major determinants in predicting marijuana use (Brook et al. 2011; Van Ryzin, Fosco, and Dishion 2012). Additional social indicators such as poor parental discipline, lack of parental monitoring, poor social relationships (Brook et al. 2011; Van Ryzin et al. 2012), delinquent school peers, and low socioeconomic status (SES) (Lemstra, et al. 2008) have also been linked to habitual marijuana use among adolescents. Each of these factors highlights the link between social and economic factors on potential marijuana use. However, when partnered with biological/genetics factors, the likelihood of marijuana use is expected to increase. For instance, one study found that a combination of biological and social factors associated with marijuana use in adolescence predicts marijuana use in later adulthood until around age 30 (Brook et al. 2011). These studies imply that the moderating effect of biological and social factors can greatly influence an individual's chance of engaging in substance use.

Other studies reveal that biosocial components explain a significant association between low self-control and substance use (Boisvert et al. 2013; Chang, Lichtenstein, and Larsson 2012). Self-control is considered a significant marker for biosocial approaches as low self-control can be impacted by both biological (i.e., prenatal care and poor nutrition) and social (i.e., poor parenting, negative home and/or school environments) factors that impact antisocial tendencies and illicit behavior. Another study found that marijuana use was significantly influenced by low self-control and delinquent peers (Ragan and Beaver 2010). It is expected that a moderating relationship between biological and social factors influences self-control, which in turn affects substance use.

Marijuana use is the most common form of drug use in the United States and is currently legal and decriminalized in several states. However, there are still several negative impacts associated with marijuana use, including higher school dropout rates (Roebuck, French, and Dennis 2003), cardiovascular issues, and mental health problems. Biosocial theories help explain the predictors of marijuana use and how these correlates were established. Some of the predictors surrounding substance use include several biological and environmental factors such as prenatal care, chemical imbalances, poor social relationships, low self-control, and low SES. Overall, the current research supports the idea that biosocial factors can greatly impact adolescent marijuana use and chronic marijuana use throughout the lifetime.

Kristen N. Sobba and Lauren Waldrop

See also: Conflict and Labeling Theories; Control Theories; Social Bonding Theory/Social Control Theory.

Further Reading

Bava, Sunita, and Susan F. Tapert. "Adolescent Brain Development and the Risk for Alcohol and Other Drug Problems." *Neuropsychology Review* 20 no. 4 (2010): 398–413.

Beaver, Kevin M., Matt DeLisi, John Paul Wright, and Michael G. Vaughn. "Gene—Environment Interplay and Delinquent Involvement: Evidence of Direct, Indirect, and Interactive Effects." *Journal of Adolescent Research* 24 no. 2 (2009): 147–168.

Boisvert, Danielle, Brian B. Boutwell, J. C. Barnes, and Jamie Vaske. "Genetic and Environmental Influences Underlying the Relationship between Low Self-Control and Substance Use." *Journal of Criminal Justice* 41 no. 4 (2013): 262–272.

Brook, Judith S., Chenshu Zhang, and David W. Brook. 2011. "Developmental Trajectories of Marijuana Use from Adolescence to Adulthood: Personal Predictors." *Archives of Pediatrics & Adolescent Medicine* 165 no. 1 (2011): 55–60.

Chang, Zheng, Paul Lichtenstein, and Henrik Larsson. "The Effects of Childhood ADHD Symptoms on Early-Onset Substance Use: A Swedish Twin Study." *Journal of Abnormal Child Psychology* 40 no. 3 (2012): 425–435.

Lemstra, Mark, et al. "A Meta-Analysis of Marijuana and Alcohol Use by Socio-Economic Status in Adolescents Aged 10–15 Years." *Canadian Journal of Public Health* 99 no. 3 (2008): 172–177.

Patrick, Megan E., et al. "Reasons High School Students Use Marijuana: Prevalence and Correlations with Use across Four Decades." *Journal of Studies on Alcohol and Drugs* 80 no. 1 (2019): 15–25.

Ragan, Daniel T., and Kevin M. Beaver. "Chronic Offenders: A Life-Course Analysis of Marijuana Users." *Youth & Society* 42 no. 2 (2010): 174–198.

Roebuck, M. Christopher, Michael T. French, and Michael L. Dennis. "Adolescent Marijuana Use and School Attendance." *Economics of Education Review* 23 no. 2 (2004): 133–141.

Van Ryzin, Mark J., Gregory M. Fosco, and Thomas J. Dishion. "Family and Peer Predictors of Substance Use from Early Adolescence to Early Adulthood: An 11-year Prospective Analysis." *Addictive Behaviors* 37 no. 12 (2012): 1314–1324.

Blunts

A "blunt" is a crumbled cannabis flower rolled in a hollowed-out cigar wrapping, which is then smoked. While the use of blunts has become common throughout cannabis culture, its origins lie in New York City in the mid-1980s (Sifaneck et al.

2003). Researchers believe that Caribbean immigrants to the city brought with them the culture of smoking spliffs, the Rastafarian method of smoking cannabis rolled in tobacco, or "fronto" leaves. The subsequent spread of this method of consumption was likely a reaction to the tight market for marijuana in New York during this period. These market conditions created an increase in cost of cannabis flowers, meaning that for inner-city residents with limited resources multiple people (three to five, on average) would have to pool their resources to afford to purchase a small quantity of marijuana, which would then have to be shared among the contributors. The smoking of blunts facilitated this shared consumption and helped to ensure that all participants consumed roughly equal amounts of the cannabis. A typical blunt or Jamaican spliff is larger than a standard joint—1–1.5 grams compared to the 0.3–0.5 of a gram in most joints. This larger size allowed the cannabis to be consumed in a shorter period of time, thus reducing the risk for smokers of being caught in the illegal act (Sifaneck et al. 2003). In addition, the nature of the remains was easier to dispose of in the outdoor environment, where consumption typically occurred (Kelly 2012).

As the popularity of this consumption method spread from the ethnic enclaves where fronto leaves were available, adaptations in the creation process became necessary. The tobacco leaves were replaced with emptied shells of cheap cigars, particularly those of Philly Blunts, a brand of smaller, inexpensive cigars that could be easily bought from convenience stores and bodegas. It is from this particular brand that the term "blunts" originated (Sifaneck et al. 2003). The process of rolling a blunt involves the splitting of the cigar lengthwise and the emptying of the contents. The hollow shell is then filled with crumbled cannabis flower, rolled up, and resealed.

The spread of blunt smoking from the Northeast to cannabis culture nationally is largely attributed to its popularity in the hip-hop subculture. During the 1990s, it was common to hear New York–based rappers mention blunts or phillies in their music. Rappers from other areas of the country picked up the habit and even altered some of the nomenclature that had originated in New York. By the late 1990s and early 2000s, rappers from California's Bay Area were some of the most notable promoters of blunt use on the West Coast—but they preferred to use Backwoods brand cigars as opposed to Philly Blunts. Judging by the lyrics in modern hip-hop music, this brand preference has taken hold nationwide. It has been argued that the use of Backwoods or other cigars that utilize a more tobacco leaf-style wrap (as opposed to the pulverized tobacco paper-style wrap of other brands) is preferred because of the more difficult rolling process involved. Being able to roll a blunt from this style of wrap is indicative of a higher skill level and thus can boost one's social status within the cannabis subculture (Dunlap et al. 2006). Additionally, around this same time period premanufactured blunt wraps, which are cigar wrappers without the tobacco filling, became commonly available in nonspecialized stores. These products were embraced by marijuana smokers who were not skilled enough to roll a blunt from a split cigar.

Within cannabis culture, blunt smokers tend to be younger (Kelly 2012), although those who were adolescents during the 1990s would be now in their late thirties or early forties and may still use this method (Murphy et al. 2012).

Research has shown that true to its origins blunt smoking is primarily a communal process, although individual blunt smoking is not uncommon (Kelly 2012).

Common settings for blunt consumption include, but are not limited to sessions, cyphers and parties (Dunlap et al. 2006). Sessions are preplanned gatherings where all parties contribute to the purchase of the marijuana and often pair smoking with other activities such as watching sports or playing video games. These activities keep participants entertained during the extended time they are socializing. The cannabis purchased for such an event is typically fully consumed before participants leave the event. Cyphers, a term originally associated with impromptu rap competitions occurring in small groups, is also used to refer to blunt use that, unlike sessions, are not planned in advance and usually involve less people. Typically, a cypher forms when users are attending some event that is not about cannabis but decide to split off from the larger group to partake in blunt smoking. Often, only one or two people contribute the cannabis used in this way, but others familiar to this individual are often invited to join in. This decision of who is to be included is left to those who have contributed to the blunt. Parties, as a setting for consumption, are merely a setting where a cypher is highly likely to occur. The term "parties" here refer to the typical definition of a gathering of people getting together to celebrate or socialize. These events are not directly geared toward cannabis consumption but provide the impetus for people to gather together. Once the party is underway, however, some participants might decide that a blunt would be an enjoyable addition to the activities and separate from the crowd to form a cypher (Dunlap et al. 2006).

Jebadiha E. Potterf

See also: Bongs and Water Pipes; Dabbing; Edibles; Gravity Bongs; Joints; Single-Use Devices.

Further Reading

Dunlap, Eloise, Bruce D. Johnson, Ellen Benoit, and Stephen J. Sifaneck. "Sessions, Cyphers, and Parties: Settings for Informal Social Controls of Blunt Smoking." *Journal of Ethnicity in Substance Abuse* 4, no. 3–4 (2006): 43–80.

Kelly, Brian C. "Bongs and Blunts: Notes from a Suburban Marijuana Subculture." In *The Cultural/Subcultural Contexts of Marijuana Use at the Turn of the Twenty-first Century*, edited by Andrew Golub. Oxfordshire, UK: Routledge, 2012, 89–106.

Murphy, Fiona, et al. "Baby Boomers and Cannabis Delivery Systems." *Journal of Drug Issues* 45, no. 3 (2015): 293–313.

Sifaneck, Stephen J., Charles D. Kaplan, Eloise Dunlap, and Bruce D. Johnson. "Blunts and Blowtjes: Cannabis Use Practices in Two Cultural Settings and Their Implications for Secondary Prevention." *Free Inquiry in Creative Sociology* 31, no. 1 (2003): 3–14.

Soldz, Stephen, Dana Joy Huyser, and Elizabeth Dorsey. "The Cigar as a Drug Delivery Device: Youth Use of Blunts." *Addiction* 98, no. 10 (2003): 1379–1386.

Bongs and Water Pipes

The simplest definition of a bong is a device used to smoke marijuana in which the smoke is filtered through water before it is inhaled. The purpose of the water is to cool the smoke and filter harmful chemicals before it is inhaled. By this definition, all

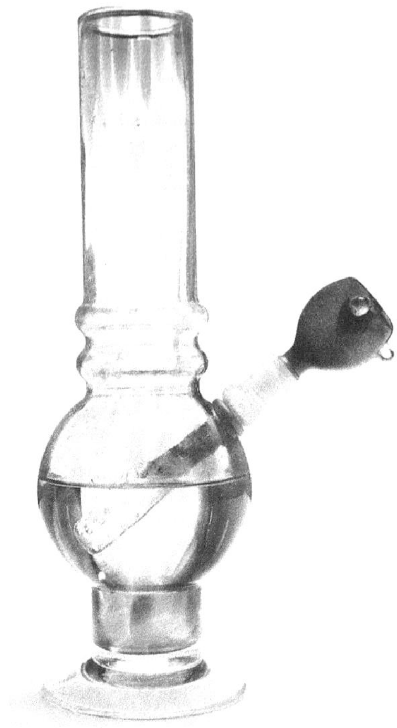

Bongs are water-cooled smoking devices commonly used to smoke cannabis. The water cools the smoke making it smoother and easier to inhale. (Suppersppy/Dreamstime.com)

bongs are water pipes but not all water pipes are bongs. Many different types of water pipes exist, such as hookahs and nargiles, and they have been used for centuries to smoke tobacco and other materials throughout Asia and the Middle East. As bongs are specific to water pipes used to smoke cannabis, they are illegal in many parts of the country, whether they have been used or not. The term "bong" originates from the Thai word *baung*, referring to a cylindrical pipe made from bamboo used to smoke tobacco (Weedmaps dictionary 2020).

Modern bongs can be made from a wide variety of materials, but glass or plastic are the most common, followed by ceramics and natural materials. Regardless of the material they all share certain features in common. They are primarily vertically oriented with an enclosed base that holds the water and an opening at the other end for the user's mouth. Toward the bottom, there is a down stem that goes through the side and into the water and a separate bowl for the cannabis to be burned in. While bongs can display a mind-boggling array of designs, mechanically they can be divided into two distinct types, depending on how the smoke gathered in the chamber is released. Carburetor bongs are the simplest; their design includes a small hole drilled somewhere above the water that is covered when inhaling from a lit bowl and uncovered to release the smoke. A pull carb bong does not have a hole, but rather the bowl piece is removed, and air is drawn in the same way as the smoke would be with the bowl in place (Franciosi 2020).

The oldest water pipes ever discovered were found by J.C. Dombroski in Ethiopia in 1971. Dated between 1100 and 1400 BCE, these pipes contained traces of cannabis along with other herbs. They were constructed directly in the ground and consisted of buried pottery used to hold the water and smoke and two wooden stems, one for the user's mouth and the other where the smoking material was placed with burning embers. While earth pipes have also been discovered in Asia, those in Africa have been dated to be older (Weedmaps dictionary 2020).

Arthur Dunhill, an archaeologist who has studied smoking devices throughout history, argues that the first portable water pipes were created by the San people of South Africa, a wooden tube pipe with water in one end and connected by a tube to the bowl on top (Weedmaps dictionary 2020). The first recorded use of a water pipe as a way to filter tobacco smoke, which was not introduced from the new world until the early 1500s, was from India when a sixteenth-century physician named Hakim Abul Fath created one using a coconut as the water reservoir and bamboo shoots as the stems. It was his contention that filtering tobacco smoke through water would reduce the harmful nature of the smoke (WHO 2015). Regardless of the exact origin of the water pipe, the device spread throughout the Middle East and Asia by traders traveling the Silk Road. And as the popularity of tobacco spread, so did their use (Weedmaps dictionary 2020).

One of the reasons for the popularity of bongs in cannabis smoking is the belief that they produce a more intense "high" than smoking from a pipe or joint. Although a 2000 study conducted by the National Organization for the Reform of Marijuana Laws (NORML) and the Multidisciplinary Association for Psychedelic Studies (MAPS) did not support this belief (Weedmaps dictionary 2020), research from the literature on tobacco smoking with water pipes has shown that it can produce higher concentrations of nicotine and other chemicals in the blood than cigarette smoking (Fakhreddine, Kanj, and Kanj 2014).

The popularity of bongs within cannabis culture grew exponentially during the late twentieth century. Bob Snodgrass, often called the godfather of bongs, was a glass blower who toured with the Grateful Dead and brought the modern glass bong to the hippie subculture. When he settled in Oregon and started teaching glassblowing, the availability of such smoking utensils expanded and their use blossomed (Weedmaps dictionary 2020). With this popularity came a dizzying array of new styles and designs, from low-cost plastic carbureted units to artisanal blown glass sculptures costing tens of thousands of dollars.

Within the variety of different bong types, several distinct subtypes should be recognized. The first big advancement was the creation of multichamber/percolator bongs, where the vertical tube is divided into two or more separate chambers, each with their own water chamber that the smoke passes through. Prized for their "cool" appearance, the multiple chambers of water in such bongs are thought to better filter and cool the smoke (Franciosi 2020). Additionally, bongs are among the most popular DIY (do-it-yourself) smoking devices that people make at home. All that is necessary is a vessel with an opening at one end that can hold water and have its side punctured for addition of the bowl and down stem. The honey bear bong, made from the bear-shaped honey bottles, is a well-known example of this type of bong.

Bubblers are smaller, easily transported bongs. Traditional bongs range from half a foot to several feet in height, but a bubbler is typically less than a foot tall. One feature that distinguishes a bubbler from a bong is that with a bubbler the bowl/down stem are a fixed part of the piece going directly into the water and the mouthpiece is the appendage piece (as opposed to the bowl/down stem being the appendage piece, as with bongs). Gas mask bongs are created when a bong is attached to the intake vent of a gas mask. When used, the individual attaches the mask to his or her face and breathes. The major difference between a gas mask and any other type of bong is that there is no break between hits. One will simply inhale and exhale in a normal fashion until the bowl has burned out and there is no more smoke left.

Lastly, whereas a traditional bong is activated by the user inhaling and pulling smoke from the bowl through the water and into the chamber, in a gravity bong, the user uses air pressure to accomplish this. This type of device has only two holes, one at the top for the bowl and one at the bottom to drain the water. After filling the chamber with water, the bowl is sealed to one hole and the water is then allowed to slowly drain, which creates the suction necessary to fill the chamber with smoke (Franciosi 2020).

Jebadiha E. Potterf

See also: Blunts; Dabbing; Edibles; Gravity Bongs; Joints; Single-Use Devices.

Further Reading

Fakhreddine, Hisham M. Bou, Amjad N. Kanj, and Nadim A. Kanj. "The Growing Epidemic of Water Pipe Smoking: Health Effects and Future Needs." *Respiratory Medicine* 108, no. 9 (2014): 1241–1253.

Franciosi, Anthony. "Different Types of Bongs and Their Benefits Explained." *Honest Marijuana*, 2020. https://honestmarijuana.com/types-of-bongs/

Weedmaps dictionary. "Bong." Weedmaps, 2020. https://weedmaps.com/learn/dictionary/bong/

WHO Study Group on Tobacco Product Regulation. *Advisory Note: Waterpipe Tobacco Smoking: Health Effects, Research Needs and Recommended Actions by Regulators*. Geneva, Switzerland: World Health Organization. 2015.

Bush (George H.W.) Administration "War on Drugs"

George H. W. Bush (1924–2018) served as the forty-first president of the United States from January 20, 1989, to January 20, 1993. Some of the most momentous issues President Bush faced as president included leading an international coalition of nations in response to Iraq's invasion of Kuwait in the first Gulf War (1990–1991), the reunification of East and West Germany, the signing of the Americans with Disabilities Act of 1990, the strengthening of the Clean Air Act, and the initial negotiations of the North American Free Trade Agreement (NAFTA). With respect to marijuana and broader drug policies, the Bush administration largely followed the precedents set by the Reagan administration (1981–1989), in which Bush had served as vice president. These policies included the "re-launch" and expansion of the so-called "War on Drugs" during the 1980s.

President Richard M. Nixon had officially declared America's first "War on Drugs" in June of 1971, but federal antidrug efforts had foundered during the turbulent political environment of the late 1970s. The Reagan/Bush administration reenergized the antidrug campaign. Although marijuana, cocaine, and other drug use began declining before Reagan took office and continued to decline substantially throughout the Reagan/Bush years, illegal drug use and its association with violent crime were central issues during the 1988 presidential election, during which time Bush secured the Republican nomination. Buoyed by public concerns about the issue of illicit drug use and its alleged impact on American society, Vice President Bush's support for the War on Drugs provided him with a competitive advantage over Democratic challenger Michael Dukakis. Bush ultimately won the election with 53.7 percent of the popular vote and 426 electoral votes (Morrison 2020).

When Bush assumed the presidency, public concern over drug use was widespread (Hawdon 2001). President Bush responded to this concern by quickly establishing his staunch antidrug position. In his first television address from the Oval

Office, President Bush held up a bag of crack cocaine in front of the camera and explained how it had been seized by Drug Enforcement Administration (DEA) agents in Lafayette Park, which is across the street from the White House. He then stated, "It's as innocent looking as candy, but it's turning our cities into battle zones." Although the sale and seizure of the cocaine had been arranged by his own administration, President Bush made it clear that the War on Drugs launched by President Reagan was going to continue under his administration because, as he said, "everyone who uses drugs" was causing "the gravest threat" toward America (Bush 1989). While the "war" specifically targeted cocaine, especially crack cocaine, it also resulted in increased enforcement of anti-marijuana laws.

President Bush's anti-marijuana policies were spearheaded by William Bennett (1943–), who he appointed as the first director of the Office of National Drug Control Policy (ONDCP) in March 1989. ONDCP was created by the Anti-Drug Abuse Act of 1988, and its director became known as the "drug czar." Director Bennett was known for his support for tough antidrug policies and his consistently staunch anti-marijuana position:

> As far as marijuana is concerned, let me say this: I didn't have to become drug czar to be opposed to legalized marijuana. As Secretary of Education I realized that, given the state of American education, the last thing we needed was a policy that made widely available a substance that impairs memory, concentration, and attention span. Why in God's name foster the use of a drug that makes you stupid? (Bennett 1992, 224)

In addition to continuing the traditional strategies of enforcing marijuana laws, President Bush increased federal efforts to combat the expanding indoor marijuana cultivation industry. In October 1989, President Bush launched Operation Green Merchant, a nationwide investigation of businesses advertising hydroponic and other horticultural equipment believed to be used to grow cannabis indoors. Specifically, the operation focused on advertisements in the marijuana-oriented magazines *High Times* and *Sinsemilla Tips*, traced United Parcel Service records to find customers who had purchased the equipment, and raided their homes. The DEA led raids of hydroponics stores in 46 states. The raids led to the closing of numerous indoor grow shops, the seizing of thousands of marijuana plants, and the arrest of over 100 individuals (Boyd 2005).

Another Bush administration antidrug initiative became known as "Smoke a joint, Lose your license." Beginning in 1990, the Bush administration called for states to increase punishments associated with drug offenses, including relatively minor offenses involving cannabis possession. One of the punishments recommended by the administration was suspension of drivers licenses for offenders for six months. States that did not comply with the administration's request for tougher enforcement risked losing federal highway funding (Boire 1996).

The Bush administration also reversed earlier decisions to expand the number of patients who could obtain federally produced cannabis under the Compassionate Investigational New Drug program, or Compassionate IND. Originally established by the Carter administration (1977–1981) in 1978, the Compassionate IND allows select patients suffering from serious or life-threatening conditions to use unapproved drugs or medical devices. Initially, people in the program were allowed to use cannabis under the program if they suffered from conditions such as glaucoma. The program was expanded to include those with AIDS in the mid-1980s. While very few people were ever approved to receive cannabis from the federally administered medicinal marijuana farm in Mississippi, the Bush administration closed the program to new applications in 1992 (Lee 2012).

During his tenure, President Bush saw rates of marijuana use decrease dramatically. Although rates of use had been declining significantly since 1979, they continued to decline during his presidency. The percentage of high school seniors who used marijuana annually was the lowest ever recorded in the *Monitoring the Future* data that began collecting data in 1975. While annual marijuana prevalence among twelfth graders peaked in 1979 at 51 percent, by 1992, the last full year of President Bush's term, only 21.9 percent of high school seniors used marijuana annually (Johnston et al. 2021, 14). Public concern over drug use also decreased substantially during President Bush's term. In his first year in office, over 30 percent of Americans believed drug abuse was the most important problem facing the nation; this figure declined to 8 percent by the time President Bush left office (Hawdon 2001).

James Hawdon

See also: American Presidents; Anti-Drug Abuse Acts of 1986 and 1988; Reagan Administration "War on Drugs."

Further Reading

Bennett, William. "Mopping Up After the Legalizers: What the 'Intellectual' Chorus Fails to Tell You." In *Drug Legalization: For and against*, edited by Rod Evans and Irwin Berent. Chicago: Open Court, 1992, 221–228.

Boire, Richard Glen. *Marijuana Law.* Berkeley, CA: Ronin Publishing, 1996.

Boyd, Ray. "Operation Green Merchant." *Cannabis Culture*, October 14, 2005.

Bush, George H.W. Test of President's Speech on National Drug Control Strategy. New York Times, September 6, 1989. https://www.nytimes.com/1989/09/06/us/text-of-president-s-speech-on-national-drug-control-strategy.html

Hawdon, James. "The Role of Presidential Rhetoric in the Creation of a Moral Panic: Reagan, Bush, and the War on Drugs." *Deviant Behavior* 22, no. 5 (2001): 419–445.

Johnston, Lloyd, Richard Miech, Patrick O'Malley, Jerald Bachman, John Schulenberg, and Megan Patrick. *Monitoring the Future: National Survey Results on Drug Use 1975–2020: Overview, Key Findings on Adolescent Drug Use.* Ann Arbor: Institute for Social Research, University of Michigan, 2021.

Lee, Martin A. *Smoke Signals: A Social History of Marijuana-Medical, Recreational and Scientific.* New York: Simon and Schuster, 2012.

Morrison, Donald. "United States Presidential Election of 1988." *Encyclopedia Britannica*, 2020. https://www.britannica.com/event/United-States-presidential-election-of-1988

Bush (George W.) Administration "War on Drugs"

George W. Bush (1946–), son of the forty-first president, George H. W. Bush, served as the forty-third president of the United States from January 20, 2001, to January 20, 2009. Bush faced several momentous national security and foreign policy challenges as president including the September 11 terrorist attacks, creation of the Department of Homeland Security, the "War on Terror," and the wars in

Afghanistan and Iraq. In Bush's second term, he faced growing criticism not only for his administration's foreign policy record but also for his response to Hurricane Katrina and the 2008 financial crisis. With respect to marijuana and broader drug policies, the Bush administration continued strict drug control policies including raids on medical marijuana clinics, depictions of marijuana as a dangerous "gateway" drug, and assertions that marijuana trafficking might be a source of money for terrorist groups such as Al Qaeda (Dreyfuss 2005).

In the run-up to the 2000 presidential election, George W. Bush avoided directly answering questions about his drug use earlier in his life. In a secretly recorded conversation later released and taking place before the 2000 presidential election, Bush indicated the reason he would not answer the marijuana question. On the tape, he states: "Do you want your little kid to say, 'Hey daddy, President Bush tried marijuana, I think I will'" (BBC News 2005). In addition to marijuana, it is also suggested he likely used cocaine in his younger years. When asked about his illegal drug use back in 1999 (at age 53), he indicated he had not used any illegal drugs in the past 25 years, or since 1974. According to this time table, Bush seemed to implicitly acknowledge that he used drugs on at least an occasional basis until his late twenties (Carroll 1999). During this time period in his life, he was also known for his struggles with alcohol abuse including a DUI in 1976. In 1977, he married Laura Welch, who provided what he characterized as a stabilizing element in his life. In 1986, Bush gave up using alcohol entirely.

Drug Czar John Walters served as the director of the Office of National Drug Control Policy (ONDCP) for the majority of George W. Bush's two terms, from December 7, 2001, to January 20, 2009. He adamantly opposed drug decriminalization, legalization, and medical marijuana. During his tenure, he refocused the War on Drugs on marijuana and launched a major campaign to promote student drug testing. During the Bush administration, an estimated $35 billion a year was spent on the War on Drugs (Dreyfuss 2005) despite stable rates of drug use (although narcotic deaths increased). During this time period, the Bush administration oversaw an increased militarization of domestic drug law enforcement. By the end of Bush's term, about 40,000 paramilitary-style SWAT raids were being conducted per year in the United States—many for nonviolent drug law offenses (Balko 2013; Hawdon 2019).

Walters aggressively launched efforts to depict marijuana as a gateway drug, arguing that marijuana inevitably leads to other drug use and is linked with other problems: "Marijuana use, especially during the teen years, can lead to depression, thoughts of suicide and schizophrenia" (Dreyfuss 2005). In addition to the gateway argument, Walters also played on fears of terrorism, linking drugs to terror and airing ads that suggested money spent on marijuana is used to fund terrorist groups such as Al Qaeda.

Critics of Bush administration drug policies claimed that Walters' focus on marijuana was wrongheaded. According to Graham Boyd, director of the Drug Law Reform Project of the American Civil Liberties, "For Walters, it's all marijuana, all the time. He is reinforcing the atmosphere that marijuana is the drug we should care about, and that the government will do everything it can, including locking everyone up, if that's what it comes to" (Dreyfuss 2005).

During Walters time as Drug Czar, an estimated $4 billion a year was spent arresting and prosecuting marijuana crimes. During congressional testimony in 2005, Walters testified that this focus was having a deterrent effect on teen use of other drugs.

Additional attempts to crack down on marijuana use during the Bush administration included a nationwide effort to pressure schools to conduct drug tests on student athletes, those engaged in extracurricular activities, and in some cases the entire student population. These efforts were aided by the 2002 Supreme Court ruling in *Board of Education of Pottawatomie v. Earls*. This decision upheld a lower court ruling that school districts are permitted to drug test students participating in any competitive or extracurricular activity. "Extracurricular activity" was further stretched to include students who parked at the school.

In 2005, the Supreme Court affirmed the federal government's powers to enforce federal drug laws even in states that had legalized medical marijuana in its *Gonzalez v. Raich* decision. During the Bush administration, 13 states legalized medical marijuana. From the onset of the Bush administration, federal raids (often with heavily armed agents) of state-legal medical marijuana growers and dispensaries were common with over 100 raids from 2001 to 2003. In 2006, DEA agents arrested 594 medical marijuana users in California alone, seizing business owners' assets and confiscating property (Trumble and Kasai 2017).

Bryan Lee Miller

See also: Bush (George H.W.) Administration "War on Drugs"; Gateway Drug Hypothesis; *Gonzalez v. Raich* (2005); Medical Marijuana and the Law; Office of National Drug Control Policy.

Further Reading

Balko, Radley. *Rise of the Warrior Cop: The Militarization of America's Police Forces.* New York: PublicAffairs, 2013.

BBC News. "Bush Hinted at Use of Marijuana." February 21, 2005. http://news.bbc.co.uk/2/hi/americas/4282799.stm

Carroll, Joe. "Bush Fails to Convince on Question of Cocaine." *The Irish Times*, August 21, 1999. https://www.irishtimes.com/news/bush-fails-to-convince-on-question-of-cocaine-use-1.218905

Dreyfuss, Bob. "Bush's War on Pot." *RollingStone Magazine*, August 11, 2005. https://www.rollingstone.com/culture/culture-news/bushs-war-on-pot-62338/

Hawdon, J. "Crises of Security and Crises of Legitimacy: Organizational Evolution in American Policing, 1860–2017." In *On These Mean Streets... People Are Dying: Police & Citizen Brutality in America,* edited by Lisa Eargle and Ashraf Esmail. Lake Charles, LA: Green Legacy Publishing, 2019, 40–70.

Heisele, Kenneth J. "Board of Education of Independent School District No. 92 of Pottawatomie County v. Earls." *Ohio Northern University Law Review* 29 (2002): 459.

Somin, Ilya. "Gonzales v. Raich; Federalism as a Casualty of the War on Drugs." *Cornell Journal of Law and Public Policy* 15 (2005): 507.

Trumble, Sarah, and Nathan Kasai. "The Past—and Future—of Federal Marijuana Enforcement." Third Way, May 12, 2017. https://www.thirdway.org/memo/the-past-and-future-of-federal-marijuana-enforcement

Butane Hash Oil

Butane hash oil (BHO), commonly known as "wax," "budder," "honey oil," or "shatter," is the resin-like remains after chemical extraction of tetrahydrocannabinol (THC) from the flower of the cannabis plants. Butane hash oil has a higher concentration and potency of THC than can be derived from the traditional smoking of marijuana, thus offering a faster and longer "high" conveyed in a single dose. Another attractive aspect of BHO, from the user perspective, is the ability to use trimmings and leftover fragments of marijuana plants that otherwise would not be converted into consumable product. Butane hash oil is to marijuana what crack is to powder cocaine, but is a direct derivative of the marijuana plant, so drug control policy legislation regarding marijuana almost categorically applies to butane hash oil.

"Dabbing" is the most common form of consuming the vapors from waxy butane hash residue, frequently with a blowtorch to heat a few small droplets (a "dab") of the resin that has been placed on a ceramic or titanium surface attached to a typical water bong. When the resin is vaporized, users inhale the concentrated marijuana extraction, but BHO can also be consumed through a vaporizer, offering a more controlled release that can be used for medical applications. BHO is now commonly sold in marijuana dispensaries in all states offering recreational and medical marijuana.

Dangers associated with the use of butane hash oil often involve the manufacturing process, as is the case with methamphetamine. "Blasting" is the process of passing or pouring butane through a steel or hard plastic tube packed with marijuana. As the butane seeps through the marijuana, it dissolves the THC in the plant matter that is then collected in some type of receptacle. Butane hash oil is the substance that remains after the butane evaporates, posing a risky practice of using a highly combustible compound that may result in fires or physical harm from exploding glass shrapnel. Creating butane hash oil in unsafe home workshops can also create an accumulation of noxious compounds that can be ignited by static electricity or an open flame.

An increase in fires related to butane hash oil production has been noted in states that have legalized the use of marijuana for medical and recreational use (Bell et al. 2015). Such incidents are more common among users under the age of 18 who are precluded from making purchases at legal markets. Injuries also derive from use, especially with homemade BHO that, unlike legal lab-produced concentrates, has uneven butane distribution that often results in "sparks" that break glass pipes. Injuries can be limited by legislation that requires a standardization of the manufacturing process. Most states have outlawed home laboratories for creation of butane hash oil and carry a prison sentence for this practice, but the extent of home production is not really known.

Potential health risks for butane hash oil as compared to smoking marijuana are not clear either. It is theorized that consuming butane hash oil may be safer than conventional pot-smoking as it removes the combustible aspect, tar, and other carcinogens and therefore reduces the likelihood of lung damage. Further, bacteria, mold, and fungi are destroyed in the manufacturing process. Still, health experts and law enforcement have expressed concern that loss of consciousness, accidents, and falls are speculated to be more common after dabbing.

Stephanie M. Koskinen and J. Mitchell Miller

See also: Dabbing; Tetrahydrocannabinol (THC); Vaporizers.

Further Reading

Bell, Cameron, et al. "Butane Hash Oil Burns Associated with Marijuana Liberalization in Colorado." *Journal of Medical Toxicology* 11, no. 4 (2015): 422–425.

Miller, Bryan Lee, John M. Stogner, and J. Mitchell Miller. "Exploring Butane Hash Oil Use: A Research Note." *Journal of Psychoactive Drugs* 48, no. 1 (2016): 44–49.

Porter, C. J. W., and J. R. Armstrong. "Burns from Illegal Drug Manufacture: Case Series and Management." *The Journal of Burn Care & Rehabilitation* 25, no. 3 (2004): 314–318.

Stogner, John M., and Bryan Lee Miller. "Assessing the Dangers of 'Dabbing': Mere Marijuana or Harmful New Trend?" *Pediatrics* 136, no. 1 (2015): 1–3.

C

California

California has long had a progressive attitude when it comes to the legalization of marijuana. In 1996, it was the first state to legalize medicinal marijuana in the United States thanks to a voter-approved state ballot. In 2015, California passed legislation to create a state licensing and regulatory system for medical marijuana. However, in 2016 that legislation was repealed when voters approved legalization of recreational marijuana use. This law went into effect in January 2018. Over the next two years, recreational marijuana use generated $1.03 billion in tax revenue for California (Jagielski 2020).

In 1996, California voters approved Proposition 215, or the Compassionate Use Act (CUA), which allowed for the possession and cultivation of medical marijuana by licensed patients and caregivers. According to California's state cannabis portal, this was the first initiative for medical marijuana that became law by virtue of a voter-approved state ballot in the United States. The CUA paved the way for many other states to pass their own medical marijuana laws and ultimately contributed to the legalization of recreational marijuana in several states.

In 2015, California passed the Medical Cannabis Regulation and Safety Act (MCRSA). This act, comprising three separate bills, helped to establish a licensing and regulatory system for medical marijuana. In that effort, the MCRSA established the Bureau of Cannabis Control, CalCannabis Cultivation Licensing, and Manufactured Cannabis Safety Branch. However, with the passage of the MAUCRSA in 2017, these bills were repealed ("Department of Cannabis Control, California" 2020).

In 2016, Proposition 64, or the Adult Use of Marijuana Act (AUMA), was passed in California. Under AUMA, adults 21 years of age or older could use, possess, and give away up to an ounce of marijuana for recreational use. Adults were also allowed to grow no more than six marijuana plants for recreational use at their residence. This act also legalized the commercial sale and distribution of marijuana through state-licensed businesses beginning in January 2018. Marijuana also remained legal for all patients who have a prescription under the CUA of 1996. Lastly, under AUMA, adults are not allowed to use marijuana in any public place, or nonsmoking area, or consume or possess an open container of marijuana while driving.

In 2017, Senate Bill 94 was passed by the state legislature in California. This was a budget trailer bill that combined MCRSA with AUMA to create the Medicinal and Adult-Use Cannabis Regulation and Safety Act (MAUCRSA). In January 2019, the Office of Administrative Law (OAL) in California approved

MAUCRSA, and it was signed into law. This provided the regulatory framework for both commercial medicinal and adult recreational use of marijuana across the state.

D. Tyler Love

See also: Alaska; Colorado; Compassionate Use Act (1996); Decriminalization; Taxation; Vermont; Washington D.C.; Washington State.

Further Reading

Department of Cannabis Control, California "Laws & Regulations." *CA.gov*, 2020. https://cannabis.ca.gov/laws-regulations/

Jagielski, David. "It's Been Just over Two Years since Legal Recreational Marijuana Sales Started in the Golden State." *The Motley Fool*, March 11, 2020. https://www.fool.com/investing/2020/03/11/californias-cannabis-tax-revenues-top-1-billion.aspx

Cannabichromene (CBC)

Cannabichromene (CBC) is one of many cannabinoids found in cannabis plants. It is structurally similar to various other well-known natural cannabinoids, including tetrahydrocannabinol (THC), cannabidol (CBD), and cannabinol (CBN). CBC stems from cannabigerolic acid, which is produced by cannabis plants. CBC is nonpsychoactive, meaning that ingesting it will not cause a euphoric "high." This is because, unlike the THC in marijuana that causes users to get "high," CBC does not bind well to the CB1 cannabinoid receptors in the brain. However, CBC does bind to other receptors in the brain, particularly those linked to pain perception. Therefore, lab research has begun to examine the pharmaceutical properties of CBC (Turner et al. 2017). It is believed that CBC has the potential to benefit both individuals on its own and in combination with other cannabinoids.

Hope has emerged for the numerous medical benefits of CBC, including its potential as a cancer-fighting tool. A 2013 study showed CBC might be effective at fighting tumor inflammation and growth in mice (Nakajima et al. 2013). A 2006 study also suggested CBC might be effective at combating breast cancer (Ligresti et al. 2006). Another emerging area of medical interest is the potential for CBC to reduce pain. CBC has been shown to have significant anti-inflammatory effects in animals, while avoiding many of the negative side effects of nonsteroid anti-inflammatory drugs (DeLong et al. 2010). Another study, again looking at mice, found CBC had a positive effect on brain cells, promoting healthy brain function (Shinjyo and Di Marzo 2013). Moreover, research shows CBC might likewise be effective at fighting acne by acting as an anti-inflammatory and also suppressing excessive lipid production in the sebaceous glands (Oláh et al. 2016). Finally, initial studies indicate CBC might also serve to reduce depressive symptoms. Indeed, a 2010 study found CBC, in conjunction with THC and CBD, can reduce depressant properties (El-Alfy et al. 2010).

In sum, knowledge of the medicinal properties of CBC continues to emerge. While numerous studies have examined the effects of CBC in animals, more work is needed to understand the potential medical veracity of CBC in humans. Moreover, additional research on the effect of CBC in conjunction with other cannabinoids is needed to gain a fuller understanding of the potential interactive effects on humans.

Matthew Costello

See also: Cannabidiol (CBD); CBD Wellness Beverages; Chronic Pain; Medical Uses; Tetrahydrocannabinol (THC).

Further Reading

DeLong, Gerald T., Carl E. Wolf, Alphonse Poklis, and Aron H. Lichtman. "Pharmacological Evaluation of the Natural Constituent of Cannabis sativa, Cannabichromene and Its Modulation by Δ9-Tetrahydrocannabinol." *Drug and Alcohol Dependence* 112, no. 1–2 (2010): 126–133.

El-Alfy, Abir T., et al. "Antidepressant-like Effect of Δ9-Tetrahydrocannabinol and Other Cannabinoids Isolated from Cannabis Sativa L." *Pharmacology Biochemistry and Behavior* 95, no. 4 (2010): 434–442.

Ligresti, Alessia, et al. "Antitumor Activity of Plant Cannabinoids with Emphasis on the Effect of Cannabidiol on Human Breast Carcinoma." *Journal of Pharmacology and Experimental Therapeutics* 318, no. 3 (2006): 1375–1387.

Nakajima, Jun'ichi, Dai Nakae, and Ken Yasukawa. "Structure-dependent Inhibitory Effects of Synthetic Cannabinoids Against 12-O-tetradecanoylphorbol-13-acetate -induced Inflammation and Skin Tumour Promotion in Mice." *Journal of Pharmacy and Pharmacology* 65, no. 8 (2013): 1223–1230.

Oláh, Attila, et al. "Differential Effectiveness of Selected Non-psychotropic Phytocannabinoids on Human Sebocyte Functions Implicates Their Introduction in Dry/Seborrhoeic Skin and Acne Treatment." *Experimental Dermatology* 25, no. 9 (2016): 701–707.

Shinjyo, Noriko, and Vincenzo Di Marzo. "The Effect of Cannabichromene on Adult Neural Stem/Progenitor Cells." *Neurochemistry International* 63, no. 5 (2013): 432–437.

Turner, Sarah E., Claire M. Williams, Leslie Iversen, and Benjamin J. Whalley. "Molecular Pharmacology of Phytocannabinoids." In *Phytocannabinoids*. Cham: Springer, 2017, 61–101.

Cannabidiol (CBD)

CBD is the second most widely used cannabinoid extracted from the cannabis plant. Depending on how it is manufactured, it can be ingested orally, smoked, or topically applied. Scientists have developed synthetic versions of CBD. The U.S. Food and Drug Administration (FDA) approved Epidiolex in 2018. Epidiolex is an oral synthetic form of CBD used to treat epilepsy. Natural CBD can be found in health, food, beauty, and bath products.

CBD does not contain a large amount of Delta-9 tetrahydrocannabinol (THC), which is the psychoactive ingredient in cannabis that gives the intoxicating effect. As such, CBD users experience a different effect than the "high" that is normally experienced in THC users. Effects most frequently reported by CBD users are feelings of relaxation and drowsiness.

Different types of CBD exist. CO_2 extraction is a method used to extract the raw material to manufacture CBD. The term used to describe CBD with zero THC is

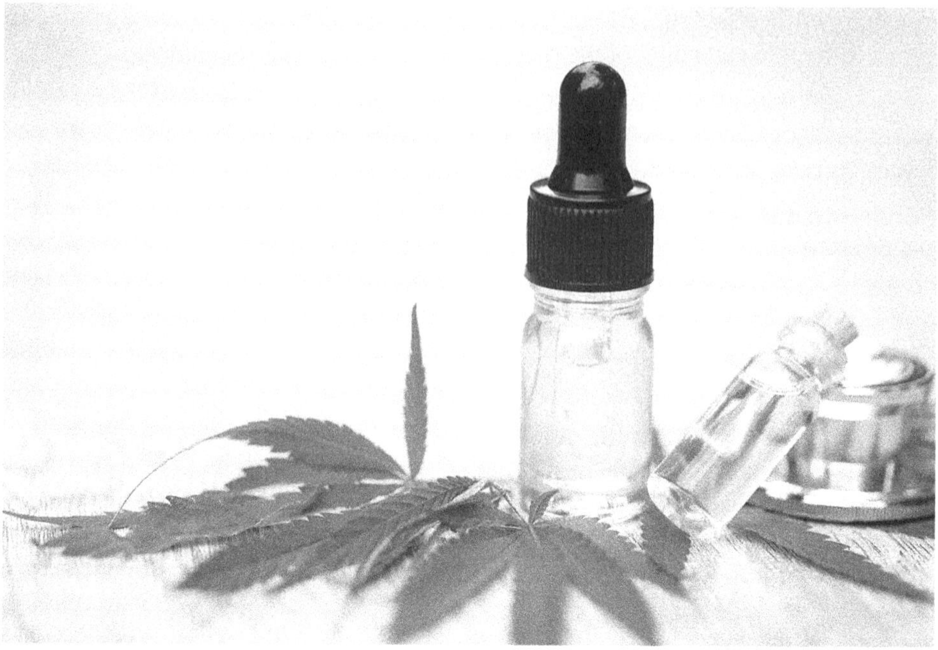

Cannabidiol (CBD) is the second most prevalent active ingredient in cannabis, derived directly from the hemp plant. It is non-intoxicating and is found in a number of common products. (Tinnakorn Jorruang/Dreamstime.com)

called CBD isolate. This means the consumer is getting 99 percent CBD. Consuming true CBD isolate will not show up with drug testing. Different definitions for full spectrum and broad spectrum exist. CBD full-spectrum oil contains THC. Broad-spectrum CBD has additional cannabinoids. Broad spectrum has the same qualities as full spectrum, with the exception of a few compounds. It is believed that CBD full-spectrum oil has a more powerful effect as compared to CBD isolate. This is because CBD and THC work together in a complementary fashion. When both THC and CBD are consumed together—as is the case with CBD full spectrum—a product with both antidepression and antianxiety properties is produced.

A major problem with purchasing CBD is that unless the contents have been tested, a consumer cannot verify that the CBD contains the compound that the package claims. In the United States, the Food and Drug Administration (FDA) is currently completing hearings for the regulation of the CBD industry. It is believed by many stakeholders in the CBD industry that the regulations that will be enforced by the FDA will allow consumers to have more certainty that the CBD they are purchasing actually contains what sellers say it does. As of 2020, there is no certified organic certificate for CBD in the United States.

Research suggests that CBD might have a number of health benefits, including reducing pain, nausea, anxiety, and infection and alleviating ADHD and immune disorder symptoms. Promising results are observed with using CBD for the treatment of opioid drug addiction and addiction to alcohol and tobacco. Researchers also have speculated that the anti-inflammatory properties of CBD might be useful to those with arthritis. It is also a highly effective sleep aid. Despite the personal stories often shared online, however, no long-term clinical trial in humans has shown that CBD can cure cancer. Consumers should be cautious of products that overstate the health benefits of CBD on packaging.

Accurate dosage of CBD is a concern. Since growing cannabis is not a standardized method, and CBD is ingested in different ways, a uniform dosing strategy does not yet exist. It is up to the consumer to gauge what quantity of CBD works best for their particular needs or wants. The water solubility of CBD is also a factor, since water-soluble CBD has a higher "bioavailability" (level of absorption into the circulatory system) as compared to oil-based CBD.

Cannabis products are not allowed in professional or college athletics. However, as of 2019 the American National Football League (NFL) announced plans to study the benefits of cannabis for pain. Currently, CBD is allowed for pain management in the Big3 American basketball league, a three-on-three professional league established in 2017.

Although human studies are limited, scientists do not consider CBD dangerous or addictive. Adverse reactions have been identified in patients taking antiepileptic drugs. No human or animal has ever overdosed on CBD, which is marketed for both human and veterinarian health.

Margot Gage Witvliet

See also: Casual Users, Health Effects; CBD Wellness Beverages; Medical Marijuana and the Law.

Further Reading

Brown, Maury. "Ice Cube and Jeff Kwatinetz Talk Use of CBD in Big3 Basketball." *Forbes*, Last modified August 2, 2018. https://www.forbes.com/sites/maurybrown/2018/08/02/ice-cube-and-jeff-kwatinetz-talk-use-of-cbd-in-big3-basketball/#456a6dd86cad

Grotenhermen, Franjo, Ethan Russo, and Antonio Waldo Zuardi. "Even High Doses of Oral Cannabidiol Do not Cause THC-Like Effects in Humans: Comment on Merrick et al. *Cannabis and Cannabinoid Research* 2016; 1 (1): 102–112; DOI: 10.1089/can. 2015.0004." *Cannabis and Cannabinoid Research* 2, no. 1 (2017): 1–4.

Iffland, Kerstin, and Franjo Grotenhermen. "An Update on Safety and Side Effects of Cannabidiol: A Review of Clinical Data and Relevant Animal Studies." *Cannabis and Cannabinoid Research* 2, no. 1 (2017): 139–154.

Iversen, Leslie L. *The Science of Marijuana.* New York: Oxford University Press, 2001.

Mechoulam, Raphael, Linda A. Parker, and Ruth Gallily. "Cannabidiol: An Overview of Some Pharmacological Aspects." *The Journal of Clinical Pharmacology* 42, no. S1 (2002): 11S–19S.

Russo, Ethan, and Geoffrey W. Guy. "A Tale of Two Cannabinoids: The Therapeutic Rationale for Combining Tetrahydrocannabinol and Cannabidiol." *Medical Hypotheses*66, no. 2 (2006): 234–246.

USADA. "Marijuana FAQ Your Questions Answered." n.d. Accessed January 3, 2020. https://www.usada.org/athletes/substances/marijuana-faq/

World Health Organization. "Cannabidiol (CBD) Pre-Review Report Agenda Item 5.2." Last modified November, 2017. https://www.who.int/medicines/access/controlled-substances/5.2_CBD.pdf

Cannabis Drinks

Cannabis-infused drinks, also referred to as a liquid edibles or drinkables, are products that contain cannabinoids, especially THC (the psychoactive ingredient in marijuana) and CBD, which can be consumed for recreational or medical purposes. The cannabis-infused beverage market is on a steady rise and accounted for $89 million in U.S. sales in 2018 (Kovacevich 2019). Marketed to consumers looking for alternatives to smoking cannabis, these products often contain alcohol or caffeine and are sold as cannabis-infused tonics, beers, sparkling water, sparkling fruit beverages, soft drinks, lemonades, teas, and coffee.

Although cannabis drinks have become popular in medical marijuana and recreational marijuana dispensaries, ingesting cannabis in a liquid form has a much longer history. Bhang lassi is a cannabis-infused drink made with bhang, an Indian edible product that has been used in food and drink products as early as 1000 BC (Courtwright 2009). The leaves of the cannabis plant are ground into a paste using a mortar and pestle and mixed with milk and filtered. A variety of sugar, fruit, and spices are added to flavor the beverages. Variants of bhang beverages are associated with traditional festivals and as medicinal products. For example, Bhang beverages are popular during the Hindu festival of spring (i.e., Holi festival).

At the end of the 1800s, a Swedish cannabis-based drink, Maltos-Cannabis, became popular in Norway and Denmark and was marketed more for its medical value and pleasant taste than psychoactive properties (Potter, Bouchard, and Decorte 2016). Similarly, in the United States a variety of products emerged in the late 1800s and early 1900s as part of the patent medicine industry. Many of these products sold as cures for a variety of ailments contained psychoactive drugs including heroin, cocaine, alcohol, and marijuana. Several of these elixirs, soft drinks, and cough syrups contained marijuana as a main ingredient, including popular remedies such as Pronto Grippe, Colds, Coughs, Nervous or Bilious Headaches and Sore Throat; Bees Laxative B Cough Syrup; Security Cough, Cold and Distemper Remedy; Dr. Hands Pleasant Physic for Children; and Gray's Balsam for the Throat and Lungs. Regulation of the patent medicine industry brought about with the passage of the Pure Food and Drug Act of 1906 required these products to list ingredients; banned misleading, overstated, and fraudulent claims; and forced the pharmaceutical industry to adopt scientific standards in manufacturing its products. Nevertheless, by 1937, there were at least 2000 cannabis medicinal products sold by 280 manufacturers (*Antique Cannabis Book* 2018).

More recently, a variety of cannabis-infused beverages have emerged as medical marijuana dispensaries have sought to develop options for consumers less comfortable with smoking. These products fall into two main categories: those mainly with THC and those with CBD. Similarly to marijuana, THC-dominated drinks are consumed primarily for their psychoactive properties and produce a "high" similar to THC edibles. Alternatively, CBD beverages are primarily consumed for medicinal or wellness value. Research has not specifically evaluated cannabis-infused drinks as an alternative form of medical marijuana administration, and the FDA has yet to approve the claims of CBD products. Some medical marijuana patients may be more comfortable consuming products in a liquid form, and with effects similar to other edible products, cannabis drinks may offer a suitable alternative.

Bryan Lee Miller

See also: Cannabidiol (CBD); CBD Wellness Beverages; Dispensaries; Edibles; Tetrahydrocannabinol (THC).

Further Reading

The Antique Cannabis Book. 2nd ed. January 2018. antiquecannabisbook.com.

Courtwright, David T. *Forces of Habit: Drugs and the Making of the Modern World*. Cambridge, MA: Harvard University Press, 2009.

Kovacevich, Nick. "Drink Up: The Next Frontier in Cannabis Is Beverages." *Forbes*, April 15, 2019.

Potter, Gary R., Martin Bouchard, and Tom Decorte. "The Globalization of Cannabis Cultivation." In *World Wide Weed*. New York: Routledge, 2016, 21–40.

Cannabis indica

Cannabis indica is a type of cannabis plant found in the family Cannabaceae. The *C. indica* plant contains high levels of tetrahydrocannabinol (THC), which is the psychoactive constituent of cannabis. The plant has been cultivated for centuries for religious, recreational, and medicinal reasons. In addition to its psychoactive qualities, it has served as a source of food, fuel, fiber, medicine, and building material.

About three decades after Carl Linnaeus had classified European hemp as *Cannabis sativa*, biologist Jean-Baptiste de Lamarck discovered the plant had more than one type (Watts 2006). Writing in 1785, he described the samples brought to him originating from the Hindu Kush Mountains of the Indian subcontinent, which differed from other samples of sativa in many significant ways. Naming the species *C. indica*, Lamarck noted that it had a thicker stem, broader leaves, and differently shaped flowers (Schultes et al. 1974). Later examinations would reveal a plant that grew less tall than the *C. sativa* plant and was denser and more conical in shape. Moreover, Lamarck maintained that *C. indica* was more psychoactive than the *C. sativa*, but inferior to sativa in its fiber quality.

In the 1970s, cannabis growers sought to improve the quality of their product, which had become widely popular in the United States, despite being illegal. Genetic variations of cannabis from around the world found their way to the United States, but *C. indica* seeds smuggled from Afghanistan and Pakistan proved especially important (Rendon 2012). Rather than smoke-dried cannabis flowers, the people of the Indian subcontinent tended to cultivate the plant in order to produce a form of hashish known as "charas" (Bradford and Mansfield 2019). Regardless, its origin in a harsh mountain climate made *C. indica* well suited to growing in temperate climates with shorter growing seasons, and the "Emerald Triangle" of Northern California—a center of domestic production of illicit marijuana crops—proved optimal. Growers there revolutionized the American marijuana trade by significantly increasing the tetrahydrocannabinol (THC) content of marijuana available to consumers (Rendon 2012).

Today, the consensus is that while individual strains vary widely, indica and sativa produce roughly the same amounts of THC, the compound responsible for the euphoric and intoxicating effects of the plant (Rahn 2018). Most consumers use a shorthand to predict the psychoactive effects, with *C. indica* thought to be more physically sedating and relaxing while *C. sativa* was more cerebrally invigorating and more suitable for physical activity. This rule of thumb has, however, been called into question by researchers examining the chemical makeup of the two species (Piomelli and Russo 2016). Rather than these differences being innate to the two species, many researchers believe that different levels of cannabinoids are responsible for the distinctiveness of the intoxication. Nevertheless, the shorthand is ubiquitous, especially now with legal dispensaries typically lumping their stock into three categories: *C. sativa*, *C. indica*, and hybrids.

Robert Perdue

See also: *Cannabis sativa*; Synthetic Cannabinoids; Tetrahydrocannabinol (THC).

Further Reading

Bradford, James, and David Mansfield. "Known Unknowns and Unknown Knowns: What We Know about the Cannabis and the Hashish Trade in Afghanistan." *Echo-Geo* 48 (April/June 2019): 1–11.

Clarke, Robert C., and Mark D. Merlin. *Cannabis: Evolution and Ethnobotany*. Oakland: University of California Press, 2013.

Piomelli, Daniele, and Ethan B. Russo. "The Cannabis sativa Versus Cannabis Indica Debate: An Interview with Ethan Russo, MD." *Cannabis and Cannabinoid Research* 1, no. 1 (2016): 44–46.

Rahn, Bailey. "Indica vs. Sativa? What's the Difference Between Cannabis Types?" *Leafly*, September 20, 2018. https://www.leafly.com/news/cannabis-101/sativa-indica-and-hybrid-differences-between-cannabis-types

Rendon, Jim. *Super-Charged: How Outlaws, Hippies, and Scientists Reinvented Marijuana*. Portland, OR: Timber Press, 2012.

Schultes, Richard Evans, Klein, William M., Plowman, Timothy, and Tom E. Lockwood. "Cannabis: An Example of Taxonomic Neglect." *Botanical Museum Leaflets, Harvard University* 23, no. 9 (1974): 337–367.

Watts, Geoff. "Cannabis Confusion." *BMJ* 332, no. 7534 (2006): 175–176.

Cannabis Oils

Cannabis oils are extracted from marijuana and can be used in a variety of ways, including in vaporizer devices for medical and recreational purposes. The use of hash oil and other marijuana extracts is not a new phenomenon, but with medical and recreational marijuana expanding in the early 2000s in the United States, these products are increasingly becoming commercially available and in more concentrated forms. Often referred to as "budder," "honey oil," and "wax," cannabis concentrates offer higher levels of tetrahydrocannabinol (THC) (the psychoactive ingredient in marijuana) and allow users to vaporize the product instead of smoking through traditional combustion (Miller, Stogner, and Miller 2016).

Although the consumption of cannabis oils is often portrayed as a new trend by the popular media, its origins among American substance users can be traced to the 1960s (Booth 2015). It is believed that some U.S. soldiers serving in Vietnam extracted tetrahydrocannabinol (THC) into a liquid concentrate by using solvents such as acetone or petrol. These users then either smeared the product onto a rolling paper or saturated tobacco with the liquid concentrate (Booth 2015). Another form of hashish oil became popular back in the United States during this time. Allegedly manufactured in Mexico, "smash" was a marijuana product cooked with acetone. Modern concentrates are made through a variety of methods including using CO_2 and butane for extraction. Butane Hash Oil (BHO) has become popular since the production process for BHO is relatively simple for both amateur and commercial manufacturers and the product is far more potent than flower cannabis (Al-zouabi et al. 2018).

Aiding in the popularity of these products, manufacturing techniques used to create BHO allow for an easier method of utilizing once-wasted parts of the cannabis plant. Consumer movement toward vaporizing as a means of marijuana consumption, combined with increased efficiency in the production process, has made these products more popular with both medical and recreational users. However, commercial products available in states with legal recreational markets have created a demand and prompted amateur production of cannabis oils. Some of these processes, such as using butane in amateur manufacturing labs (referred to as "blasting"), have resulted in numerous fires and injuries and drawn increased law enforcement concern (Al-zouabi et al. 2018).

Some cannabis oils that have extremely high THC concentration levels, and can be consumed through novel methods of consumption (such as dabbing), have become an increased health concern. There is little research available on the harmful effects of the rapid consumption of high quantities of THC, but a number of adverse effects have been attributed to dabbing (Stogner and Miller 2015b). Along with the hazards involved in manufacturing, these more potent forms of marijuana consumption have prompted concern and led to increased regulation of these products in some states (Stogner and Miller 2015a). Other forms of cannabis oils with lower THC levels have become popular and used in vaporizer pens for both medical and recreational purposes.

Bryan Lee Miller

See also: Butane Hash Oil; Dabbing; Edibles.

Further Reading

Al-Zouabi, Ihsan, John M. Stogner, Bryan Lee Miller, and Elizabeth S. Lane. "Butane Hash Oil and Dabbing: Insights into Use, Amateur Production Techniques, and Potential Harm Mitigation." *Substance Abuse and Rehabilitation* 9 (2018): 91.

Booth, Martin. *Cannabis: A History*. New York: Macmillan, 2015.

Miller, Bryan Lee, John M. Stogner, and J. Mitchell Miller. "Exploring Butane Hash Oil Use: A Research Note." *Journal of Psychoactive Drugs* 48, no. 1 (2016): 44–49.

Stogner, John M., and Bryan Lee Miller. "Assessing the Dangers of "Dabbing": Mere Marijuana or Harmful New Trend?" *Pediatrics* 136, no. 1 (2015a): 1–3.

Stogner, John M., and Bryan Lee Miller. "The Dabbing Dilemma: A Call for Research on Butane Hash Oil and Other Alternate Forms of Cannabis Use." *Substance Abuse* 36, no. 4 (2015b): 393–395.

Cannabis sativa

An herbaceous flowering plant native to central and southern Asia, *Cannabis sativa* has been used since the beginning of human history. The list of uses of the plant is remarkable, with cultivation yielding fiber, oil, food, medicine, building materials, and most famously, psychoactive substances. It has been used in religious rituals, as medicine, and for recreational purposes for centuries, and it continues to be used in these ways today.

Cannabis has proven difficult to classify because of its genetic plasticity; before landing in the Cannabaceae family, it had been classified in the nettle family (Urticaceae) and the mulberry family (Moraceae) (Duvall 2014). Carl Linnaeus, geneticist and developer of the taxonomic nomenclature, believed cannabis to be monotypic (a single species) and therefore classified all hemp plants as *C. sativa* in 1753 (Hartsel et al. 2016). Sativa means *cultivated* in Latin, a term typically used to label plants that promote wellness and/or for crops that are domesticated for food production. Linnaeus was only examining fiber-type hemp specimens common in Europe at the time, however, and he was unaware of cultivars native to Asia (Hartsel et al. 2016). Comparing European and Indian cannabis plants led Jean-Baptiste Lamarck to classify Asian hemp as a different species, *Cannabis indica*, in 1785 (Duvall 2014). *C. sativa* was taller and allegedly better for fiber, while *C. indica* allegedly had more powerful psychoactive properties. About 150 years later, Soviet botanist D.E. Janischevsky noticed that Russian hemp plants did not fit the characteristics of *C. sativa* or *C. indica* and contended the existence of a third species, *C. ruderalis* (Schultes et al. 1974).

C. sativa plants are woody and can grow up to 20 feet tall, markedly taller and rangier than *C. indica*. Thriving in equatorial climates, landrace *C. sativa*, a variety of cannabis that is grown in and adapted to the environment of its native land, requires a combined growing and flowering period of six months, with a long flowering period of up to 16 weeks to maturity (Reichard n.d.). This timeline has been compressed in commercial growing operations, sometimes to as little as 90 days. Flowers most often have both male and female parts, but it is the plants with female parts that are cultivated for psychoactive purposes. Male plants are removed to prevent fertilization and induce parthenocarpy, or the production of seedless fruits, commonly referred to as "sin semilla" (Duvall 2014). Most commercially available psychoactive cannabis is a result of cross breeding of *C. sativa* and *C. indica* to yield more desirable strains of what is typically thought of as "marijuana."

C. sativa contains more than 500 compounds. The most famous of these compounds is tetrahydrocannabinol (THC), sought for the euphoric "high" feeling it can produce. More than 100 cannabinoids (CBDs) have also been identified, which are increasingly being studied for their medicinal benefits (Walker, Strangman, and Huang 2002). Not psychoactive like THC, CBDs are being evaluated for their promise to reduce anxiety and depression (Linares et al. 2019), relieve pain (Walker et al. 2002), alleviate cancer-related symptoms (Johnson et al. 2010), among other potential benefits.

Robert Perdue

See also: *Cannabis indica*; Synthetic Cannabinoids; Tetrahydrocannabinol (THC).

Further Reading

Duvall, Chris. *Cannabis*. London, UK: Reaktion Books Ltd., 2014.

Hartsel, Joshua A., et al. "Cannabis Sativa and Hemp." In *Nutraceuticals: Efficacy, Safety and Toxicity*, edited by Ramesh C. Gupta. Cambridge, MA: Academic Press, 2016, 735–754.

Johnson, Jeremy R., et al. "Multicenter, Double-blind, Randomized, Placebo-Controlled, Parallel-Group Study of the Efficacy, Safety, and Tolerability of THC: CBD Extract and THC Extract in Patients with Intractable Cancer-Related Pain." *Journal of Pain Symptom Management* 39, no. 2 (2010):167–179.

Linares, Ila M., et al. "Cannabidiol Presents an Inverted U-Shaped Dose-Response Curve in a Simulated Public Speaking Test." *Brazilian Journal of Psychiatry* 41, no. 4 (2019): 9–14.

Reichard, Zach. "Cannabis Sativa." MedicalJane, n.d. https://www.medicaljane.com/2013/07/22/cannabis-sativa-as-explained-by-medical-jane/

Schultes, Richard Evans, William M. Klein, Timothy Plowman, and Tom E. Lockwood. "Cannabis: An Example of Taxonomic Neglect." *Botanical Museum Leaflets, Harvard University* 23, no. 9 (1974): 337–367.

Walker, J. Michael, Nicole M. Strangman, and Susan M. Huang. "Cannabinoids as Analgesics." In *Biology of Marijuana: From Gene to Behavior*, edited by Emmanuel S. Onaivi. New York: Taylor & Francis, 2002, 573–589.

Casual Users, Health Effects

Marijuana has complex and varied interactions with the human brain. Numerous studies highlight the importance of understanding the effects of marijuana on its users. Those who use cannabis may experience different reactions depending on factors such as age and personal genetics, as well as the length of use, quantity, and quality of the substance. Some of the most common effects noted by experts are mood and appetite changes and pain relief, as well as cardiovascular complications, dissociation, stroke, and lapses in critical reasoning. Scientists believe the casual use of marijuana is not safe and therefore is not recommended without medical supervision. More studies are necessary to reach a consensus about the physical and emotional impacts of marijuana on casual users.

Marijuana can be classified as legal or illegal in public policy and law. Legal marijuana has a regulatory process similar to the pharmaceutical industry: it must comply with varied standard requirements and pass sanitation inspections. On the other hand, illegal marijuana has no such legally mandated safety and quality standards. The main difference between legal and illegal marijuana for the user resides in the control of production, packaging, commercialization, and quality of the products. Researchers note that samples of secondhand marijuana often contain additional toxic substances such as fungus, bacteria, pesticides, and mold.

Marijuana users can be classified as recreational (or social), casual, and frequent (or heavy). Most studies treat those who use marijuana one to three times per week as casual users, while those who use cannabis more frequently are treated as frequent users and those who do it less frequently as recreational users. Social, or recreational, use is often confused with casual use; it is important to note that the qualifying aspect of this classification is the regularity of the use.

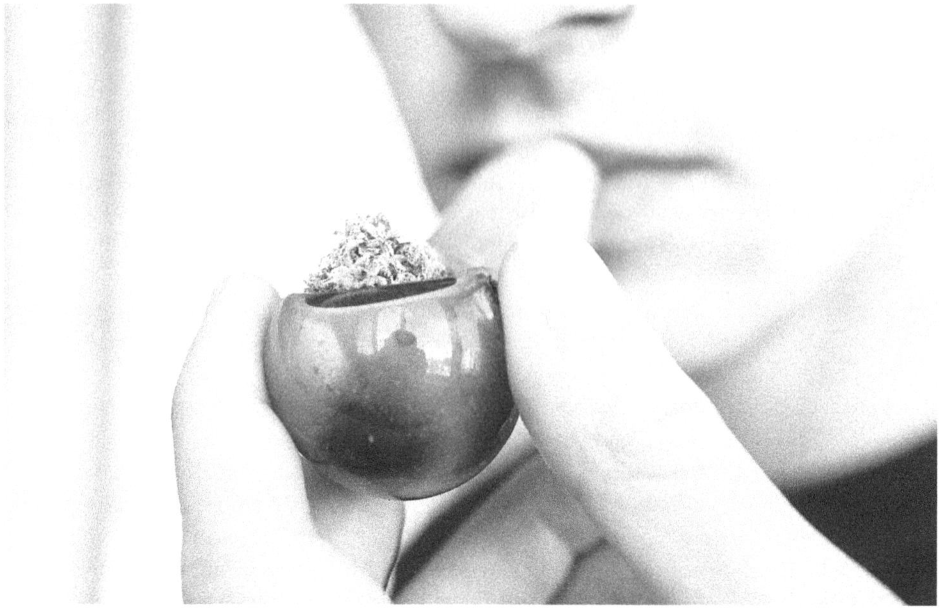

A man holds a glass pipe filled with marijuana buds. Pipes are often used to smoke marijuana and come in a variety of shapes, sizes, and materials. (Kyrylo Vasilev/ Dreamstime.com)

Researchers typically regard "casual users" as people who consume marijuana on a regular basis, generally at least once per week.

The methods of marijuana use also vary. Although smoking is the most common way of consuming cannabis, it is possible to find a wide range of marijuana-based products, including food "edibles," drinks, and "vaping." A number of studies have found that regardless of marijuana form, it contains more than 500 different substances, among them tetrahydrocannabinol (THC). Evidence suggests that THC directly affects memory, motor coordination, reaction time, information processing, motor performance, and attention and can increase the risk of road accidents if users drive while under its influence (Cohen, Weizman, and Weinstein 2019). Other psychotropic substances contained in cannabis have also been linked to thought disruption, impairment of recent memory, cognitive alterations, time distortion, and poor academic performance. According to research (e.g., Pope and Yurgelun-Todd 1996), a casual use of just one time per week is detrimental to the user. As such, it was found that students who never used marijuana had a GPA of 0.429 higher than students who used cannabis at least once per week (Jones, Jones, and Peil 2018).

The question of whether marijuana use can be a cause of various psychiatric disorders remains controversial. Despite abundant research linking marijuana with the development of schizophrenia and paranoia, some studies suggest that this effect is likely to happen on individuals with a genetic predisposition to develop schizophrenia (Power et al. 2014). Nonetheless, in Portugal, almost 600 marijuana users are hospitalized per year with psychotic episodes (Gonçalves-Pinho, Bragança, and Freitas 2020).

The casual use of marijuana has been associated with high risks of heart diseases. Researchers observe an increase of cardiovascular activity, increase of heart rate, and decrease of blood pressure when marijuana is used. A study reported that within minutes, the pulse rate of an individual increased from a mean of 66 to 89 beats per minute after using marijuana. Cases of stroke during the use of marijuana have also been observed. Evidence supports that marijuana increases the vascular resistance and velocity in users compared to nonusers (Thomas, Kloner, and Rezkalla 2014).

Another potentially negative effect of marijuana use concerns how cannabis may interact with other drugs and medications. Cases were reported linking the interaction of cannabis with alcohol and cocaine, as well as many commonly used medicines. Interaction reports list the following medicines as the most affected: diphenhydramine (Benadryl), escitalopram (Lexapro), morphine, tramadol (Ultram), and alprazolam (Xanax), among others. Further studies are needed to determine whether it is safe to use marijuana with these or other medicines or substances.

In spite of some studies suggesting that marijuana can impact the fertility of users, there is evidence associating the legalization of marijuana with baby booms. The use of marijuana has been linked to an increase in casual sexual activities and birth rates. According to research, individuals under the influence of marijuana are more likely to have multiple partners and less likely to use contraception (Baggio, Chong, and Simon 2019).

There also have been a number of clinical studies suggesting positive effects associated with marijuana use, such as better sleep and pain management as well as relief of seizures and stress. Researchers found that the majority of adolescents seek the use of medical marijuana to treat seizures, while pain management was the most frequent reason cited for prescription or self-medication among adults. It should be noted that although some studies suggest certain medical benefits of marijuana, there are controversies regarding the quantity of cannabis that can have positive effects, age of users, and side effects.

A debate also still rages as to whether marijuana use can grow into dependence. A significant number of research works have not found evidence of physical dependence caused by the use of marijuana, but the possibility of psychological dependence has not been discarded and appears to be fairly common (Abood and Martin 1992; Flores Mosri 2017). Both casual and heavy users may be psychologically dependent in specific situations, surroundings, or when socializing. Additionally, the development of tolerance to cannabis has been largely documented. Studies show that most users need to increase the use of marijuana to achieve the same effects over time (Bresin and Mekawi 2019).

Joao Fasolino De Menezes and Stan Korotchenko

See also: Neurological Effects; Recreational Marijuana Laws.

Further Reading

Abood, Mary E., and Billy R. Martin. "Neurobiology of Marijuana Abuse." *Trends in Pharmacological Sciences* 13 (1992): 201–206.

Baggio, Michele, Alberto Chong, and David Simon. "Sex, Marijuana and Baby Booms." *Journal of Health Economics* 70 (2020): 102283.

Bresin, Konrad, and Yara Mekawi. "Do Marijuana Use Motives Matter? Meta-analytic Associations with Marijuana Use Frequency and Problems." *Addictive Behaviors* 99 (2019): 106102.

Cohen, Koby, Abraham Weizman, and Aviv Weinstein. "Positive and Negative Effects of Cannabis and Cannabinoids on Health." *Clinical Pharmacology & Therapeutics* 105, no. 5 (2019): 1139–1147.

Flores Mosri, Daniela. "A Neuropsychoanalytic Understanding and Treatment for a Borderline Patient Who Used Cannabis." *Neuropsychoanalysis* 19, no. 1 (2017): 87–101.

Gonçalves-Pinho, Manuel, Miguel Bragança, and Alberto Freitas. "Psychotic Disorders Hospitalizations Associated with Cannabis Abuse or Dependence: A Nationwide Big Data Analysis." *International Journal of Methods in Psychiatric Research* 29, no. 1 (2020): 1–6.

Jones, Jacob, Nicole Jones, and Jenny Peil. "The Impact of the Legalization of Recreational Marijuana on College Students." *Addictive Behaviors* 77 (2018): 255–259. https://doi.org/10.1016/j.addbeh.2017.08.015

Kalant, Oriana Josseau. "Report of the Indian Hemp Drugs Commission, 1893–94: A Critical Review." *International Journal of the Addictions* 7, no. 1 (1972): 77–96.

Meyer, Roger, Richard Pillard, Leo Shapiro, and Steven Mirin. "Administration of Marijuana to Heavy and Casual Marijuana Users." *American Journal of Psychiatry* 128, no. 2 (1971): 198–204.

Palamar, Joseph, et al. "A Comparison of Self-Reported Sexual Effects of Alcohol, Marijuana, and Ecstasy in a Sample of Young Adult Nightlife Attendees." *Psychology & Sexuality* 9, no. 1 (2018): 54–68. https://doi.org/10.1080/19419899.2018.1425220

Pope, Harrison G., and Deborah Yurgelun-Todd. "The Residual Cognitive Effects of Heavy Marijuana Use in College Students." *JAMA* 275, no. 7 (1996): 521–527.

Power, Robert, et al. "Genetic Predisposition to Schizophrenia Associated with Increased Use of Cannabis." *Molecular Psychiatry* 19, no. 11 (2014): 1201–1204. https://doi.10.1038/mp.2014.51

Sachs, Jane, Erin McGlade, and Deborah Yurgelun-Todd. "Safety and Toxicology of Cannabinoids." *Neurotherapeutics* 12 (2015): 735–746.

Thomas, Grace, Robert Kloner, and Shereif Rezkalla. "Adverse Cardiovascular, Cerebrovascular, and Peripheral Vascular Effects of Marijuana Inhalation: What Cardiologists Need to Know." *The American Journal of Cardiology* 113, no. 1 (2014): 187–190. https://doi.org/10.1016/j.amjcard.2013.09.042

Volkow, Nora, et al. "Effects of Cannabis Use on Human Behavior, Including Cognition, Motivation, and Psychosis: A Review." *JAMA Psychiatry* 73, no. 3 (2016): 292–297.

CBD Wellness Beverages

CBD (cannabidiol) wellness beverages have emerged as a specific type of cannabis-infused drink. The long history of cannabis-based drinks consumed for their reputed medical or wellness properties dates back to ancient India as early as 1000 BC (Courtwright 2009). The Swedish cannabis-based drink, Maltos-Cannabis, which became popular in Scandinavia in the late 1800s, was marketed for its medical value and pleasant taste (Potter, Bouchard, and Decorte 2016). Although the broader category of liquid edibles or drinkables also includes tetrahydrocannabinol

(THC)-rich products, CBD beverages are able to be sold more broadly and not subject to the same restrictions as THC products. For example, they can be sold outside of dispensary locations and sold even in states that have not legalized medical or recreational marijuana.

In the late 2010s, CBD products, including wellness beverages, emerged in large quantity in both marijuana prohibitionist states and states with legal medical and recreational marijuana industries. Although CBD wellness products still have an ambiguous legal status, they are commercially available throughout the United States. The 2018 Agriculture Improvement Act of 2018 legalized hemp, which in turn paved the way for the sale of hemp-derived CBD, although the legal status of CBD wellness products remains unclear. If a plant contains less than 0.3 percent THC (the psychoactive ingredient in marijuana), then it is no longer classified as a "marijuana" plant, but classified instead as a legal hemp plant, and this legality extends to CBD oils derived from the plant. The Drug Enforcement Administration (DEA) has made it clear that the Farm Bill legalizing hemp with less than 0.3 percent THC means that hemp-derived CBD is no longer a drug and no longer under their purview.

However, the Food and Drug Administration (FDA) prohibits the sale and advertisement of CBD in food or drink and as a wellness product if it has not been approved by the agency. As of October 2020, the FDA only lists the drug Epidiolex as an agency-approved CBD product, meaning that all other CBD wellness products, including wellness beverages, are in violation of the FDA (Akpan and Leventhal 2019). Although FDA enforcement has only involved issuing warning letters to violators, however, these products remain widely available in many parts of the country. Some individual states, however—including Iowa, Ohio, and Texas—have outlawed these products and have more aggressively enforced these bans (Akpan and Leventhal 2019). Another complication concerning the legal status of CBD is that these products can be sold without violating FDA regulations if they are sold without making any health claims, are not put in food, and are not added to a dietary supplement.

With more states allowing recreational marijuana, CBD products have become increasingly popular and have recently been sold outside dispensaries and specialty shops. This includes wellness beverages, with CBD being sold at major grocery stores in California and Colorado (Reiley 2019). Additionally, CBD drinks can be found in gas stations and "head shops" in states that still prohibit recreational marijuana. Looking to the future, it is unclear how CBD wellness beverages will be regulated and where and how they will be permitted to be sold.

Bryan Lee Miller

See also: Cannabidiol (CBD); Cannabis Drinks; Dispensaries; Drug Enforcement Administration (DEA); Edibles; Head Shops.

Further Reading

Akpan, Nsikan, and Jamie Levental. "Is CBD Legal? Here's What You Need to Know, According to Science." *PBS News Hour, Science*, July 12, 2019.

Courtwright, David T. *Forces of Habit: Drugs and the Making of the Modern World.* Cambridge, MA: Harvard University Press, 2009.

Potter, Gary R., Martin Bouchard, and Tom Decorte. "The Globalization of Cannabis Cultivation." In *World Wide Weed*. New York: Routledge, 2016, 21–40.

Reiley, Laura. "CBD-Infused Food and Beverages Are Still Illegal under U.S. Law. So Why Are They Everywhere?" *Washington Post*, June 24, 2019.

Central Asia

Central Asia stretches from the Caspian Sea to China and from Russia to Afghanistan, and it consists of the former Soviet republics of Kazakhstan, Kyrgyzstan, Tajikistan, Turkmenistan, and Uzbekistan. Cannabis has a long history in the region. One of the oldest cultivated plants in Central Asia, it was grown for grain and fiber as well as for recreational, medical, and ritual purposes. The region is known for its use of hashish, which is made from the resin extracted from cannabis plants.

Based on 2018 United Nations (UN) data, Central Asia has the highest average marijuana use rate among any regions on the Asian continent. Approximately 2.6 percent of the adult population use marijuana annually across Central Asia. This rate is higher than the average for Asia as a whole, but lower than the global average of 3.9 percent of the adult population (defined by the UN as ages 15–64). Among the Central Asian nations reporting to the United Nations, Kyrgyzstan and Uzbekistan have the highest rates of use, with 4.2 percent of the adult population reportedly using marijuana annually. Armenia, Azerbaijan, and Georgia all report that approximately 3.5 percent of their adult populations use cannabis. Marijuana is currently the major drug of choice in these areas; however, at least according to official data, the use of the drug is relatively rare when compared to other nations. For example, the same UN report indicates that approximately 17 percent of adults in the United States are annual marijuana users (UNODC 2018).

Although official statistics indicate cannabis use is relatively rare in Central Asian nations, there is anecdotal evidence that its use may be far more common than these governments admit. For example, in the Armenian town of Martuni, "Hemp Monday" is celebrated every Easter by stuffing traditional dolmas (rice balls wrapped in vine leaves) with the flowering tops of marijuana plants. Marijuana use is also allegedly prevalent in the Lake Evan region and in the rural villages near Yerevan (Hawdon 2005). Although the reported rates of marijuana use in Central Asia are slightly below the global average, use is believed to be stable or increasing in every reporting nation of the region. As in other Islamic cultures, marijuana use often exceeds the use of alcohol. This pattern is especially true in Tajikistan and Uzbekistan, where alcohol consumption is among the lowest in the world. It is also true in Turkmenistan, despite the relatively low rate of marijuana consumption found there.

Throughout the region, cannabis is illegal and its use often carries harsh penalties. Many of the strict laws regulating cannabis date to at least the Soviet era, but the new governments continued these antidrug policies even after independence. For example, Uzbekistan's Criminal Code states that any "involvement in use" with cannabis can be punished with three years of correctional labor or a three-year prison sentence. In Tajikistan, the production, sale, and possession of marijuana for either medicinal or recreational purposes is punishable with up to five years in prison for possession and capital punishment or 25-year sentence for smuggling (Veldman 2020). Yet, other Central Asian nations are considering alternative approaches toward cannabis. For example, Deputy Prime Minister of Kyrgyzstan Tolkunbek Abdygulov recommended legalizing cannabis to improve tourism in the country in 2017 (Weinberg 2017).

James Hawdon

See also: Africa; China and Southeast Asia; Europe; Hashish; India and South Asia; Latin America; Middle East.

Further Reading

Hawdon, James. *Drug and Alcohol Consumption as Functions of Social Structures: A Cross-Cultural Sociology*. No. 47. Lewistown, NY: Edwin Mellen Press, 2005.

Ren, Meng, et al. "The Origins of Cannabis Smoking: Chemical Residue Evidence from the First Millennium BCE in the Pamirs." *Science Advances* 5, no. 6 (2019): eaaw1391.

United Nations Office on Drugs and Crime (UNODC). *World Drug Report 2018*. New York: Oxford University Press, 2018.

Veldman, Maurice. "Cannabis in Tajikistan—Laws, Use, and History." *Sensi Seeds*, 2020. https://sensiseeds.com/en/blog/countries/cannabis-in-tajikistan-laws-use-history/

Wee, Rolando Y. "Marijuana Use by Region of the World." *WorldAtlas,* April 25, 2017. worldatlas.com/articles/marijuana-use-by-region-of-the-world.html

Weinberg, Bill. "Kyrgyzstan Could Bring Legal Cannabis to Central Asia." *High Times,* September 20, 2017. https://hightimes.com/news/kyrgyzstan-could-bring-legal-cannabis-to-central-asia/

Cheech and Chong

During the 1970s, the comedy duo "Cheech" and "Chong" emerged as well-known symbols of America's marijuana counterculture, relying on routines in television appearances, movies, and comedy records that leaned heavily into stoner humor and personas. Trailblazers of the American stoner film genre, Richard "Cheech" Marin and Tommy Chong made getting high as an exciting and, at times, rewarding lifestyle choice to the American public. Their unconventional act (and their later advocacy for legalization) helped normalize the use of marijuana in mainstream film and music. Today, Cheech and Chong are remembered as symbols of the zeitgeist of the irresponsible, longhaired, wildly clothed, but essentially good-natured pot enthusiast in the 1970s.

Richard Anthony Marin was born on July 13, 1946, in South Los Angeles, California, to parents of Mexican descent. As a newborn, Marin earned his notorious nickname "Cheech" by an uncle who said he looked like a chicharron (e.g., deep-fried pigskin). He attended college at California State University, Northridge, but prior to completion, he relocated to Canada to avoid the Vietnam War draft. In 1968, Cheech met Canadian-born musician Thomas B. Kin Chong (b. 1938) and joined his Improv comedian group to give performances at Chong's family-owned strip club in Vancouver. Shortly thereafter, Lou Adler, a reputable director in the entertainment industry on the West Coast, noticed their act and soon became their agent.

With Adler's support, the two young men released a comedy album, *Cheech & Chong*, in August 1971. The album included 11 tracks of not-so-politically-correct social

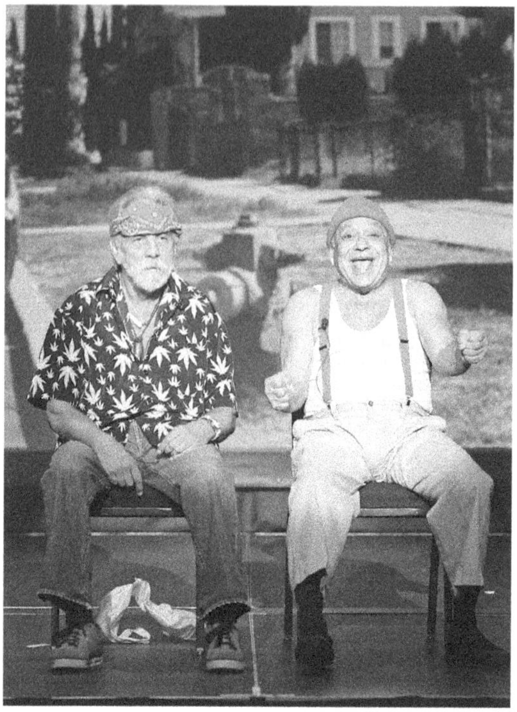

Cheech Marin and Tommy Chong performing together. The movie stars and comedians are icons of the marijuana subculture and are best known for movies such as *Up in Smoke* and *Cheech and Chong's Next Movie*. Tommy Chong also starred in the TV series *That '70s Show.* (Michael Bush/Dreamstime.com)

commentary and musical shorts to make the audience laugh out loud. Marin and Chong's liberation of marijuana as the forbidden fruit on the musical (and later, screen) stage was embraced by American youth and the drug culture. Marin and Chong followed up with a second recording, *Big Bambu* (1972), which earned them a Grammy nomination for Best Comedy Album. *Big Bambu* was the highest selling comedy album in history to that point in time. In 1974, Marin and Chong captured the Grammy Award for Best Comedy Album for their third album, *Los Cochinos* (1973). They ultimately collaborated on nine albums, the last of which was *Get Out of My Room: Cheech and Chong* in 1985.

Cheech and Chong are best known for their series of archetypal "stoner" movies. Cowritten and codirected by Chong, *Up In Smoke* (1978) was an instant hit at the box office, grossing $41.5 million and ranking eleventh in domestic films for the year. The comedy's plot orbited around extreme acts of marijuana consumption and the pot-smoking lifestyle, with Cheech and Chong at various points puffing on burrito-sized joints and smuggling a van made of marijuana from Mexico into Los Angeles. Barriers continued to be broken with more pot-smoking shenanigans in *Cheech and Chong's Next Movie* (1980), *Nice Dreams* (1981), *Things Are Tough All Over* (1982), and *Cheech and Chong: Still Smoking* (1983) and concluded with *The Corsican Brothers* (1984).

Following their final film in 1985, Cheech and Chong embarked on solo careers in America's entertainment industry and other creative ventures. Cheech diverted from stoner films and the stoner persona to play a variety of roles in film and television, including roles in the *Spy Kids* series, *Beverly Hills Chihuahua*, and the Disney series, *Cars*. He also became known for his expansive collection of Chicano art, some of which he made available for traveling exhibitions. His philanthropic efforts in promulgating Chicano artworks span to his authorship of children's books (six in total) and an honorary Doctorate of Fine Arts from Otis College of Art & Design in Los Angeles (awarded in 2007).

Contrary to Cheech, Chong continued to rely on the onscreen stoner persona in movies such as *Far Out, Man!* (1990) and *National Lampoon's Senior Trip* (1995), as well as a recurring role on *That '70s Show* (1998–2006). He also became a visible crusader for decriminalization of marijuana. The crusade heightened in 2003 when Chong was arrested and served nine months in Taft Correctional Institution in Taft, California, for distributing illegal drug paraphernalia through his family-owned business, Chong Glass. Code-named Operation Pipe Dreams and Operation Headhunter, the federal investigation crackdown on marijuana nationwide led to hundreds of arrests. Undeterred, Chong used his incarceration as a platform to bring further public attention to what he described as the beneficial effects and multiple uses of cannabis. In 2005, the documentary film *A/k/a Tommy Chong* told the story of his arrest and the time he spent incarcerated while also exploring why federal law enforcement lacks control over the billion-dollar "illegal" marijuana industry.

In September 2008, Cheech and Chong reconnected after 25 years for a reunion stand-up comedian tour called "Light Up America." In 2010, they partnered with the Marijuana Policy Project (MPP) for another tour in North America ("Cheech & Chong: Get It Legal") that combined material from their old routines with new material, all for the cause of raising awareness and support for legalizations. They also collaborated on a production line of pot-related paraphernalia and *Cheech & Chong* memorabilia. In 2016, Chong and his family launched a line of medicinal cannabis available at dispensaries and online. Chong also maintains a social media presence in the fight for legalization of marijuana.

Courtney B. Ross

See also: Marijuana Policy Project (MPP); Stoner Films.

Further Reading

Bibliography.com, eds. *Cheech Marin Biography.* Stamford, CT: A&E Television Networks, April 2014.

Chong, Tommy. *Cheech & Chong: The Unauthorized Autobiography.* New York: Gallery Books. 2009.

Chong, Tommy. *The I Chong: Meditations from the Joint.* New York: Gallery Books, 2007.

Gilbert, Josh, dir. *A/k/a Tommy Chong.* London, UK: Blue Chief Entertainment, 2006. DVD.

Kory, Grow. "Cheech and Chong on 40 Years of 'Up in Smoke': 'Real Life Drove Everything.'" *Rolling Stone,* Last modified April 20, 2018. https://www.rollingstone.com/movies/movie-features/cheech-and-chong-on-40-years-of-up-in-smoke-real-life-drove-everything-629983/

Marin, Cheech. *Cheech Is not My Real Name: ...But Don't Call Me Chong.* New York: Grand Central Publishing, 2017.

Meltzer, Marisa. "Leisure and Innocence: The Eternal Appeal of the Stoner Movie." *Slate.com,* Last modified June 26, 2007. https://slate.com/news-and-politics/2007/06/the-eternal-appeal-of-the-stoner-movie.html

China and Southeast Asia

South East Asia is perhaps better known for the production and use of opiates, but cannabis is one of the oldest cultivated plants in the region and is by far the region's most widely used illegal drug. The United Nation's World Drug Report estimates that approximately 9.7 million people in the region use marijuana at least once a year while approximately 3.2 million use opiates and prescription opioids (UNODC

2018). Yet compared to other regions of the world, marijuana use is rare in East and South East Asia. According to the best and most recently available data, only 0.6 percent of the adult population (defined by the UN as people ages 15–64) in the region used marijuana in 2016. To put this rate of use in perspective, approximately 3.9 percent of the world's adult population use marijuana, and approximately 17 percent of the population in the United States use marijuana.

Low rates of marijuana use are reported for several nations in the region. For example, Indonesia, Japan, Lao People's Democratic Republic, Myanmar, and the Republic of Korea all report rates of marijuana use that range from approximately 0.3 percent of the adult population to 0.8 percent of the adult population. The Philippines and Malaysia both report rates of use of approximately 1.6 percent of the adult population. Although these are relatively high rates of use for the region, they are well below the global average. Cambodia, with a rate of marijuana use of 3.5 percent, is the only South East Asian nation that approaches the global average of 3.9 percent of the adult population using marijuana annually (UNODC 2004, 2018).

MARIJUANA USE IN CHINA

The pattern of relatively low rates of use is seen when we look at marijuana use in specific South East Asian nations. For example, rates of use are low in China despite the fact that the earliest direct evidence of human consumption of cannabis was recently found in western China, in a 2,500-year-old Jirzankal cemetery in the Pamirs Mountains (Ren et al. 2019). Hemp and cannabis were widely used as food in ancient China and considered a major grain, along with millet, rice, barley, and soybean. Cannabis was also widely used medicinally as early as the Neolithic era, and it played an important role in religious rituals in ancient China. Despite marijuana's long history in China, its use is inconsistent with the Chinese family-based social system (Li 1975).

More recently, however, as China continues to rise in international stature, there is evidence that marijuana use among Chinese youth has been increasing. According to China's National Narcotics Control Commission, marijuana is the most popular drug among Chinese youth, and approximately 70 percent of the nation's marijuana users are between the ages of 18 and 35.

Given the size and diversity of China, it is unsurprising that rates of use vary across the country's regions. For example, rates of use in Macao SAR (Special Administrative Region) are nearly twice that of Hong Kong's rates. Still, illegal production of marijuana has been found in all 23 provinces, 4 municipalities, 5 autonomous regions, and 2 SARs that comprise China. Chinese authorities have expressed concern about how legalization of recreational use in Canada and some U.S. states may adversely affect their attempts to combat cannabis use among the nation's young.

MARIJUANA USE IN OTHER SOUTH EAST ASIAN NATIONS

Nations such as Singapore and Brunei Darussalam report some of the lowest rates of marijuana use in the world. Although the available data from these nations date to the mid-2000s, these nations report that less than one-tenth of 1 percent of the adult population use marijuana annually (UNODC 2004). Similarly, North

Korea reported a marijuana use rate of only 0.05 percent of the adult population in the early 1990s, but more recent data regarding marijuana use in that notoriously secretive nation is unavailable. The low rates of use in Singapore, Brunei Darussalam, and North Korea may be a result of the extremely harsh penalties associated with drug possession. For example, Singapore's Misuse of Drugs Act defines cannabis and its derivatives as Class A—Part 1 drugs, the same classification as cocaine, heroin, fentanyl, and methamphetamine. Possession of 15 grams of cannabis or cannabis resin or 30 grams of cannabis mixture is considered as "trafficking," and 100 grams of resin or 500 grams of cannabis or cannabis mixture results in a mandatory death sentence.

Like the rest of East Asia, Japan was a relatively latecomer in the recreational marijuana market. Despite an active illicit drug scene, marijuana did not become popular in Japan until the late 1960s, when cannabis offenses more than doubled between 1969 and 1972. Yet, even after marijuana use began to increase among Japanese youth, Japan did not experience major problems with marijuana abuse (Hawdon 2005). Laws regulating cannabis use are far less harsh than in nations such as Singapore, but penalties for marijuana offenses can nonetheless be significant. Illegal since 1948, marijuana possession is punishable by up to five years' imprisonment, and cultivation, transportation, and distribution are punishable by up to 10 years' imprisonment and a fine.

Thailand is another South East Asian nation with a storied marijuana history. Although the rate of marijuana use among the adult population of Thailand is only 1.2 percent according to one early 2010s' estimate, Thailand is famous for producing highly potent marijuana sold in the form of "Thai sticks" (Maguire 2013). While recreational marijuana use is illegal in Thailand—and possession or use carried a death sentence until 2017—Thailand is embracing the use of medical marijuana. They became the second nation in South East Asia to legalize medical marijuana in 2018 (Somerset 2018).

Other South East Asian nations have or are considering legalizing medical marijuana. South Korea was the first nation in the region to legalize medical marijuana. Japan, Malaysia, China, and even Singapore are researching medical applications for cannabis. While recreational marijuana use is relatively rare and is unlikely to be legalized in South East Asia in the foreseeable future, cannabis may again become a medicinal staple in the region, as it was centuries ago.

James Hawdon

See also: Africa; Central Asia; Europe; India and South Asia; Latin America; Middle East.

Further Reading

Hawdon, James. *Drug and Alcohol Consumption as Functions of Social Structures: A Cross-Cultural Sociology*. Lewistown, NY: Edwin Mellen Press, 2005.

Li, Hui-Lin. "The Origin and Use of Cannabis in Eastern Asia: Their Linguistic-Cultural Implications." In *Cannabis and Culture*, edited by Vera Rubin. Chicago: Aldine, 1975, 51–62.

Maguire, Peter. *Thai Stick: Surfers, Scammers, and the Untold Story of the Marijuana Trade*. New York: Columbia University Press, 2013.

Ren, Meng, et al. "The Origins of Cannabis Smoking: Chemical Residue Evidence from the First Millennium BCE in the Pamirs." *Science Advances* 5, no. 6 (2019): eaaw1391.

Somerset, Sara Brittany. "Thailand Legalizes Medical Marijuana and Kratom." *Forbes*, December 25, 2018. https://www.forbes.com/sites/sarabrittanysomerset/2018/12/25/thailand-legalizes-medical-marijuana-and-kratom/#7114d3bd2bb9

United Nations Office on Drugs and Crime (UNODC). *World Drug Report 2004.* Oxford, UK: Oxford University Press, 2004.

UNODC. *World Drug Report 2018.* Oxford, UK: Oxford University Press, 2018.

Chronic Pain

Medical marijuana is a potential treatment for chronic pain. Over 50 million adults in the United States experience chronic pain, according to estimates from the Centers for Disease Control (CDC). Some medical conditions associated with chronic pain include fibromyalgia, migraine, arthritis, multiple sclerosis, and cancer, and effective pain management is an essential part of treatment plans for all of these diseases and maladies.

Most states with medical marijuana laws have approved marijuana for the treatment of severe, chronic, or intractable pain. Chronic pain is the most common condition for those seeking and using medical marijuana, either as prescribed or for self-medication. For example, physicians in nine California assessment clinics indicated pain was the most common condition for prescribing medical marijuana (Reinarman et al. 2011). Likewise, over half of respondents using marijuana for medical use indicated they did so to address pain interference—i.e., pain that interfered with engagement in one's daily life (Wall et al. 2019). Medical marijuana patients are roughly 33 percent more likely to indicate they used marijuana for pain relief than non-patient marijuana users.

Is medical marijuana effective for treating pain? Substantial evidence indicates cannabis substantially reduces chronic pain (Hill et al. 2017) with a 30 percent reduction in pain across studies. Cannabis most successfully manages chronic pain, neuropathic pain, and spasticity associated with multiple sclerosis. Less is known about the most effective methods to administer cannabis and the proper dosages. However, both smoking and vaporizing cannabis significantly reduce neuropathic pain intensity even at low dosages (Wilsey et al. 2013). Additionally, cannabis appears to improve the lives of patients with chronic pain, as cannabis used to treat pain is weakly associated with improved health-related quality of life.

Another key question in chronic pain treatment is how medical marijuana compares to opioids in terms of effectiveness and the risks of problematic use (e.g., abuse and dependence). Problematic use is of particular concern for opioids, since opioid-related mortality rates have tripled from 2000 to 2015 (Bradford et al. 2018). Cannabis appears to be equally effective with opioids for reducing pain severity and pain interference (Shah, Craner, and Cunningham 2017), and studies indicate marijuana has a lower risk for addiction and little risk of overdose (Wen and Hockenberry 2018). For instance, based upon DSM-IV criteria for dependence, patients treated with prescription opioids have over twice the odds of problematic use compared to those treated with medical marijuana (Feingold et al. 2017). Furthermore, medical marijuana to treat pain may reduce opioid use in the population. For example, states with legalized medical marijuana have shown a reduction in opioid prescriptions filled by Medicaid and Medicare for the treatment of pain (Bradford et al. 2018; Wen and Hockenberry 2018). Also, states with medical marijuana laws have lower annual opioid overdose mortality rates (Bachhuber et al. 2014).

Researchers, however, have documented adverse effects of using medical marijuana as well among some users. Studies indicate that roughly 10 percent of marijuana users will develop cannabis abuse or dependence over a year regardless of whether they use marijuana for recreational or medical purposes (Lin et al. 2016; Volkow et al. 2014). Nevertheless, one-third of medical marijuana users use cannabis daily, compared to 11 percent of recreational users (Lin et al. 2016). It has been estimated that 25–50 percent of daily cannabis users may become addicted, with a higher risk of addiction for individuals who first began using marijuana in early adolescence (Volkow et al. 2014). Therefore, even though medical marijuana has lower risk of problematic use than opioids, medical marijuana still poses a potential risk for abuse or dependence, especially with daily usage.

Anastasia S. Vogt Yuan

See also: Medical Marijuana and the Law; Medical Uses.

Further Reading

Bachhuber, Marcus A., et al. "Medical Cannabis Laws and Opioid Analgesic Overdose Mortality in the United States, 1999–2010." *JAMA Internal Medicine* 174, no. 10 (2014): 1668–1673.

Bradford, Ashley C., W. David Bradford, Amanda Abraham, and Grace Bagwell Adams. "Association between US State Medical Cannabis Laws and Opioid Prescribing in the Medicare Part D Population." *JAMA Internal Medicine* 178, no. 5 (2018): 667–672.

Feingold, Daniel, et al. "Problematic Use of Prescription Opioids and Medicinal Cannabis among Patients Suffering from Chronic Pain." *Pain Medicine* 18, no. 2 (2017): 294–306.

Hill, Kevin P., Matthew D. Palastro, Brian Johnson, and Joseph W. Ditre. "Cannabis and Pain: A Clinical Review." *Cannabis and Cannabinoid Research* 2, no. 1 (2017): 96–104.

Lin, Lewei A., Mark A. Ilgen, Mary Jannausch, and Kipling M. Bohnert. "Comparing Adults Who Use Cannabis Medically with Those Who Use Recreationally: Results from a National Sample." *Addictive Behaviors* 61 (2016): 99–103.

Reinarman, Craig, Helen Nunberg, Fran Lanthier, and Tom Heddleston. "Who Are Medical Marijuana Patients? Population Characteristics from Nine California Assessment Clinics." *Journal of Psychoactive Drugs* 43, no. 2 (2011): 128–135.

Volkow, Nora D., Ruben D. Baler, Wilson M. Compton, and Susan RB Weiss. "Adverse Health Effects of Marijuana Use." *New England Journal of Medicine* 370, no. 23 (2014): 2219–2227.

Wall, Melanie M., Jun Liu, Deborah S. Hasin, Carlos Blanco, and Mark Olfson. "Use of Marijuana Exclusively for Medical Purposes." *Drug and Alcohol Dependence* 195 (2019): 13–15.

Wen, Hefei, and Jason M. Hockenberry. "Association of Medical and Adult-Use Marijuana Laws with Opioid Prescribing for Medicaid Enrollees." *JAMA Internal Medicine* 178, no. 5 (2018): 673–679.

Wilsey, Barth, et al. "Low-Dose Vaporized Cannabis Significantly Improves Neuropathic Pain." *The Journal of Pain* 14, no. 2 (2013): 136–148.

Clinton, Bill (1946–)

William (Bill) Jefferson Clinton (1946–present) was the forty-second president of the United States, serving from 1993 to 2001. Clinton, a Democrat, defeated incumbent Republican President George H. W. Bush in 1992 and won a second term when he turned back Republican challenger Bob Dole in 1996. Before becoming president, Clinton served as the governor of Arkansas from 1979 to 1981 and from 1983 to 1992, as well as the attorney general of Arkansas from 1977 to 1979.

Clinton's terms as president were marked by several noteworthy achievements. Among them was when Clinton presided over the longest economic expansion in American history, passed the North American Free Trade Agreement (NAFTA), and ushered in a new crime-control act, the Violent Crime Control and Law Enforcement Act. Clinton also passed welfare reform and the State Children's Health Insurance Program and appointed two justices to the Supreme Court.

Clinton's presidency was also marked by controversy, though. Notably, in 1998 Clinton became only the second president in U.S. history to be impeached. He was accused of committing perjury and obstruction of justice as part of an effort to conceal his extramarital affair with Monica Lewinsky, a White House intern. He was acquitted by the Senate, however, and left office with the highest approval rating in decades.

While campaigning for his first term as president, Clinton admitted to smoking marijuana when he was a Rhodes Scholar at Oxford University. In response to a question about past drug use, Clinton stated, "I've never broken a state law. But when I was in England, I experimented with marijuana a time or two, and I didn't like it. I didn't inhale it, and never tried it again." This remark was largely interpreted lightheartedly and seemingly had little effect on Clinton's presidential ambitions. In fact, it even became a source of ribbing and mockery for late-night comics. For instance, Johnny Carson subsequently joked, "That's the trouble with the Democrats. Even when they do something wrong, they don't do it right" (Waxman 2017). Even years later, the comment's cultural legacy was noticeable. For example, when then-Democratic presidential candidate Barack Obama was asked if he had ever smoked marijuana, he replied, "I did." He called that decision a mistake, but also confessed to being confused by Clinton's claim that he didn't inhale it when he experimented with marijuana himself. "I never understood that line," said Obama. "The point was to inhale. That was the point" (CNN 2007).

As president, Clinton took a firm stance on drugs. He frequently warned the public of the dangers of drug use, including marijuana use. In 1998 and 1999, Barry McCaffrey, Clinton's Drug Czar, paid $25 million to major television networks to include antidrug messages in their prime-time shows. The White House was allowed to sign off on the scripts in advance of their airing (Siff 2014). Moreover, the 1994 Violent Crime Control and Law Enforcement Act, passed during Clinton's first term, provided funding for the construction of new prisons and community police and drug courts, banned certain assault weapons, and instituted a three-strikes law whereby criminals convicted of a violent felony would be mandated to serve a life sentence in prison if they had two or more previous state or federal felony convictions, including drug-related convictions (Farley 2016).

The bill was seen, in part, as a continuation of the long-standing "War on Drugs" in America, first initiated by President Nixon in 1971. Indeed, the number of individuals incarcerated in state and federal prisons rose more rapidly under Clinton than any other previous president (Murch 2016). While Clinton long defended the legislation during his tenure, citing falling rates of both violent and overall crime rates, others criticized the bill for contributing to mass incarceration in the United States. The law's provisions for imprisoning individuals who engaged in relatively minor crimes, including crimes involving marijuana, received some of the most heated condemnation from critics. Clinton's defense of the bill finally relented in 2016. At an NAACP convention in Philadelphia, he admitted the 1994 crime bill exacerbated the incarceration problem in America, saying, "I signed a bill that made the problem worse, and I want to admit it" (Farley 2016).

Matthew Costello

See also: American Presidents, Anti-Drug Abuse Acts of 1986 and 1988; Obama, Barack (1961–); Reagan Administration "War on Drugs"; Trump, Donald (1946–).

Further Reading

CNN. "Obama: Yes, I Inhaled—That Was the Point." 2007. https://politicalticker.blogs.cnn.com/2007/11/26/obama-yes-i-inhaled%E2%80%94that-was-the-point/

Farley, Robert. "Bill Clinton and the 1994 Crime Bill." *Factcheck Posts,* April 12, 2016. https://www.factcheck.org/2016/04/bill-clinton-and-the-1994-crime-bill/

Murch, Donna. "The Clinton's War on Drugs: When Black Lives Didn't Matter." *The New Republic*, February 9, 2016. https://newrepublic.com/article/129433/clintons-war-drugs-black-lives-didnt-matter

Siff, Stephen. "The Illegalization of Marijuana: A Brief History." *Origins: Current Events in Historical Perspective*, 7, no. 8 (2014). https://origins.osu.edu/article/illegalization-marijuana-brief-history

Waxman, Olivia B. "Bill Clinton Said He 'Didn't Inhale' 25 Years Ago—But the History of U.S. Presidents and Drugs Is Much Older." *Time,* March 29, 2017. https://time.com/4711887/bill-clinton-didnt-inhale-marijuana-anniversary/

Coffeeshops

Coffeeshops refer to Dutch sales outlets for cannabis products, which mainly include cannabis herb and resin (hash), but they also include cannabis edibles to a lesser extent. While not technically legal, these sales outlets have been tolerated since the revision of the Dutch Opium Act in 1976.

Part of the rationale of the 1976 revision was the growing emphasis of Dutch drug policy on public health and the aim to separate "soft" and "hard" drug markets. Cannabis was viewed as posing an acceptable risk for consumers while hard drugs were associated with unacceptable risks. Cannabis-friendly coffeeshops thus came to be seen as a means to keep cannabis consumers at a greater distance from scenes and settings where more addictive and destructive drugs such as heroin are consumed (Grund and Breeksema 2013).

Coffeeshops evolved in three phases. They first appeared as an underground market in the 1960s and 1970s as part of the rising youth counterculture. The second phase was marked by the emergence of "house dealers" in community youth

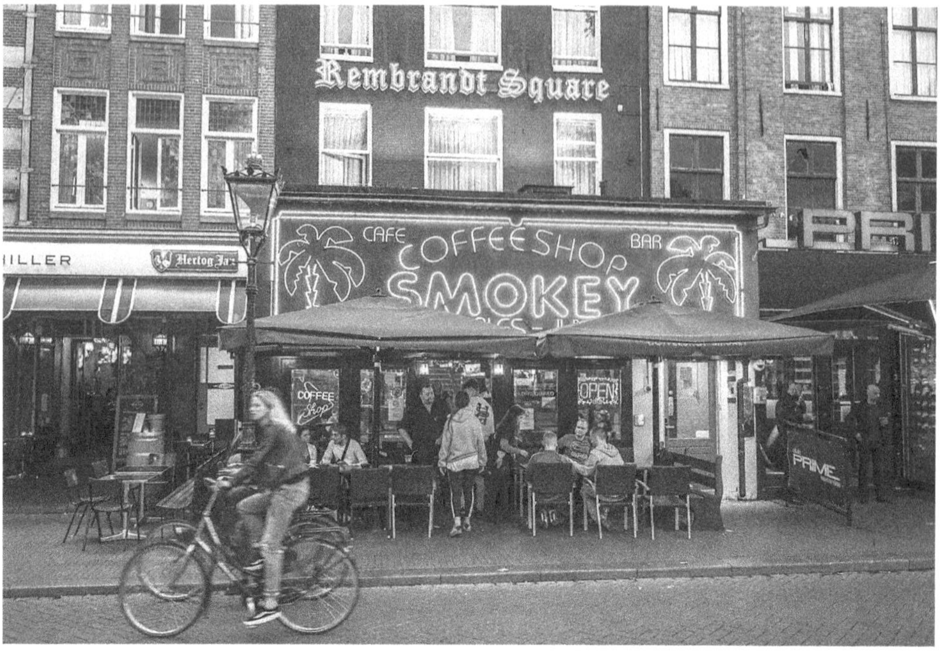

Coffeeshops are stores in the Netherlands where marijuana is openly sold. The sale of marijuana is illegal, but not punishable. Most coffeeshops are located in Amsterdam, as they have been closed in most other towns. (Erik Lattwein/Dreamstime.com)

centers and music venues in cities such as Amsterdam, Rotterdam, and The Hague. The final third phase formalized this emerging "house dealer" system and started the current period of tolerated coffeeshops when national regulations governing their operations were officially formalized in 1979 (Korf 2019).

Today, coffeeshops are required to have a license from the mayor of the local municipality, and keeping this license requires strict adherence to operational rules and regulations. These rules are referred to as the national AHOJ-G(I) criteria. (A) refers to a ban on advertising, apart from a minor reference to the establishment's cannabis offerings on the physical shop itself. (H) refers to strict regulations forbidding possession of any other hard drugs in these establishments. O (which is short for a Dutch term "overlast") refers to provisions to make sure that the coffeeshop establishments are not a nuisance to the wider community by, for example, generating litter, excessive noise, or parking problems. J ("jongeren") refers to regulations that do not permit young people under the age of 18 to be in the establishment. G ("grote hoeveelheden") refers to limitations on transactions to ensure that no large quantities are sold to individuals and that sales are for personal use only. Maximum selling stock is also set at 500 grams (17.6 ounces) per coffeeshop at any given moment. I, meanwhile, stands for *ingezetenen*, meaning that access to coffeeshops is only for Dutch residents. The last criteria (I) has been implemented in some but not all Dutch coffeeshop municipalities, mainly the ones bordering Germany, Belgium, and France (e.g., in the southern city of Maastricht).

Other restrictions imposed on coffeeshop operations include no alcohol sales (officially since 1996) and guidelines ensuring that all coffeeshops are at least 250 meters (0.15 miles) away from secondary education schools. Municipalities can also implement local criteria such as requiring coffeeshops to employ security staff and restrict opening hours. In the beginning of 2017, there were 567 coffeeshops operating in the Netherlands across 103 municipalities—about 30 percent of the nation's total number of municipalities. The remainder of the 390 municipalities that constitute the Netherlands had had a zero-tolerance policy toward cannabis coffeeshops (Bieleman, Mennes, and Sijstra 2017).

A paradox of the Dutch coffeeshop system is that while selling cannabis is tolerated through these establishments under the AHOJ-G(I) criteria, large-scale cultivation of cannabis has remained illegal. This means that coffeeshops rely on the illegal black market to procure cannabis for sale. Amendments to this so-called "back door" problem were made in 2017 when the parliament passed the Closed Coffeeshop Circuit Act (*Wet Gesloten Coffeeshopketen*) with a small majority vote. This act will set up an experiment in a total of 10 Dutch municipalities in which, under strict conditions, professional or commercial cannabis growers can operate without prosecution.

At the time of writing, the experiment is transferring from the *preparation phase*, where the implementation of the Experiment Act and the underlying Administrative Decree is agreed upon, to the actual *experiment phase*, where cannabis can be produced for, delivered to and sold in coffeeshops of the participating municipalities. The experiment phase is meant to run for four years, potentially followed by a *run-down phase,* which would bring the situation back to where it was before the experiment. This run-down phase, planned to take place in 2025, was criticized by the appointed experiment advisory committee in its 2018 report (Adviescommissie Experiment Gesloten Cannabisketen 2018) as illogical, especially if the experiment proves to be successful (Korf 2019, 12–15).

Aleksi Hupli

See also: Decriminalization; Europe.

Further Reading

Bieleman, Bert, Ralph Mennes, and Maurits Sijstra. *Coffeeshops in Nederland 2016. Aantallen Coffeeshops en gemeentelijk beleid 1999–2016.* Groningen: Intraval, 2017.

Grund, Jean-Paul, and Joost Breeksema. *Coffee Shops and Compromise—Separated Illicit Drug Markets in the Netherlands.* New York: Open Society Foundations, 2013.

Jacques, Scott. *Grey Area—Regulating Amsterdam's Coffeeshops.* London, UK: UCL Press, 2019.

Korf, Dirk. *Cannabis Regulation in Europe: Country Report Netherlands.* Amsterdam: Transnational Institute, 2019.

Colonial America

Hemp, which is a variety of the *Cannabis sativa* plant, was the most important raw good produced in the American colonies, and against the wishes of the British Crown, colonists used it to manufacture their own finished products. This led to a boom in the American textile industry. Hemp was also cultivated as marijuana and was commonly used medicinally and recreationally when tobacco and alcohol were unavailable.

Colonial American farmers began growing hemp to fill an obligation to England. King James I expected every property owner in the New World colony to export at least 100 plants each. Although tobacco became the primary crop in Virginia, farmers continued growing hemp to generate extra income. English farmers grew their own hemp, but as immigration to the colonies increased, a labor shortage negatively affected English hemp farms. At the same time, Americans began to produce finished goods (e.g., rope, paper, cloth) made of hemp. This was against British colonial policy, and the American hemp industry started to compete with that of the English.

Hemp became the most economically important crop in America, especially after farmers started "large scale spinning operations, thus establishing America's fledgling textile industry" (Deitch 2005). Hemp was also used to produce paper for newspapers and books. Other colonial American industries that benefited indirectly from hemp cultivation include shipbuilding, cabinetry, and furniture making. Hemp was so important to the colonies that several towns were named after the crop.

Colonial Americans also knew that marijuana could be used medicinally, and it was one of the only medicines available to them. Farmers intentionally cultivated marijuana with a high tetrahydrocannabinol content, and it was regularly smoked, brewed, or ingested to treat aches and pains.

Marijuana was also smoked recreationally because it was abundant and free, unlike tobacco. All classes of Americans from all over the colonies smoked marijuana, but only Virginians smoked tobacco. Americans smoked recreationally until after the Civil War. After the war, hemp production declined, and the collective knowledge of smoking marijuana was lost among white people. However, enslaved African Americans brought knowledge of the uses of marijuana from Africa and passed it down to their descendants.

Amanda M. Burroughs

See also: Europe; Latin America.

Further Reading

Deitch, Robert. *Hemp—American History Revisited: The Plant with a Divided History.* New York: Algora Publishing, 2005.

Lee, Martin A. *Smoke Signals: A Social History of Marijuana—Medical, Recreational and Scientific.* New York: Simon and Schuster, 2012.

Colorado

During the general election of November 6, 2012, the people of the state of Colorado voted on a groundbreaking ballot initiative, called Amendment 64, to fully legalize recreational cannabis in the state. In putting recreational legalization on the ballot, Colorado became one of the first two states to vote on and legalize recreational cannabis in the United States (the state of Washington held a similar successful vote on the same day). A slight majority (55 percent) of Colorado's voting public opted to legalize recreational marijuana, culminating a controversial, lengthy, but ultimately successful campaign to put state regulations on the sale of cannabis (see Ingold 2012). Although the vote was groundbreaking in many ways, overcoming the legal,

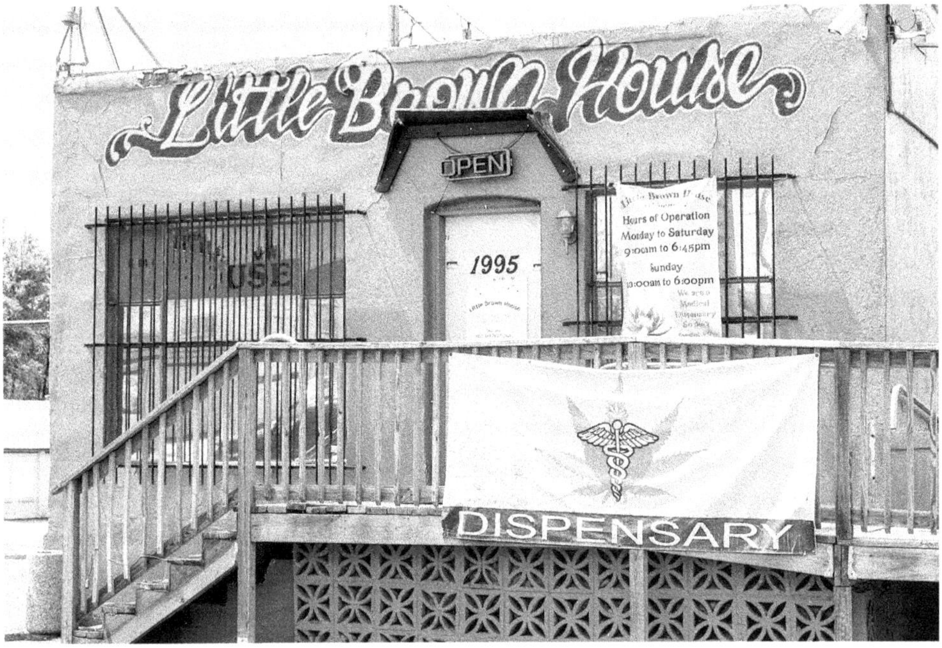

Little Brown House Pot Dispensary in Colorado. Colorado legalized medical marijuana in 2000 and became the first state to legalize recreational marijuana in 2012. Marijuana can now be purchased legally in marijuana dispensaries located throughout the state. (Freetraders/Dreamstime.com)

logistical, and economic issues surrounding recreational legalization provided daunting challenges to state lawmakers. Despite this, the Colorado legislature passed legislation governing the recreational market. On January 1, 2014, Colorado became the first state in the United States to allow for recreational cannabis sales.

Colorado's decision to put recreational cannabis legalization on the general election ballot marked the culmination of a long series of historical trends and events. Dating back to the conclusions of the Indian Hemp Drug Commission in 1894 and other historical research showing very few deleterious effects of cannabis use on the body (Allentuck and Bowman 1942, 250), Colorado's recreational vote also drew from a precedent that had been established in several states that already regulated cannabis sales for medical purposes. While proponents of the ballot measure often voiced their support for the measure by referencing empirical research on cannabis and prior medical legalizations across the United States, concerns about the potential impact of legalization were also widely expressed. In particular, opponents were concerned that recreational legalization would detrimentally impact the state's children and present insurmountable legal challenges and conflicts with federal authorities (Blair 2012; Ingold 2012).

The latter of these issues—legal challenges—was the most immediately problematic following the vote to recreationally legalize in Colorado. Article VI of the U.S. Constitution establishes the Supremacy Clause and the Preemption Doctrine, a set of related legal doctrines that establish the enforceable principle that state law cannot contradict federal law. In the event where a state law does come into conflict with federal statute, the federal government can "preempt," or nullify, the state law. Since cannabis remained a federally illegal Schedule I substance at the time when Colorado legalized recreational use, Colorado's state statutes conflicted with federal statutes on the issue of recreational marijuana legalization. Despite this, the Obama-era Justice Department and Attorney General Eric Holder emphasized the state's new law would not be preempted by the federal government. The lack of preemption was noteworthy because it demonstrated the federal government was open to reinterpreting the DEA Schedule and federal legalization status of cannabis.

Despite the political controversy surrounding it, there have been a number of benefits associated with the legalization of recreational cannabis. As of June 2019, Colorado had generated over $1 billion in tax revenue from cannabis sales (Associated Press 2019). This revenue comes from two sources. First, there is the state's general sales tax, which taxes each cannabis transaction at 2.9 percent. Second, and most beneficial for state revenue, is a 15 percent special sales tax on all cannabis that is sold in the state. Collectively, this income is redistributed to three entities—the Colorado Department of Education, the state's general fund, and a sizable, special marijuana tax fund, which is nearly entirely spent on education in a broad capacity. As a result of this tax structure, the state has been able to support general school funds as well as school construction, behavioral health programs, bullying prevention efforts, dropout prevention programs, and literacy initiatives.

Colorado's private sector has also seen sizable economic growth since the amendment was passed, and proponents of legalization say that the state's stance on marijuana use is one reason why. For example, two of Colorado's private industries—real estate and tourism—have enjoyed some of the most notable economic benefits. Since legalizing recreational cannabis, there has been a population influx across the state. In relation to this, home values have risen at a statewide average of 6 percent annually, an increase that is likely due to growing demand for housing (Cheng, Mayer, and Mayer 2018). However, residential housing is not the only segment of the real estate market that has experienced a property value increase. Due to harsh Colorado winters, cannabis growing is primarily an indoor enterprise. Therefore, commercial real estate, and especially warehouse space, is coveted by growers, and rent has increased two- to threefold for cannabis grow houses since legalization (CBRE 2017, 3). These increases in property values and population size have coincided with increases in travel industry revenue.

In addition to the economic gains from recreational cannabis legalization, a number of social benefits have transpired since the vote of 2012. Despite public concern about the effects of legalized cannabis on youth, there are several indicators that children and adolescents in Colorado have actually reaped advantages from legalization. Most notably, school dropout rates have declined while graduation rates have risen post-legalization. Furthermore, the number of students who reported trying cannabis before the age of 13 decreased from 2015 to 2017 (Colorado Division of Criminal Justice, Department of Public Safety 2018, 104). Similar findings suggest that the youth rate of cannabis consumption has been trending downward since 2013 (Colorado Division of Criminal Justice, Department of

Public Safety 2018, 121). Finally, in 2018, the Colorado Division of Criminal Justice reported that the number of felony cannabis court case filings has decreased.

While the overall cannabis-related arrest rate has subsided, racial disparities in arrest patterns for marijuana remain. Specifically, data from 2016 and 2017 show that Blacks are almost twice as likely as whites to be arrested (Colorado Division of Criminal Justice, Department of Public Safety 2018, 5) and 27 percent more likely to be booked into jail instead of being ticketed for cannabis violations (25–26).

Although there are a number of other advantages Colorado gained from legalizing recreational cannabis (e.g., medical research funding has expanded dramatically), there have been documented instances where legalization negatively impacted both public health and crime. For example, the Rocky Mountain Poison and Drug Center detected a notable and prolonged spike in cannabis-related exposures that plateaued between 2014 and 2017 (Colorado Division of Criminal Justice, Department of Public Safety 2018, 80). Additionally, traffic fatalities where drivers tested positive for any cannabinoid (alone or in combination with other substances) increased from 18 percent to 32 percent from 2013 to 2017 (Colorado Division of Criminal Justice, Department of Public Safety 2018, 50). Though Colorado State Patrol data suggest that total impaired driving citations decreased by 15 percent during the same time frame, there was an increase in cases where cannabis (alone or in combination) was identified as the impairing substance (Colorado Division of Criminal Justice, Department of Public Safety 2018, 2). Colorado's legalization has also impacted federal agencies, as evidenced by a steady increase in cannabis seizures by the U.S. Postal Inspection Service in the region (Colorado Division of Criminal Justice, Department of Public Safety 2018, 3).

Despite having some negative repercussions, several adverse consequences that were predicted to happen appear to have been entirely avoided. Overall, evidence suggests that the estimated number of high school students using cannabis appears to have decreased since legalization (Colorado Division of Criminal Justice, Department of Public Safety 2018). Although this could also be the result of other policy changes that happened around the same time (notably changes to zero-tolerance school policies), school-based suspensions, expulsions, and referrals to law enforcement remain at a similar level as they were prior to legalization (Colorado Division of Criminal Justice, Department of Public Safety). Accordingly, pre-legalization concerns about the impact of recreational cannabis on Colorado's youth appear to be largely unfounded. Instead, it seems likely that Colorado's education-focused tax revenue model has protected students from anticipated negative consequences and has even improved their education and quality of life in a variety of ways.

Though there was intense opposition to Amendment 64, Colorado's legalization of recreational cannabis has put strict state regulations on a substance that has relatively few negative health effects (see Allentuck and Bowman 1942) and legitimized an industry that previously existed primarily on the black market. In the process, Colorado's model of recreational legalization has proven to be a successful economic venture for both the public and private sectors. By demonstrating its fiscal feasibility, the tax revenue system that Colorado has created has been replicated in other states and serves as a national model for how to generate revenue from recreational cannabis sales. However, the key beneficiary of Colorado's recreational cannabis legalization is the state's education system and—by extension—children and adolescents in Colorado. If the Colorado model of recreational legalization serves as any indication, regulating recreational cannabis sales can ease the burden on the criminal justice system while simultaneously bolstering state coffers and private sector economics, improving schools, supporting research, and benefiting the greater public good.

Cori Pryor and John H. Boman, IV

See also: Alaska; California; Comprehensive Drug Abuse Prevention and Control Act (1970); Decriminalization; Vermont; Washington D.C.; Washington State.

Further Reading

Allentuck, Samuel, and Karl M. Bowman. "The Psychiatric Aspects of Marijuana Intoxication." *American Journal of Psychiatry* 99 no. 2 (1942): 248–251.

Associated Press. "Colorado Has Made over $1 Billion from Legal Marijuana." *New York Post* June 13, 2019.

Blair, Christina. "Protect Our Kids, Vote No on 64." *Huffington Post,* September 26, 2012.

CBRE. "Three Years after Legalization … Marijuana Real Estate in Denver." June 5, 2017.

Cheng, Cheng, Walter J. Mayer, and Yanling Mayer. "The Effect of Legalizing Retail Marijuana on Housing Values: Evidence from Colorado." *Economic Inquiry* 56, no. 3 (2018): 1585–1601.

Colorado Division of Criminal Justice, Department of Public Safety. "Impacts of Marijuana Legalization in Colorado: A Report Pursuant to Senate Bill 13-283." 2018. https://cdpsdocs.state.co.us/ors/docs/reports/2018-SB13-283_Rpt.pdf

Dean Runyan Associates. *Colorado Travel Impacts.* Last modified June 2018. https://industry.colorado.com/sites/default/files/DeanRunyan%20EconomicImpact2017.pdf

Ginsburg, Brett C. "Strengths and Limitations of Two Cannabis-Impaired Driving Detection Methods: A Review of the Literature." *The American Journal of Drug and Alcohol Abuse* 45, no. 6 (2019): 610–622.

Ingold, John. "Colorado Marijuana Legalization: The Strategy behind the Victory." *The Denver Post,* December 28, 2012.

Kalant, Oriana Josseau. "Report of the Indian Hemp Drugs Commission, 1893–94: A Critical Review." *International Journal of the Addictions* 7 no. 1 (1972): 77–96.

Compassionate Use Act (1996)

Proposition 215, Section 11362.5—better known as the CUA (Compassionate Use Act)—was added to the California Health and Safety Code in 1996. Proposition 215 was the first voter-approved initiative to protect rights for the use of medical marijuana within the United States, passing by a 56 percent vote. Conflicting with federal law, the Compassionate Use Act assured California residents the ability to be prescribed medicinal marijuana without threat of legal prosecution. The CUA legalized the use and cultivation of medical marijuana across the state of California. The CUA allows eligible patients or caregivers the right to possess and cultivate marijuana with orders prescribed by a physician. The act ensures that severely ill citizens of California are given the right to obtain medicinal marijuana as a way to relieve pain. These ailments include cancer, anorexia, AIDS, chronic pain, glaucoma, arthritis, migraines, and any other illness that may cause pain that impacts quality of life.

The CUA also provides protections to physicians prescribing medical marijuana to patients or caregivers. Under Proposition 215, physicians will not suffer legal punishment or prosecution for recommending or prescribing medical marijuana. Patients, patient's caregivers, those who have a prescription for possession of medicinal marijuana, and those who cultivate medicinal marijuana are protected from Sections 11357 and 11358 of the state's Health and Safety Code, associated with the possession and cultivation of marijuana, respectively. Along with providing legal protections to physicians, users, and cultivators of medical marijuana, the Compassionate Use Act also laid the groundwork for secure and inexpensive distribution of medicinal marijuana to all patients in need of marijuana.

Dennis Peron, a San Francisco marijuana legalization activist, led the efforts to place Proposition 215 on the ballot and get it passed. Peron fought for the use of marijuana for medical purposes in memory of his late partner Jonathan West, who alleviated symptoms of AIDS with marijuana. Before the Compassionate Use Act, in 1991, Peron organized efforts to pass the San Francisco medical marijuana initiative, also known as Prop P. With sweeping success, Prop P passed with 79 percent of the vote. Prop P did not enforce or change legislation but represented the city's support of the use of medicinal marijuana for treatment of symptoms of severe ailments and illnesses.

As the popularity of bills similar to Prop P grew across the state of California, attention turned to legalizing medical marijuana statewide. In 1995, the California legislature approved a bill legalizing medical marijuana, but the measure was later vetoed by Governor Pete Wilson. Peron worked with Dr. Tod Mikuriya, seen as an architect of Proposition 215, to form foundational roots in promoting a statewide legalization of medicinal marijuana. This movement focused on voters' approval of Proposition 215, which also became known as the Compassionate Use Act. A petition drive to gain more than 400,000 signatures necessary to qualify on the ballot was created and completed after wealthy donors donated more than $1 million dollars to the signature-gathering campaign. Elected officials and other Californians opposed to Proposition 215 argued that the bill would allow marijuana to be grown in volumes far exceeding the necessary amount for patients and that the excess would inevitably find its way to recreational users. Despite these concerns, Prop 215, the Compassionate Use Act, was enacted on November 5, 1996.

Anne McNutt Patrick

See also: Comprehensive Drug Abuse Prevention and Control Act (1970); Medical Uses.

Further Reading

Bergstrom, Allison L. "Medical Use of Marijuana: A Look at Federal & State Responses to California's Compassionate Use Act." *DePaul Journal of Health Care Law* 2 (1997): 155–182.

Compassionate Use Act. *California Health & Safety Code* section 11362.5, 2009. https://leginfo.legislature.ca.gov/faces/codes_displaySection.xhtml?sectionNum=11362.5.&lawCode=HSC

Feldman, Harvey W., and Jerry Mandel. "Providing Medical Marijuana: The Importance of Cannabis Clubs." *Journal of Psychoactive Drugs* 30, no. 2 (1998): 179–186.

Fox, Margalit. "Tod H. Mikuriya, 73, Dies; Backed Medical Marijuana." *The New York Times*, May 29, 2007.

Goldberg, Carey. "Wealthy Ally for Dissidents in the Drug War." *The New York Times*, September 11, 1996.

Ludlum, Marty, and Darrell Ford. 2010. "Three Lessons from California's Compassionate Use Act." *Academy of Health Care Management Journal*, 7 no. 2 (2010): 22–26.

Sloman, Larry. *Reefer Madness: A History of Marijuana*. New York: Macmillan, 1998.

Comprehensive Drug Abuse Prevention and Control Act (1970)

The Comprehensive Drug Abuse Prevention and Control Act of 1970 is an extensive law covering drug control and regulation in the United States. Congressman Harley Staggers (D-WV) introduced the bill in the House of Representatives on September 10, 1970, and it quickly made its way through both houses of Congress. President Richard Nixon signed the bill into law on October 27, 1970, and it became effective on May 1, 1971.

The Comprehensive Drug Abuse Prevention and Control Act is split into three titles, or subsections, each with a specific focus for drug control. Title I focuses on establishing drug abuse rehabilitation programs. Title II is the Controlled Substances Act, which is frequently used to refer to the entire Comprehensive Drug Abuse Prevention and Control Act. This title is primarily responsible for regulating and classifying controlled substances within the United States. The third and final title covers both legal and illegal importing and exporting of controlled substances to and from the United States.

The Controlled Substances Act was written to replace the Marihuana Tax Act of 1937 and is enforced by the Drug Enforcement Administration (DEA) under the Department of Justice. Controlled substances are organized into five schedules by the Drug Enforcement Administration and the Food and Drug Administration (FDA) based on their harmfulness, potential for abuse and/or addiction, and their medicinal value. While some are categorized as more dangerous than others, all controlled substances are defined as easily abuseable (Gabay 2013). The five schedules range from schedule I, which contains drugs with the highest abuse potential with no accepted medical utility, to schedule V, which contains drugs with the lowest abuse potential. Examples of schedule I drugs are ecstasy, heroine, and marijuana. Schedule II drugs include morphine, fentanyl, and methadone. Included in the schedule III category are acetaminophen, aspirin, and ketamine. The schedule IV drug list includes butorphanol, diazepam, and phenobarbital. Finally, schedule V controlled substances include Robitussin AC and Phenergan. Placement in a schedule is not necessarily permanent and may shift over time, but classification changes can only occur through administrative action or the political process.

Since the passing of the Controlled Substances Act, public discourse on marijuana use has shifted, including discourse surrounding marijuana as a drug with potential medicinal benefits. State-level marijuana policies and laws have begun to reflect this shift. Marijuana is now legal as a recreational drug at the state level for those above the age of 21 in Alaska, California, Nevada, Oregon, Colorado,

Washington, Illinois, Michigan, Vermont, Massachusetts, Washington, D. C., and Maine. It has also been approved for medical use with varying rules and restrictions at the state level in 33 states. Some states have provided legal protection to medical marijuana patients without legalizing marijuana use. A significant and growing gray area exists for doctors, lawyers, and other professionals in states with legalized marijuana, as federal law still applies.

There have been many unsuccessful efforts to declassify marijuana as a schedule I drug at the federal level since the passing of the Controlled Substances Act. The attorney general is responsible for drug classification and placement among the five schedules. Federal law continues to prohibit the growing, possession, and distribution of marijuana.

Lyla Byers

See also: Decriminalization; Drug Enforcement Administration (DEA); Marijuana Opportunity Reinvestment and Expungement Act of 2019 (MORE Act of 2019); Marihuana Tax Act (1937).

Further Reading

Berke, Jeremy. "Legal Marijuana Just Went on Sale in Illinois. Here Are All the States Where Cannabis Is Legal." *Business Insider.* Last modified January 1, 2020. https://www.businessinsider.com/legal-marijuana-states-2018-1

Controlled Substances Act. Drug Enforcement Administration, 21 U.S.C. 1970. https://www.dea.gov/drug-information/csa

Gabay, Michael. "The Federal Controlled Substances Act: Schedules and Pharmacy Registration." *Hospital Pharmacy* 48, no. 6 (2013): 473–474.

Hull, Helia Garrido. "Lost in the Weeds of Pot Law: The Role of Legal Ethics in the Movement to Legalize Marijuana." *Penn State Law Review* 119, no. 2 (2014): 333–360.

Morgan, H. Wayne. *Drugs in America: A Social History, 1800–1980.* Syracuse, NY: Syracuse University Press, 1982.

Conant v. McCaffrey

Conant v. McCaffrey is a 2000 court case out of the U.S. District Court in the Northern District of California concerning the rights of physicians to discuss or recommend the use of marijuana to seriously ill patients as part of the patients' medical plans. The case was heard and decided by U.S. District Judge William Allsup.

On November 5, 1996, California voters passed the Compassionate Use Act of 1996, also known as the Medical Marijuana Initiative. The law allowed seriously ill Californians to obtain and use marijuana as recommended by their doctors as part of their treatment plans for "cancer, anorexia, AIDS, chronic pain, spasticity, glaucoma, arthritis, migraine, or any other illness for which marijuana provides relief." The law went on to state that physicians could not be punished for recommending marijuana to patients.

Federal law classifies marijuana as a Schedule I drug, the most tightly regulated class of drugs, under the federal Controlled Substances Act of 1970. The act also prohibits doctors from prescribing any Schedule I drugs as part of their routine practice, since the government views the drugs as having "no currently accepted medical use in treatment in the United States." As a result of the passage of the 1996 California law, the state was at odds with federal law.

In order to prescribe any controlled substances (Schedule 2-5 drugs, since Schedule I drugs may never be prescribed according to the Controlled Substances Act), a doctor must obtain a certificate from the U.S. attorney general. This registration, also known as a Drug Enforcement Administration (DEA) registration since the attorney general delegated this registration to the DEA, can be denied or revoked if the DEA feels the physician has committed an act against the public interest.

On December 30, 1996, the director of the Office of National Drug Control Policy responded to California's Compassionate Use Act by noting that physicians providing recommendations for the use of marijuana (a Schedule I drug) went against the public interest. As a result, the DEA would begin revoking the DEA registrations of any physicians who did so. A group of California doctors and patients filed a challenge to the federal government's position on January 14, 1997. Shortly thereafter, on February 27, 1997, a "Medical Leader Letter" to the physicians clarified the federal government's position. It stated that simply discussing marijuana with a patient was allowed, but that doctors "may not intentionally provide their patients with oral or written statements in order to enable them to obtain controlled substances in violation of federal law." This new letter did not ease the fears of neither doctors nor patients about potential prosecution, and the original lawsuit moved forward. The federal government's response, the plaintiffs argued, prevented physicians from providing accurate and comprehensive information to their patients, in fear that even writing down a discussion about the possible use of marijuana in a patient's chart might be construed by the federal government as "recommending" its use in violation of federal drug policy. They also asked the court to stop the federal government "from enforcing or threatening to enforce any federal statute, regulation or other provision of law in a manner that would punish or penalize California physicians for communicating with their patients in the context of a bona fide physician-patient relationship regarding potential risks and benefits of medical use of marijuana."

The initial case was heard on April 30, 1997, by Judge Fern Smith. She offered a preliminary injunction, pending the final outcome of the case, that said the government could only prosecute and potentially revoke the DEA registrations of physicians who recommended marijuana if the physicians then knowingly helped the patient procure the drug. Simple discussion of marijuana's possible uses, under the formal doctor-patient relationship, was not enough to revoke a DEA registration. In 1999, the court case was reassigned to Judge William Allsup.

Allsup made his final ruling on Sept. 7, 2000. He ruled that the government may not:

(1) revoke a physician's DEA registration because a physician, in their best medical judgment, recommends the drug to their patient; and

(2) begin an investigation into a physician on the grounds that they have recommended marijuana to a patient.

The ruling applies whether or not a doctor knows, or ought to know, based on the recommendation that a patient will then obtain the marijuana in violation of federal drug laws.

Katherine Ayers

See also: Medical Marijuana and the Law; Medical Uses.

Further Reading

Compassionate Use Act. *California Health and Safety Code*, Division 10, Chapter 6, Article 2, 11362.5., 1996. https://leginfo.legislature.ca.gov/faces/codes_displaySection.xhtml?sectionNum=11362.5.&lawCode=HSC

Conant v. McCaffrey. C 97-00139 WHA, 2000. https://casetext.com/case/conant-v-mccaffrey-1

Controlled Substances Act. Drug Enforcement Administration, 21 U.S.C., 1970. https://www.deadiversion.usdoj.gov/21cfr/21usc/

Lucido, Frank. "Why Doctors Can't Work with Dispensaries: Conant v McCaffrey & Conant v Walters Salient Excerpts." *Berkeley Medical Cannabis Specialist & General Practitioner*, January 20, 2011. https://drfranklucido.com/why-doctors-cant-work-infor-dispensaries-conant-v-mccaffrey-conant-v-walters-salient-exerpts/

Confidential Informants

The term "confidential informant" (CI) denotes someone who has entered into a formal interactive relationship with law enforcement, as opposed to an *informer* who simply passes on information to authorities. Confidential informants are people who, due to various circumstances and diverse motives, assist law enforcement by acquiring knowledge on suspects' criminal activities and sometimes facilitate such activities under the direction of police handlers (Madinger 2019). CIs often operate alone, but they do so also in conjunction with undercover officers in both natural and constructed drug subculture environments to effect drug enforcement casework. Informant work in drug enforcement is oriented toward arrests of suspects, seizure of illicit substances, and asset forfeiture (Miller and Selva 1994). CIs provide knowledge regarding drug-dealing practices and networks, justify requests for search warrants, and basically provide law enforcement entry to otherwise inaccessible criminal settings. While their role in buying drugs on behalf of the police to secure search warrants is the main function associated with drug informants, they also have been heavily utilized in more controversial reverse stings wherein they help negotiate drug deals with the police as the sellers rather than the buyers of illegal drugs. The controversy centers on the association of this practice with asset forfeiture-oriented operations that do not necessarily involve arrest of drug offenders or seizure of illicit drugs from society (Worrall 2001). In fact, reverse stings actually introduce illicit drugs into society to affect a more multifaceted and thus strategic style of policing.

Not surprisingly, CIs are referred to pejoratively in the popular culture due to their extensive use in U.S. drug enforcement activities since the 1960s. Snitch, stool pigeon, rat, fink, and turncoat are less common references to CIs than is *nark*—a word inducing fear and legal threat. The nark reference derives from narcotics enforcement, as CIs have been a stable of drug enforcement work since the civil rights era, peaking in the height of the War on Drugs in the 1980s and is now commonplace drug culture jargon for someone to be avoided. This disdain is evident in the growth of social movements such as Stop Snitching, an anti-police cooperation movement in many inner-city communities where drug crime enforcement and prosecution is a significant contributor to minority overrepresentation in the criminal justice system (Clampet-Lundquist, Carr, and Kefalas 2015).

A handful of studies have examined police perspectives on CIs with heavy emphasis on incidents in which they have hindered law enforcement efforts—such as by stealing police funds for purchasing illegal drugs or providing untruthful information to help law enforcement secure warrants (Dabney and Tewksbury 2016). Derived from an outdated police science-technocratic perspective, these applied works understand CIs and the process of confidential informing in terms of their casework functions and offer a "how to" approach to effect optimal informant utilization. This approach has been criticized as dehumanizing as it tends to posture CIs as tools to be managed as indicated in police training manuals that reference "informant utilization" (Harfield 2012; Lieberman 2007).

Multiple examples of police abuse of CIs also have prompted policy reforms regarding how law enforcement handles informants. Rachel's Law in Florida, for example, was named after a college student who was killed in a drug deal gone bad. In that case, police minimized involved risks and knowingly exposed a CI to danger in order to advance their own investigation. Rachel's Law also asserts the need for a CI bill of rights—a cause that was subsequently taken up in several other states as well

Only two empirical studies featuring data with actual drug informants have been conducted that explain why people are willing to become an informant for law enforcement (Miller 2011). The usual motive is that most informants are charged with or convicted of a criminal offense (usually related to drugs), and the only way for them to avoid or minimize legal penalty is to put someone else in the hot seat through *marking*, that is, helping police build a case against someone else through informant work. Other leading identified motives include revenge, drug market competition elimination, and, less frequently, informants who provide information to law enforcement in exchange for a percentage of forfeited assets linked to drug activity.

The practice of using informants has been changed in some ways by infusions of technology into law enforcement work, but opportunities to inform officials about crime increase with electronic technologies in investigation and surveillance. Toll-free telephone and text numbers, electronic mail, and even public fax machines are widely available for citizens to turn in criminals, often for a reward. Reforms to civil asset forfeiture laws undermine CI use in reverse strategies to the extent that forfeiture revenue is the objective of casework. Nonetheless, per the institutionalized dependence of law enforcement on CIs, it is likely that informing practices will remain focused on substance abuse with casework prioritization likely reflecting broader shifts in drug control policy away from marijuana and forfeiture to the ongoing opioid epidemic.

J. Mitchell Miller

See also: Drug Enforcement Administration (DEA); Law Enforcement Efforts, Marijuana Control; Law Enforcement Resources.

Further Reading

Clampet-Lundquist, Susan, Patrick J. Carr, and Maria J. Kefalas. "The Sliding Scale of Snitching: A Qualitative Examination of Snitching in Three Philadelphia Communities." *Sociological Forum*, 30 no. 2 (2015): 265–285.

Dabney, Dean A., and Richard Tewksbury. *Speaking Truth to Power: Confidential Informants and Police Investigations*. Berkeley: University of California Press, 2016.

Harfield, Clive. "Police Informers and Professional Ethics." *Criminal Justice Ethics* 31 no. 2 (2012): 73–95.

Lieberman, Brian. "Ethical Issues in the Use of Confidential Informants for Narcotic Operations." *Police Chief* 74 no. 6 (2007): 62–66.

Madinger, John. *Confidential Informant: Law Enforcement's Most Valuable Tool*. Boca Raton, FL: CRC Press, 2019.

Miller, J. Mitchell. "Becoming an Informant." *Justice Quarterly* 28 no 2 (2011): 203–220.

Miller, J. Mitchell, and Lance H. Selva. "Drug Enforcement's Double-edged Sword: An Assessment of Asset Forfeiture Programs." *Justice Quarterly* 11 no. 2 (1994): 313–335.

Williams, Jay R., and L. Lynn Guess. 1981. "The Informant: A Narcotics Enforcement Dilemma." *Journal of Psychoactive Drugs* 13(3): 235–245.

Worrall, John L. "Addicted to the Drug War: The Role of Civil Asset Forfeiture as a Budgetary Necessity in Contemporary Law Enforcement." *Journal of Criminal Justice* 29 no. 3 (2001): 171–187.

Zimmerman, Clifford S. "Toward a New Vision of Informants: A History of Abuses and Suggestions for Reform." *Hastings Constitutional Law Quarterly* 22 (1994): 81.

Conflict and Labeling Theories

Whereas most theories explaining marijuana use focus on the implications of social class in constructing social interactions, environmental settings, and drug control policy, conflict theories delineate how additional collateral effects of disparity including exploitation, social alienation, and resulting personal frustration factor as drivers of use. Heavily based on the Marxist idea that social class plays a pivotal role in social institutions, this outlook argues that societal harmony is in no way reflective of the consensus model of social order outlined by the structural-functionalist framework. Instead, the perspective asserts that social institutions, especially the criminal justice system, exacerbate and promulgate imbalances of influence and wealth in society (Miller and Miller 2014).

In the 1960s and the 1970s, a rise of critical criminology in the United States called attention to marijuana use in terms of social class and racial stratification. Historical events during this period sparked and heightened mass disillusionment with mainstream American culture, with marijuana use becoming symbolic of resistance to the nation's political and societal infrastructure. The war in Vietnam, the push for equality and civil rights, the gender equality movement, and the sexual revolution all facilitated the use of drugs recreationally, with marijuana being the most popular and common throughout the nation. Cultural shifts intensified punitive state responses to marijuana and other illicit drugs. However, these punishment-oriented drug control policies did not reduce pot use, as marijuana popularity steadily increased to the point of "cornerstoning" normative counterculture. Increased use of marijuana, in fact, has been attributed at least in part to the symbolic significance of pot using as an act of rebellion against dominant societal institutions and attitudes. Within communities of marijuana users, meanwhile, social acceptance and additional access to marijuana culture serve as reifying behavioral reinforcers. Critical sociologists led the way in investigating the origins and nature of discriminatory elements of drug policy through structural Marxist ideas that relate to social class, but other scholars have focused on studying possible relationships between drug policy and other criminal behavior. Critics asserted that these foci strayed away from controversial issues involving onerous drug policy and law enforcement procedures that poor and racial minorities identified as discriminatory and unfair. Cognizant of these charges, researchers in the fields of sociology and criminology have added themes regarding social justice, especially as evidence of the prevalence of racial and social class inequality in the criminal justice system has accumulated. Some studies have suggested that current variations in how the justice system treats virtually identical crimes are predicated at least in part on the social standing and power of the offender rather than the antisocial behavior itself (Bonger 1969). During these years of liberalization and progression, recreational marijuana consumption became a theme for "sticking it to the man" and expressing individuality. The themes that surfaced during this resistance era continue to influence cannabis culture today. Marijuana consumption emerged as a social subculture that questions or defies many aspects of the current status quo and challenges the unequal distribution of power and authority in the United States (Miller and Miller 2014).

Critical perspectives also assert that the consequences of labeling were frequently more detrimental than the original triggering behavior (Tannenbaum 1938; Lemert 1951; Becker 1963). Labeling theory contends that legal authorities assign stigmatizing labels to certain forms of conduct in order to officially designate "deviance" to socially degenerate behavior—regardless of the objective inherent harm associated with the behavior that authorities are trying to reduce or eradicate. Labeling theory also outlines that the inward acceptance of a socially negative identity deeply impacts an individual's self-perceptions going forward. For example, supporters of the theory allege that if someone accepts or even embraces their reputation as a "pothead," the label could become a sort of self-fulfilling prophecy (Miller and Miller 2014).

Whereas marijuana use was popular throughout society by the 1970s, with prohibitions against its use only intermittently and casually enforced in more affluent white suburbs, poor communities of color were often subjected to intense narcotics enforcement, even for marijuana. Public support for this selective marijuana enforcement was bolstered by associations of pot with heroin and other harder, more dangerous drugs by lawmakers, officials, schools, police, and parents. Essentially, conflict theory is a more appropriate tool for examining heroin and crack consumption in lower socioeconomic and minority communities. Marijuana remains most heavily enforced in neighborhoods with high levels of poverty and low social status that suffer from social disorganization (the deterioration of infrastructure and rent-based transition) and related limited collective efficacy (residents' collective efforts to improve the neighborhood). Notably, these communities also are more likely to display a germane and curious common willingness to engage or at least tolerate a marijuana culture—especially one with socioeconomic overtones. Critics contend that marijuana interdiction efforts are often counterproductive and include collateral consequences of deteriorated police-community relations in general and, particularly, selective enforcement that results in disproportionate minority representation in the criminal justice system. Presumably, the nationwide trend toward decriminalization and legalization of marijuana will organically relieve social justice concerns related to how cannabis "offenses" are adjudicated differently depending on the socioeconomic background of the offender.

Nathan D. Coleman and J. Mitchell Miller

See also: Cultural Identity Theories; Differential Association Theory/Social Learning Theory; Social Bonding Theory/Social Control Theory; Strain Theories; Subcultural and Learning Theories; Theories of Use.

Further Reading

Becker, Howard S. *Outsiders: Studies in the Sociology of Deviance.* New York: Free Press, 1963.

Bonger, Willem. *Crime and Economic Conditions.* Bloomington: Indiana University Press, 1969.

Lemert, Edwin. M. *Social Pathology; A Systematic Approach to the Theory of Sociopathic Behavior.* New York: McGraw Hill, 1951.

Marx, Karl. "Das Kapital." In *The Marx-Engels Reader,* edited by R.C. Tucker. New York: Norton (Original work published 1867), 1978.

Miller, J.M., and H.V. Miller. "Sociological Criminology and Drug Use." *The Nurture Versus Biosocial Debate in Criminology: On the Origins of Criminal Behavior and Criminality*, edited by Kevin M. Beaver, James Christopher Barnes, and Brian B. Boutwell. Washington DC: Sage, 2014, 315.

Tannenbaum, Frank. *Crime and Community.* New York: Ginn, 1938.

Control Theories

Social control theories address a range of behaviors relevant to activities entailing behavioral restraint. As such, they are germane to understanding a range of addictions including substance use and abuse. For example, Emile Durkheim, a giant in the field of sociology, made the role of social control in preserving stability and solidarity in a diverse, organic society a major emphasis of his research (Miller and Miller 2014). Acknowledging that criminal behaviors are largely outcomes reflecting cognitions of control, various criminological theories showcase control as a key building block (e.g., anomie, containment, social disorganization, as well as the namesake theories of social control and self-control). Crime and antisocial behavior research has long affirmed social control as a primary criminogenic factor with various forms of societal deviance, including marijuana use, viewed as a consequence of minimal exterior and internal levels of controls (Miller and Miller 2014).

Social bond theory is in essence the primary twentieth-century iteration of social control theory. It was first presented in Travis Hirschi's *Causes of Juvenile Delinquency* (1969), which identified and explained four key theoretical components: attachment, commitment, involvement, and belief. A combination and balancing of these concepts can account for why individuals are either law abiding or engage in crime and deviance—which in many parts of America still includes pot use. Per this perspective, individuals invested in prosocial behaviors and attached to prosocial others, for example, are less likely to engage in what their dominant society deems to be deviant behavior (such as marijuana use, potentially) while those without healthy social bonds have a higher likelihood of partaking in activities that the dominant culture sees as being at odds with its values (such as marijuana use, possibly). Strong bonds with the community, peers, and family serve a protective function against crime and deviance such as drug use. These observations regarding control theories were formed when marijuana use was equated with illegality; it is likely that decriminalization will subsequently effect social definitions thereby calling into need theoretical revision. Whether legal or not, there is a relationship between life activities and delinquency, crime, and substance use as captured by the involvement element of social control theory, as those less involved and committed to social norms will ostensibly be less involved in conventional activities and have more time for experimentation common to teenagers, including experimentation with drugs and alcohol. Perhaps the most recent control-based explanation of crime applicable to drug use is self-control theory (Gottfredson and Hirschi 1990). Previously Hirschi had focused on external driving factors to a greater extent than the impact of failed internal elements such as self-control. Self-control is defined as an individual's ability to regulate impulses for instant gratification and calculate probable consequences for risky behavior.

Self-control theory posits six dimensions of impulsivity: (1) preference for simple tasks, (2) enthusiasm for risk-seeking, (3) physically active, (4) lesser interest in mental exercises or activities, (5) egocentric and self-absorbed behavior, and (6) difficulty in controlling one's temper (Miller and Miller 2014). People who suffer from low self-control are more likely to engage in the use of marijuana so as "to pursue immediate pleasures that are not criminal: *they will tend to smoke, drink, use drugs, gamble, have children out of wedlock, and engage in illicit sex*" (Gottfredson and Hirschi 1990, emphasis added). The use of marijuana and other illegal drugs has been linked to lower self-control in other studies as well (Arneklev et al. 1993; Ford and Blumenstein 2013, SAGE).

Nathan D. Coleman and J. Mitchell Miller

See also: Differential Association Theory/Social Learning Theory; Social Bonding Theory/Social Control Theory; Strain Theories; Subcultural and Learning Theories; Theories of Use.

Further Reading

Arneklev, Bruce J., Harold G. Grasmick, Charles R. Tittle, and Robert J. Bursik Jr. "Low Self-Control and Imprudent Behavior." *Journal of Quantitative Criminology* 9, no. 3 (1993): 225–247.

Baker, Joseph O. "The Expression of Low Self-Control as Problematic Drinking in Adolescents: An Integrated Control Perspective." *Journal of Criminal Justice* 38, no. 3 (2010): 237–244.

Ford, Jason A., and Lindsey Blumenstein. "Self-Control and Substance Use among College Students." *Journal of Drug Issues* 43, no. 1 (2013): 56–68.

Gibbs, John J., and Dennis Giever. "Self-control and Its Manifestations among University Students: An Empirical Test of Gottfredson and Hirschi's General Theory." *Justice Quarterly* 12, no. 2 (1995): 231–255.

Gottfredson, Michael, and Travis Hirschi. *A General Theory of Crime.* Stanford, CA: Stanford University Press, 1990.

Hirschi, Travis. *Causes of Delinquency*. Berkeley: University of California Press. 1969.

Marcos, Anastasios C., Stephen J. Bahr, and Richard E. Johnson. "Test of a Bonding/Association Theory of Adolescent Drug Use." *Social Forces* 65, no. 1 (1986): 135–161.

Miller, J.M., and H.V. Miller. "Sociological Criminology and Drug Use." *The Nurture Versus Biosocial Debate in Criminology: On the Origins of Criminal Behavior and Criminality*, edited by Kevin M. Beaver, James Christopher Barnes, and Brian B. Boutwell. Washington, DC: Sage, 2014, 315.

Cultural Identity Theories

The concept of cultural identity refers to a person's sense of belonging to a particular group, place, or culture. This process entails social learning about traditions, language, religious practices, heritage, and ancestry. With respect to behavior, the perspective is important because as people internalize beliefs, values, norms, and social practices of the culture with which they identify and their own self-concept, their thinking patterns about themselves and the world around them shape their behavior (Lustig 2013).

Recreational experimentation with marijuana has been strongly associated with youth culture—at least prior to the current pattern of decriminalization across the country. It is probable that legal medical and recreational marijuana users will abandon traditional stereotypes of drug users and dichotomize themselves as mainstream versus the harder drug users with whom cannabis consumers have historically been associated, especially among Americans opposed to drug use. "Individuals belonging to the subset of users that are considered 'hard' drug users due to chronical use should be the focus of substance addiction studies," concluded one 2014 analysis. "This perspective is supported through criminological and sociological foundations of thought that impose measures of delinquent peers and subculture to address the behavioral actions of drug users, in addition to support for the direction of addiction studies towards habitual users stemming from high representation of this group in the crime-drug nexus" (Miller and Miller 2014). Though soft drug possession and distribution constitute crime according to many legal definitions, they generally do not involve threats to the property or safety of others. Accordingly, criminological and related drug researchers frequently note differences between substance abuse and moderated use, specifically when the focal point of the examination is on drug-related crime. A leading concern expressed by habitual users about maintaining their lifestyle is addiction maintenance and thus drug acquisition. Social scientists theorizing on such group-influenced behavior should remember that not all drug consumption is considered drug abuse and not all drug use is illicit, especially in regards to many emerging and novel psychoactive drugs (Miller, Miller, and Claxton 2019).

The specific cultural identity theory of drug abuse detailed by Tammy L. Anderson (1988) posits a marijuana etiology featuring a pronounced sociological criminology orientation. The terminology of core idea "drug-related identity change" in this multilayered theory serves to (1) account for geographical and environmental factors (social disorganization) on individuals, (2) differentiate between drug use and abuse while concentrating on drug abuse, (3) highlight the significance of involvement in drug subculture, and (4) directly associate chronic drug users and drug-related offenses as intertwined if not driven by identity. The theory synthesizes factors such as geographical environment, societal influences, and peer groups, which furthers the examination of drug etiology, broadly.

Overall, Anderson hypothesizes that marijuana abuse stems from internalization of drug use identity that involve three layers of examination. Microlevel (*personal marginalization*, *ego identity discomfort*, and *lack of definitional control in identity development*), mesolevel (*social marginalization* and *drug subculture immersion*), and macrolevel *(economic opportunity*, *educational opportunity*, and *popular culture reinforcement)* perspectives allow for examination of both general factors related to chronic drug use as well as individual motives stemming from environmental and social conditions that affect drug use (Anderson 1998).

Despite limited empirical support for cultural identity theory, there are still a few key contributions that advance drug etiology, including (1) the wider understanding of the root causes of drug consumption stemming from multilayer analysis of casual factors; (2) recognition that the terms "drug use" and "drug abuse" are not interchangeable; (3) importance of legitimate interaction with individuals involved in a given drug subculture as well as the culture itself; and (4) drug user "self-identities" may be created as a result of interactions with drug subcultures (Anderson 1998, Miller and Miller 2014). Though theoretically comprehensive and appropriate for thorough multilevel empirical analysis, the theory has continued to mainly lean on sociological criminology—an unfortunate reality given the perspective's applicability to the understanding of a broader range of social and behavioral phenomena.

Nathan D. Coleman and J. Mitchell Miller

See also: Conflict and Labeling Theories; Differential Association Theory/Social Learning Theory; Social Bonding Theory/Social Control Theory; Strain Theories; Subcultural and Learning Theories; Theories of Use.

Further Reading

Anderson, Tammy L. "A Cultural-Identity Theory of Drug Abuse." *Sociology of Crime, Law, and Deviance* 1, no. 262 (1998): 233–262.

Geiger-Oneto, Stephanie, and Travis Simkins. "A Social Identity Perspective on the Legalization of Marijuana in the United States." *Journal of Macromarketing* 38, no. 2 (2018): 206–217.

Lustig, M.W. *Intercultural Competence Interpersonal Communication across Cultures*, 7th ed. New York: Pearson, 2013.

Miller, J.M., and H.V. "Sociological Criminology and Drug Use." *The Nurture Versus Biosocial Debate in Criminology: On the Origins of Criminal Behavior and Criminality*, edited by Kevin M. Beaver, James Christopher Barnes, and Brian B. Boutwell. Washington, DC: Sage, 2014, 315.

Miller, J.M., H.V. Miller, and T.L. Claxton. "Theorizing Novel and Emerging Drug Use: A Motivational Typology." *Deviant Behavior* 40, no. 9 (2019): 1105–1118.

Urietta, Luis, Jr., and George W. Noblit, eds. *Cultural Constructions of Identity.* New York: Oxford University Press, 2018.

Cypress Hill

Forebears of West Coast rap/hip-hop, and the first Latinos to reach stardom in mainstream American hip-hop, Cypress Hill is known for its vocal and unapologetic blatant endorsement of marijuana. Using lyrics that depict smoking marijuana and engaging in violence as a way of life in songs such as "How I Could Just Kill a Man" and "Shoot 'Em Up," both released in 1991, Cypress Hill has had great success in the music industry, including multiplatinum sales, billboard charts, sellout concerts, and soundtrack hits. Canonical classics such as "Hits from the Bong" and "I Wanna Get High," both from their second album (*Black Sunday*, 1993), consistently rank in the top tier of greatest stoner songs. As music executive Mike Pizzo wrote, "They were the first group blunt enough—no pun intended—to openly embrace cannabis culture on a mainstream platform, making it okay for every rapper thereafter to do so" (Pizzo 2016).

Cypress Hill formed in 1988, and original members Louis "B-Real" Freese, Senen "Sen Dog" Reyes, and Lawrence "DJ Muggs" Muggerud remain the core of the group. The group first signed with Ruffhouse/Columbia Records in 1991, and its first album, *Cypress Hill*, was released in early 1992. The group's growing popularity in subsequent years has been attributed in part to its diverse sounds. Songs such as "Insane in the Brain" (1993), "Rap Superstar" (2000), and "Rock Superstar" (2000) are acknowledged by audiences across musical genres, including hip-hop, rock rap/metal rap, psychedelic rock, rap, and grunge. The group's crossover success has been continuously recognized with several Grammy nominations, and in 2018, it became the 2,660th star on the Hollywood Walk of Fame.

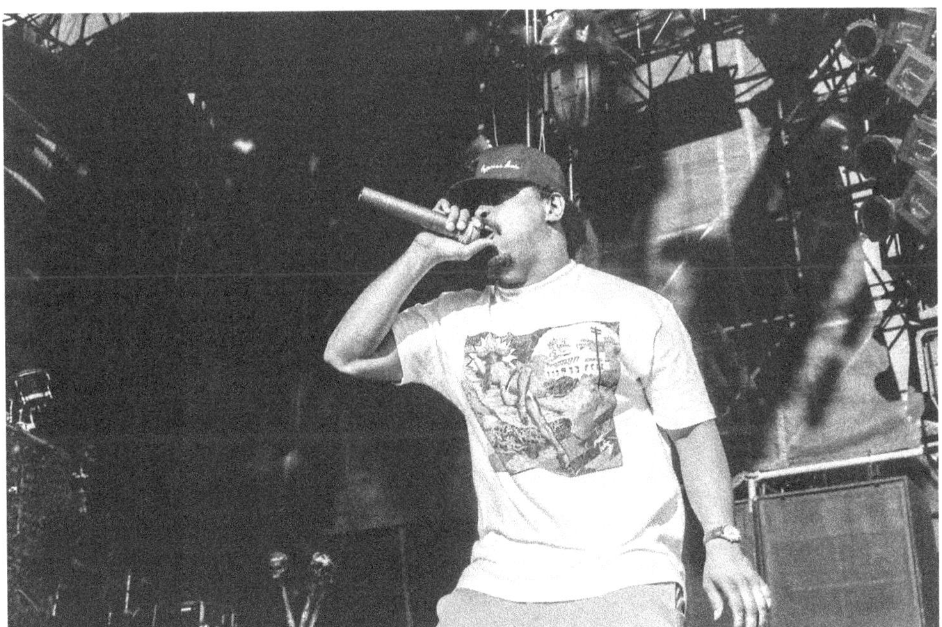

American hip-hop group Cypress Hill performing on stage. Formed in 1988 in California, the group is known for numerous pro-marijuana songs and advocacy. They have sold over 20 million albums worldwide. (Mirjana Simeunovich/Dreamstime.com)

From featuring pot leaves on its website (cypresshill.com) to recording songs that celebrate pot for more than a quarter-century—from "Legalize It" on *Black Sunday* (1993) to "The Reefer Man" on *Elephants on Acid* (2018), Cypress Hill has used its fame as a platform to endorse the legalization of recreational and medicinal marijuana. The group even discussed marijuana's purported medicinal and wellness benefits in the liner notes of *Black Sunday,* its second album. "For a long time it was a bad word; saying 'weed' was like saying 'heroin' or something," said Sen. "The fun wasn't there anymore. We just had to put a cool twist back on it like Cheech and Chong did in the 70s and get people to relax on the subject" (Pizzo 2016).

Cypress Hill's pro-marijuana stance has also been evident in its live performances. The Cypress Hill SmokeOut, for example, was a music festival featuring bands and singers across genres with a pro-pot stance. Held yearly from 1998 to 2006 and once more in 2012, the festival was particularly tailored to California-registered "green" patients (state residents legally permitted to purchase and use medical marijuana) and advocated for the safe and responsible usage of marijuana consumption. More recently, B-Real moved his advocacy into production and consumerism by opening Dr. Greenthumb's Dispensary in Sylmar, a neighborhood in Los Angeles, California. This high-end medical and recreational marketplace boasts products (including paraphernalia merchandise) crafted by experienced growers and smokers.

Courtney B. Ross

See also: Beatles, The; Garcia, Jerry (1942–1995); Marley, Bob (1945–1981); Monkees, The; Petty, Tom (1950–2017); Snoop Dogg (1971–); Woodstock.

Further Reading

Erlewine, Steven Thomas. "Cypress Hill." AllMusic.com, n.d. Accessed August 23, 2021. https://www.allmusic.com/artist/cypress-hill-mn0000147315/biography

Martin, Brittany. "Cypress Hill Rapper B-Real Is Opening an Upscale Marijuana Shop in the Valley." *Los Angeles Magazine,* August 14, 2018. https://www.lamag.com/lalifeandstyle/dr-greenthumb/

Pizzo, Mike. "How Cypress Hill Made Marijuana Mainstream." Medium.com, September 1, 2016. https://medium.com/cuepoint/how-cypress-hill-made-marijuana-mainstream-44408324ae7b

D

Dabbing

American media has often described "dabbing" as a trend that first emerged in the early 2000s, but marijuana users have engaged in the behavior since the 1960s. Dabbing refers broadly to the use of concentrated tetrahydrocannabinol, or THC, products created through the use of solvents. These products are created legally by distributers in recreational and medical marijuana states—and illegally in states where pot remains illegal. A variety of different solvents have been used to produce "dabs" or "oil," but amateurs in the production process have frequently used butane. As a result, "butane hash oil" and "BHO" have become standard terms for the product regardless of the solvent used. Other, more specific terminology that describes the product's consistency (e.g., shatter, honeycomb, crumble wax, budder, earwax) has also been used. Dabs are far more potent than traditional flower cannabis, consumed in a single inhalation rather than several breaths, and their popularity seems to be increasing.

Several factors have facilitated the spread of dabbing. First, it was seen as a novelty, a curiosity, and an advanced way of administering a new drug, all of which appealed to marijuana users eager to experiment and explore new tools and methods for getting high (Sagar et al. 2018). Users could inhale larger doses at once with impressive devices such as water pipes modified into "oil rigs" through the use of "nails" (hollow titanium or ceramic cylinder with a concave surface on one end), "swings" (a metal heating surface that moves the dab as needed with the pipe), or "skillets" (metal heating plate; Stogner and Miller 2015). Second, it was described as a way of salvaging less potent portions of the cannabis plant that were generally discarded due to THC content being too low for smoking. Curiosity and the thrill of experimentation in the production process may have also played a role, as amateur "blasting" is a simple, albeit dangerous, process that requires no prior chemical knowledge. In addition, step-by-step guidelines for the process, meanwhile, are widely available online. Third, the high achieved from dabbing has been described as more intense and qualitatively different from that achieved through traditional flower cannabis smoking (Miller, Stogner, and Miller 2016). Reports indicate that some prefer dabs after using them and act differently concerning their supply. The THC concentration of dabs can exceed 50 percent, so it is not unsurprising that substance users view them differently and experience different effects. Finally, oil products are now used in electronic devices, simplifying the process and making them easy to use in a variety of locations. These products allow for administration in a manner resembling e-cigarettes.

The creation of "dabbing" concentrates involves passing a solvent, most often liquid butane, through a tube or container of unmodified cannabis. THC and other hydrophobic compounds in the plants' trichomes dissolve into the solvent. A filter prevents the plant material from leaving the container, but the solvent and THC solution pass through into another container. The solvent either then evaporates or is removed with heat and/or a vacuum, leaving a residue with a much higher THC concentration than the material from which it was produced. Commercial/medical environments are highly regulated and must use a closed-loop system that prevents flammable solvents from accumulating in enclosed spaces. Amateurs instead use a more straightforward open system with tools such as steel tubes, window screens, and Pyrex dishes. This allows volatile and flammable compounds to accumulate and creates a genuine risk that explosions and fires may start following a spark or buildup of static electricity. Numerous fires have been connected to the production of THC concentrates via solvents in the last several years.

Many additional issues have been associated with the production of dabs. First, the number of dabbing-related fires is likely a severe underestimate of the problem. Very few fire departments are trained to distinguish these fires from those related to other sources. Further, residents of burned homes who were involved in substance distribution are unlikely to admit their involvement with THC concentration. Online discussions of dabbing promote home "blasting" without appropriately characterizing fire risk and steps that can be taken to mitigate that risk.

Additionally, blasting carries significant legal risk even in states that allow for recreation or medicinal marijuana sales (Al-Zouabi et al. 2018). Though marijuana possession may be decriminalized, the blasting process has been interpreted as the operation of a drug laboratory that may carry a sentence of three years. Finally, many products are inadequately purged of solvents. Though butane or other solvents are argued to dissipate from the dabs after extraction, experts believe that over 80 percent of THC products still contain these solvents or traces of pesticides (Raber, Elzinga, and Kaplan 2015).

Scholars and medical professionals have cautioned that it is inappropriate to assume that dabs carry no more risk than the product from which they are created. To date, there is still a lack of sufficient research to determine whether commercially or medically produced dabs are adequately safe for administration (or even equally safe compared to flower cannabis). One survey of frequent marijuana users who engage in dabbing found no indication that dabbing was associated with increased injuries, accidents, or medical issues (Loflin and Earleywine 2014). However, other studies have tied dabbing to health issues such as respiratory failure, acute lung injury, and a form of atypical pneumonia (Anderson and Zechar 2019). As these results are case studies, generalizability is a concern. Still, not enough is known about the effects of administering a high THC dose in a single breath through dabbing to make claims about safety. As one study summarized, "Patients should be advised that research is lacking, information is still largely anecdotal, and that the safest option is to refrain from use when definitive answers are lacking" (Stogner and Miller 2015, 3).

Lucas Maness and John Stogner

See also: Butane Hash Oil; Tetrahydrocannabinol (THC).

Further Reading

Al-Zouabi, Ihsan, John M. Stogner, Bryan Lee Miller, and Elizabeth S. Lane. "Butane Hash Oil and Dabbing: Insights into Use, Amateur Production Techniques, and Potential Harm Mitigation." *Substance Abuse and Rehabilitation* 9 (2018): 91.

Anderson, Ryan P., and Katie Zechar. "Lung Injury from Inhaling Butane Hash Oil Mimics Pneumonia." *Respiratory Medicine Case Reports* 26 (2019): 171–173.

Loflin, Mallory, and Mitch Earleywine. "A New Method of Cannabis Ingestion: The Dangers of Dabs?" *Addictive Behaviors* 39, no. 10 (2014): 1430–1433.

Miller, Bryan Lee, John M. Stogner, and J. Mitchell Miller. "Exploring Butane Hash Oil Use: A Research Note." *Journal of Psychoactive Drugs* 48, no. 1 (2016): 44–49.

Raber, Jeffrey C., Sytze Elzinga, and Charles Kaplan. "Understanding Dabs: Contamination Concerns of Cannabis Concentrates and Cannabinoid Transfer during the Act of Dabbing." *The Journal of Toxicological Sciences* 40, no. 6 (2015): 797–803.

Sagar, Kelly A., Ashley M. Lambros, Mary Kathryn Dahlgren, Rosemary T. Smith, and Staci A. Gruber. "Made from Concentrate? A National Web Survey Assessing Dab Use in the United States." *Drug and Alcohol Dependence* 190 (2018): 133–142.

Stogner, John M., and Bryan Lee Miller. "Assessing the Dangers of 'Dabbing': Mere Marijuana or Harmful New Trend?" *Pediatrics* 136, no. 1 (2015): 1–3.

Dazed and Confused

Dazed and Confused is a nostalgia-tinged film about U.S. youth culture set in a small, sleepy, fictitious Texas town in the mid-1970s, complete with the popular music of the day, vintage cars, tight jeans, cutting class, and plenty of marijuana use. The film, directed by Richard Linklater and released in 1993, opens on the last day of class at Buchanan High School.

In the extended, iconic first scene of the movie, set to the song "Sweet Emotion" by Aerosmith, there are over a dozen individual references to marijuana—students smoking it, buying it, drawing pictures of pot leaves, engaging in a complex dap that ends with each party pretending to puff a joint, and making plans to get together to smoke later. As the movie title—a reference to a Led Zeppelin song—would suggest, weed figures as the common, even essential, element of North American youth culture, and the film presents smoking "herb" in an overwhelmingly positive light.

The plot revolves around a coming-of-age ritual, in which the high school senior men hunt down and paddle incoming freshmen boys and senior women subject incoming first-year girls to humiliation, covering them with ketchup and mustard, commanding them to "fry like bacon," and making them propose to senior men. Other related coming-of-age rituals involve smoking grass, drinking, and sexual encounters (all of which are heterosexual). The town supports this ritual, despite its violent nature, and a lot of the youthful partying. Not everyone participates, however; only "known" or cool kids are hazed, which is like an invitation to join the partying scene. Mitch Kramer (played by Wiley Wiggins) is an incoming freshman, who is known by the seniors and singled out for a paddling. Viewers come to understand that Mitch is popular because he is a talented baseball pitcher and because his older sister is part of the cool set.

Weed is presented as normal and pervasive within the high school world, but still something to keep secret from the world at large, including parents, teachers, and other adults. And while not every teen featured in the movie smokes pot, everyone who is portrayed a "cool" seems to do so. Indeed, in one scene, a pot smoker and dealer named Slater (Rory Cochrane) asks Mitch, "You cool, man?" which another character explains means: "Do you smoke weed?" The movie is an unapologetic celebration of marijuana use, as well as a primer on the basics of weed culture—profane knowledge that titillates the initiated and initiates the curious. For example, students in shop class making a bong receive advice from Slater on how to make the carburetor airtight. Weed is represented as the pathway to fun and pleasure and social inclusion and a tool of rebellion against parental and societal authority.

The politics of the film are antiauthoritarian, anti-jerk, and pro-pleasure, with marijuana unambiguously presented as both an antidote to negative social forces and a positive symbol of fun, freedom, and a laidback approach to life. Authoritarianism and jerkiness are primarily represented by the high school football coaches, especially because they are trying to force football players to sign a pledge saying that they will not use drugs, the other major element of the plot. There are only two teen characters who are negatively represented. First there is O'Bannion (Ben Affleck), who just failed his senior year and is going to repeat. He takes sadistic pleasure in paddling the incoming freshmen. The paddling victims think he is a jerk, and O'Bannion's peers agree but still tolerate him. The young boys get the last laugh when they lure him into an open area to paddle an incoming freshman and pour white paint on his head. He leaves furious and humiliated. In one scene, O'Bannion aggressively demands drugs from Slater, who refuses him—a stand that can be easily interpreted as a form of punishment for his nasty behavior and disposition. The only other young character presented negatively is also violent—a young man who tries to pick a fight with a nerdy/intellectual character at a party.

On the surface, none of the characters seem to suffer negative consequences from their marijuana use, but upon closer inspection, the situation is more complicated. *Dazed* establishes norms with relation to the countercultural realm. The longhaired, dealer character, who wears a shirt with a marijuana leaf on it and an ascot cap on backward, is represented as friendly and cool, but is also a bit of a caricature. Perpetually high, he is in danger of flunking out of high school altogether. He is depicted as excessively preoccupied with pot, and despite the prevalence of marijuana in the youth scene, he is the only person for whom marijuana is the extent of his identity. The message is clear: pot is cool to enjoy with friends, but you should not let it become your whole life.

The laidback attitude associated with marijuana is perhaps best represented by Wooderson (Matthew McConaughey), an older character who parties with the high schoolers, but here too, we see some risks of marijuana use. Wooderson delivers the most iconic lines from the film. At one point, for example, he asks Mitch if he has a joint to share. When Mitch responds "no," Wooderson drawls that "it'd be a lot cooler if you did." He eventually makes a date with a "nerdy" redheaded sophomore girl. While the Wooderson character is depicted as cool, fun, and nonaggressive, he is also a bit of a dead-ender with no plans to go to college or embark on another career path. Wooderson is the oldest marijuana user depicted in the film, which suggests that eventually all parties must end—and that even the coolest high school graduate will eventually cease to attract the interest of high school girls.

Taken as a whole, *Dazed and Confused* promotes marijuana use during the liminal phase of life when young people are struggling to form their own identities.

Marijuana use is depicted as part of their decision to follow a less authoritarian path, but as a mainly temporary accessory. For all of the marijuana promotion, the film suggests that the time for smoking grass is finite, and you should enjoy it while you can and do so in balance with other life pursuits.

A film celebrating marijuana youth culture in the mid-1970s was a welcome offering for an early 1990s youth generation that was undergoing 1970s nostalgia and participating in their own marijuana culture, evidenced by the popularity of the marijuana theme in music and film of the day. Unlike the Cheech and Chong films of the 1970s and 1980s, which framed marijuana as a hippie, countercultural phenomenon, *Dazed and Confused* presented marijuana use as an intergenerational bond between mainstream cool kids and a quintessentially American rite of passage for youth.

Nicholas Copeland

See also: Age; Stoner Films; *That '70s Show*.

Further Reading

Hinds, Elizabeht Jane Wall. "The Devil Sings the Blues: Heavy Metal, Gothic Fiction and 'Postmodern' Discourse." *Journal of Popular Culture* 26, no 3 (1992): 151–164.

Speed, Lelsey. "The Possibilities of Roads Not Taken: Intellect and Utopia in the Films of Richard Linklater." *Journal of Popular Film and Television* 35 no. 3 (2007): 98–106.

Stewart, Kathleen. "Nostalgia: A Polemic." *Cultural Anthropology* 3 no. 3 (1988): 227–241.

Turner, Victor, Roger D. Abrahams, and Alfred Harris. *The Ritual Process: Structure and Anti-structure*. New York: Routledge Press, 2017.

Vineyard, Jennifer. "Richard Linklater on the Not-so-Inadvertent Subtext of 'Everybody Wants Some.'" Vulture, n.d. Accessed December 1, 2019. https://www.vulture.com/2016/04/linklater-on-everybody-wants-somes-gay-subtext.html

Decriminalization

Decriminalization of marijuana is not the same as legalization; instead, it treats possession of small amounts of marijuana as a civil offense, resulting in a possible fine, rather than a criminal offense that could conceivably result in jail time. Decriminalization has been defined as "reducing penalties [associated with marijuana] . . . rather than removing them altogether" (Single 1989). With decriminalization, the limit on possession is usually one ounce, although the limits differ across the various states. Possessing larger amounts of marijuana or trafficking in marijuana typically remain criminal offenses even in states that have implemented decriminalization measures, and federal laws on criminal possession of marijuana can still apply.

In 1970, President Richard M. Nixon signed the Comprehensive Drug Abuse Prevention and Control Act into law and labeled marijuana a Schedule I drug, which made possession of marijuana a criminal offense. Despite this classification, marijuana use was widespread in the 1970s, leading to calls for a variety of drug policy reforms, including decriminalization of marijuana possession (Single 1989). Because of this growing support for decriminalization, many state governments followed their own agenda by decriminalizing either the possession or consumption of marijuana despite federal directives to the contrary. In 1973, Oregon became the first state to decriminalize marijuana possession, and by the late 1970s, 10 states had enacted marijuana reforms that reduced legal consequences for possession of small amounts of pot.

Supporters of decriminalization policies say it has been an important element of overall criminal justice reform in many states. One study of the impact of decriminalization on policing, prosecution, and incarceration found that after passing marijuana decriminalization, California reported a 36 percent decline in arrests and saved over $12 million in costs related to enforcement in 1975–1976 alone (Single 1989). Another study estimated that decriminalization reduced drug arrests in Massachusetts by 1.9 percent, thereby leading to a savings of $29.5 million to the criminal justice system because of reduced prosecution and incarceration costs (Miron 2002).

Opponents of decriminalization claim lenient drug policies such as marijuana decriminalization promote illicit drug use, increase criminal behavior, and disrupt society. One researcher found that between 1973 and 1978, marijuana decriminalization was related to not only a significant increase in marijuana-related emergency room visits but also a significant reduction in emergency room episodes involving drugs other than marijuana, which may suggest some substitution may have occurred toward marijuana because its use was less severely penalized (Model 1993). However, the complex history of decriminalization, a lack of data, inconsistency on the definition of decriminalization, and the different penalties across states make it difficult to account for all of the socioeconomic impacts of decriminalization. Moreover, some researchers claim that decriminalization had no significant effect on the rate of marijuana use, the use of other drugs, or criminal activity (Single 1989).

The decriminalization movement has accelerated in recent years. As of 2019, 33 states and the District of Columbia have passed legislation in support of decriminalization of marijuana including legalization for recreational and medicinal uses (Governing Data 2019). The current trend reflects a change in public perception of marijuana, coinciding with a liberalization of public attitudes. During the 2016 presidential election, for example, Gallup polls revealed that 60 percent of adults supported marijuana legalization, compared to only 28 percent who supported such reforms in the 1970s (Ingraham 2016).

Craig A. Depken, II and Shanyn Viars

See also: Alaska; California; Colorado; Medical Uses; Pricing; Washington D.C.; Washington State.

Further Reading

Bretteville-Jensen, Anne Line. "To Legalize or Not to Legalize? Economic Approaches to the Decriminalization of Drugs." *Substance Use & Misuse* 41 no. 4 (2006): 555–565.

Governing Data. *State Marijuana Laws Map.* Last modified June 25, 2019. https://www.governing.com/gov-data/safety-justice/state-marijuana-laws-map-medical-recreational.html

Ingraham, Christopher. "Gallup: Support for Marijuana Legalization Surges to New Highs." *The Washington Post*, October 19, 2016.

Miron, Jeffrey A. "The Effect of Marijuana Decriminalization on the Budgets of Massachusetts Governments, With a Discussion of Decriminalization's Effect on Marijuana Use." In *Report to the Drug Policy Forum of Massachusetts*. 2002. http://citeseerx.ist.psu.edu/viewdoc/download?doi=10.1.1.514.7660&rep=rep1&type=pdf

Model, Karyn E. "The Effect of Marijuana Decriminalization on Hospital Emergency Room Drug Episodes: 1975–1978." *Journal of the American Statistical Association* 88, no. 23 (1993): 737–747.

Pacula, Rosalie Liccardo, Jamie F. Chriqui, and Joanna King. *Marijuana Decriminalization: What Does It Mean in the United States?* No. w9690. National Bureau of Economic Research, 2003. https://www.nber.org/system/files/working_papers/w9690/w9690.pdf

Single, Eric W. "The Impact of Marijuana Decriminalization: An Update." *Journal of Public Health Policy* 10, no. 4 (1989): 456–466.

Dependence

The alleged addictiveness of marijuana has been a contentious matter across various cultures for thousands of years (Roffman, Schwartz, and Stephens 2006). This is due in part to marijuana's long use as a folk remedy for various illnesses, as well as the fact that, until recently, there was little clear evidence of physical withdrawal symptoms such as those associated, for instance, with chronic alcohol use (Vandrey and Haney 2010). Despite its status in the United States as a patent medicine since the mid-1800s, marijuana became popularly perceived as a dangerous addictive drug upon the spread of its recreational use in the early twentieth century (Bonnie and Whitebread 1999; Roffman et al. 2006). However, the perception (both popular and among the medical establishment) of marijuana as an addictive drug has shifted significantly since then, and conflicting opinions continue to this day.

The long-standing classification of marijuana under the 1970 Controlled Substances Act as a Schedule I drug "with no currently accepted medical use" has been justified in part by what marijuana critics characterize as its "high potential for abuse." For many years, the very fact of its illegal status led to the common perception of any use of marijuana as abuse. In turn, this presumed addictiveness also contributed to the prolonged stigmatizing of cannabis by mental health practitioners (Vandrey and Haney 2010).

More recently, the modern understanding of substance dependence (or addiction) among mental health professionals usually refers to a cluster of behavioral and physiological symptoms that impel a person to repeat the use of a substance despite significant adverse consequences related to the use (Joy, Watson, and Benson 1999). Based on this diagnosis criterion, researchers have estimated rates of cannabis use disorders among Americans at about 2.9 percent of the adult population, with the highest rates (7.5 percent) found among 18- to 29-year-olds (Hasin et al. 2015).

Substance use disorders may be manifested in behavioral, psychological, or physiological symptoms (Babor 2006). Physiological dependence is diagnosed when the user of a substance develops either tolerance or withdrawal symptoms (Joy et al. 1999). Tolerance refers to the reduced response in the body to repeat doses of a drug, leading to increased dosing behavior to achieve the same psychic effect. Withdrawal refers to the adverse symptoms that emerge when repeat dosing of a drug is abruptly ended. Psychological dependence may develop independently of physical symptoms and is characterized by cravings—i.e., the intense desire for using a substance. Cravings are considered the most difficult manifestation of addiction to overcome (Gardner and David 1999).

The classification and practices for diagnosing substance dependence in use in the United States as of 2020 are coded in the fifth edition of the American Psychiatric Association (APA) *Diagnostic and Statistical Manual of Mental Disorders (DSM-V).* In this formulation, marijuana dependence is one of a group of substance use disorders that are considered psychiatric syndromes in their own right. Cannabis use disorder is thus considered a group of co-occurring symptoms related to an underlying mental disorder. Following these guidelines, drug treatment practitioners' understanding of dependence is rooted in a biomedical "disease model" of addiction—that is, the assumption that symptoms emerge from biological processes derived from the biochemical effects of the substance in the body (Earleywine 2002). Accordingly, drug and alcohol dependence develop as complex neurological phenomena; following social initiation in the use of an addictive substance, neurological mechanisms create the compulsion to use again, which then combines with cognitive mediation of substance-related behaviors (e.g., cravings) to reinforce continued use (Gardner and David 1999). In this modern understanding, addiction is then seen as an illness rather than the result of some moral character flaw. The disease model has thus contributed to deflecting some of the blame formerly attributed to individual users' depravity (Babor 2006).

Formally, the symptoms for identifying a cannabis use problem were identified in the *DSM-V* as "leading to clinically significant impairment or distress" (APA 2013, 519) based on the occurrence of 2 or more of the following 11 criteria in the last 12 months:

1. Marijuana was taken in larger amounts or over a longer period than intended.
2. There was a persistent desire or unsuccessful efforts to cut down cannabis use.
3. A great deal of time was spent in activities necessary to obtain cannabis, use cannabis, or recover from its effects.
4. There were cravings or urge to use.
5. Recurrent cannabis use resulted in a failure to meet role obligations at work, school, or home.
6. Cannabis use was continued despite experiencing social or interpersonal problems.
7. Important social, occupational, or recreational activities were given up or reduced because of marijuana use.
8. Cannabis was used recurrently in situations in which it is physically hazardous.
9. Cannabis use was continued despite knowledge of having a persistent or recurrent physical or psychological problem that is caused or exacerbated by using.
10. Tolerance was manifested by (a) a need to increase the amount of marijuana to achieve intoxication or (b) by diminishing the effect with continued use of the same amount.

11. Physical symptoms were associated with cannabis withdrawal (as specified in DSM) and/or the taking of cannabis to relieve or avoid those symptoms.

Bienvenido Ruiz

See also: Dependence, History of; Dependence, Prevalence of.

Further Reading

American Psychiatric Association. *Diagnostic and Statistical Manual of Mental Disorders*. 5th ed. Washington, DC: APA, 2013.

Babor, Thomas F. "The Diagnosis of Cannabis Dependence." In *Cannabis Dependence: Its Nature, Consequences and Treatment*, edited by Roger A. Roffman and Robert S. Stephens. Cambridge, MA: Cambridge University Press, 2006, 21–36.

Bonnie, Richard J., and Charles H. Whitebread, II. *The Marijuana Conviction: A History of Marijuana Prohibition in the United States*. 2nd ed. New York: The Lindesmith Center, 1999.

Earleywine, Mitch. *Understanding Marijuana: A New Look at the Scientific Evidence*. Oxford, UK: Oxford University Press, 2002.

Gardner, Eliot L., and James David. "The Neurobiology of Chemical Addiction." In *Getting Hooked: Rationality and Addiction*, edited by. Jon Elster and Ole-Jørgen Skog. Cambridge, UK: Cambridge University Press, 1999, 93–136.

Hasin, Deborah S., Tulshi D. Saha, Bradley T. Kerridge, et al. "Prevalence of Marijuana Use Disorders in the United States between 2001–2002 and 2012–2013." *JAMA Psychiatry* 72, no. 12 (2015): 1235–1242.

Joy, Janet E., Stanley J. Watson, and John A. Benson. "Marijuana and Medicine." *Assessing the Science Base*. Washington DC: National Academy, 1999.

Roffman, Roger A., Sam Schwartz, and Robert S. Stephens. "Themes in the History of Cannabis Dependence." In *Cannabis Dependence: Its Nature, Consequences and Treatment*, edited by Roger A. Roffman and Robert S. Stephens. Cambridge, MA: Cambridge University Press, 2006, 3–20.

Vandrey, Ryan, and Margaret Haney. "How Real Is the Risk of Addiction?" In *The Pot Book: A Complete Guide to Cannabis. Its Role in Medicine, Politics, Science, and Culture*, edited by Julie Holland. New York: Simon and Schuster, 2010, 187–195.

Dependence, History of

The very existence of marijuana dependence has long been the subject of many public, medical, legal, and policy debates. Far from being a mere "scientific" matter, cultural and political factors have contributed to defining the concept of marijuana dependence, and they can be expected to do so in the future.

The medical establishment (including the American Psychiatric Association-APA and the American Medical Association-AMA) initially objected to the harsh prohibitions against marijuana use contained in the Marijuana Tax Act of 1937, given that it was at the time a fairly common practice to prescribe and dispense marijuana through legitimate apothecaries (Bonnie and Whitebread 1999). At the time, the scientific consensus was that marijuana users did not show the tolerance and dramatic withdrawal symptoms then associated with alcoholism or opiate addiction. However, the image of marijuana as addictive was reinforced in 1930s and 1940s in part because federal enforcement agencies such as the Federal Bureau of Narcotics began to regulate cannabis in a manner similar to "narcotic opiates" (Bonnie and Whitebread 1999). In addition, during this time period pop culture depictions of marijuana as a menace to American families cast an increasingly dark shadow over the drug's reputation.

The medical profession responded to these trends by becoming more ambivalent about marijuana. With a few exceptions, physicians and psychiatrists did not dispute allegations that marijuana could induce psychosis among users—a claim that became increasingly widespread in the press, in law enforcement communications, and even in popular culture of the time. A few attempts were made before the 1950s to test the assumption that marijuana was a psychologically addictive drug (Bonnie and Whitebread 1999).

In the 1960s and 1970s, government commissions reporting on illegal drug use vacillated in their designation of marijuana as a dependence-inducing narcotic. The 1967 presidential Commission on Law Enforcement and Administration of Justice and the 1972 National Commission on Marihuana and Drug Abuse separately concluded that marijuana does not lead to physical dependence and even implied that the limited risk to public health deriving from its psychological dependence did not warrant the same level of user criminalization as opiates (Roffman, Schwartz, and Stephens 2006). Following the publication of the federal commission reports, it was common to categorize the difficulties faced by marijuana users as "habituation," "misuse," or problem use, which were considered less severe conditions than outright addiction (Hall and Pacula 2003). This was prompted in part by the assumption that only physiological symptoms such as withdrawal and tolerance were considered hard evidence for dependence, and these were short-lived, if ever observed, among marijuana users—and even thought by many to be nonexistent. This view also encouraged an influential reform movement in the 1970s seeking (and in part achieving) the reduction of marijuana-related penalties (Roffman et al. 2006)

Beginning in the early 1980s, compulsion to use and other related behaviors associated with "harmful use" became relatively more important in defining marijuana dependence among drug rehabilitation practitioners, and this shift was reflected in the revised third edition of the APA's *Diagnostic and Statistical Manual of Mental Disorders (DSM)* and subsequent editions (Hall and Pacula 2003). Similarly, a 1981 World Health Organization (WHO) report calling for improved understanding of drug dependence recommended the use of more cognitive and behavioral criteria in diagnosing substance abuse, such as subjective awareness of cravings and "a desire to stop drug use in the face of continued use" (Edwards, Arif, and Hadgson 1981, 210). Nevertheless, when the APA published the fourth edition of *DSM* in 1994, cannabis was not considered to be physiologically addictive, mainly because withdrawal symptoms "have not yet been reliably shown to be clinically significant" (APA 1994, 216). As more clinical evidence began to accumulate, however, this view was increasingly criticized (Babor 2006).

Although indeed most cannabis users report no withdrawal problems upon stopping, in clinical settings, abruptly stopping dosing with delta-9-tetrahydrocannabinol (THC) or smoked marijuana has been documented to cause symptoms such as mood fluctuations, sleep disturbance, decreased appetite, stomach pain, nausea, runny nose, sweating and cramping, and/or anxiety among chronic daily users

(Budney, Novy, and Hughes 1999). The physiological effects of marijuana were also becoming much better understood since the 1980s because of neurological studies identifying the brain mechanisms that contribute to its dependence, such as a cannabinoid receptor in brain cells and a cannabinoid antagonist—i.e., a drug that inhibits the neurological effects of THC. The development of tolerance to the mood-enhancing effect of marijuana was also confirmed by other researchers (Haney et al. 1999). Marijuana was long assumed to be potentially addictive because its use is pleasurable to many people. This trait is now thought of as capable of triggering psychological reinforcements in the reward systems of the brain that are so common with use of other psychoactive substances (Koob and Le Moal 1997). Similarly, marijuana tolerance is now linked to the neurological changes that develop with frequent use (González, Cebeira, and Fernández-Ruiz 2005).

A 2002 survey reported that up to 30 percent of regular marijuana users report withdrawal symptoms when they stop using (Teesson et al. 2002). Among the subgroup of chronic marijuana users who seek treatment, most report withdrawal symptoms (Budney and Hughes 2006). The physiological symptoms of dependence to marijuana, and their relation to using behaviors, are now clearly established in the fifth edition of the DSM (2013), where one of the diagnostic criteria is "withdrawal, and the fact that for some chronic users, withdrawal symptoms may contribute to difficulty quitting or relapse among those trying to abstain" (APA 2013, 519). Although the quantity and the frequency of marijuana use are no longer recommended measurements for diagnosing dependence, both are observed to correlate with symptoms of cannabis use disorders (Compton et al. 2009).

If the DSM-V approach simplifies the diagnosing of addiction in practice, the issue of marijuana's addictiveness is an altogether different one. Its relative addictiveness (whether based on its ability to produce withdrawal symptoms, tolerance, or dependence) is considered low compared to most other illegal substances. It has been compared to caffeine, although still ranked more addictive than hallucinogens such as MDMA, LSD, or mescaline. Addictiveness also varies widely in the population because, like many other psychoactive substances, genetic factors are associated with marijuana dependence (Kendler and Prescott 1998); this association seems to be related to individual genetic differences in how THC interacts with the person's neurological reward system.

Bienvenido Ruiz

See also: Dependence; Dependence, Prevalence of.

Further Reading

American Psychiatric Association. *Diagnostic and Statistical Manual of Mental Disorders*. 4th ed. Washington, DC: APA, 1994.

American Psychiatric Association. *Diagnostic and Statistical Manual of Mental Disorders*. 5th ed. Washington, DC: APA, 2013.

Babor, Thomas F. "The Diagnosis of Cannabis Dependence." In *Cannabis Dependence: Its Nature, Consequences and Treatment,* edited by Roger A. Roffman and Robert S. Stephens. Cambridge, MA: Cambridge University Press, 2006, 21–36.

Bonnie, Richard J. and Charles H. Whitebread, II. *The Marijuana Conviction: A History of Marijuana Prohibition in the United States*. 2nd ed. New York: Lindesmith Center, 1999.

Budney, Alan J., and John R. Hughes. "The Cannabis Withdrawal Syndrome." *Current Opinion in Psychiatry* 19, no. 3 (2006): 233–238.

Budney, Alan J., Pamela L. Novy, and John R. Hughes. "Marijuana Withdrawal among Adults Seeking Treatment for Marijuana Dependence." *Addiction* 94, no. 9 (1999): 1311–1322.

Compton Wilson M., Tulshi D. Saha, Kevin P. Conway, and Bridget F. Grant. "The Role of Cannabis Use within a Dimensional Approach to Cannabis Use Disorders." *Drug and Alcohol Dependence* 100 (2009): 221–227.

Edwards, Griffith, Awing Arif, and R. Hadgson. "Nomenclature and Classification of Drug-and Alcohol-Related Problems: A WHO Memorandum." *Bulletin of the World Health Organization* 59, no. 2 (1981): 225–242.

González, Sara, Maribel Cebeira, and Javier Fernández-Ruiz. "Cannabinoid Tolerance and Dependence: A Review of Studies in Laboratory Animals." *Pharmacology Biochemistry and Behavior* 81, no. 2 (June 2005): 300–318.

Hall, Wayne, and Rosalie Liccardo Pacula. *Cannabis Use and Dependence: Public Health and Public Policy.* Cambridge, UK: Cambridge University Press, 2003.

Haney, Margaret, et al. "Abstinence Symptoms Following Oral THC Administration to Humans." *Psychopharmacology* 141, no. 4 (1999): 385–394.

Kendler, Kenneth S., and Carol A. Prescott. "Cannabis Use, Abuse, and Dependence in a Population-Based Sample of Female Twins." *American Journal of Psychiatry* 155, no. 8 (1998): 1016–1022.

Koob, George F., and Michel Le Moal. "Drug Abuse: Hedonic Homeostatic Dysregulation." *Science* 278, no. 5335 (1997): 52–58.

Roffman, Roger A., Sam Schwartz, and Robert S. Stephens. "Themes in the History of Cannabis Dependence." In *Cannabis Dependence: Its Nature, Consequences and Treatment,* edited by Roger A. Roffman and Robert S. Stephens. Cambridge, MA: Cambridge University Press, 2006, 3–20.

Teesson, Maree, Michael Lynskey, Barry Manor, and Andrew Baillie. "The Structure of Cannabis Dependence in the Community." *Drug and Alcohol Dependence* 68, no. 3 (2002): 255–262.

Dependence, Prevalence of

Despite a relatively low estimated risk of users ever experiencing dependence, the status of marijuana as the most common illicit drug of choice for Americans accounts for the fact that, after nicotine and alcohol, marijuana is still the most frequently diagnosed drug dependence in the United States (Smith and Borden 2020). A national study from 2019 found that 11.5 percent of Americans age 12 or older (31.6 million) were current marijuana users—i.e., have used in the past month (Substance Abuse and Mental Health Services Administration (SAMHSA) 2020). The global rate of DSM-IV cannabis dependence in the U.S. population age 12 or older was estimated in that study to be 1.8 percent. However, realistic estimates of marijuana use, abuse, and dependence in the general population have fluctuated broadly across the decades, in good measure due to shifting definitions and diagnosing practices (Anthony 2006). Beyond matters of definition, estimate variations are introduced by the methods used to assess the prevalence of problem marijuana use, which range from self-reports of use frequency to survey questionnaires designed to measure cognitive, mood or medical concerns, or even cost/benefit scales (Asbridge et al. 2014).

The measured incidences of dependence and treatment success in the United States are further complicated by the fact that an unknown proportion of those counted as seeking treatment do so only to avoid criminal sanctions or to comply with court-mandated treatment (Earleywine 2002). Prescribing drug treatment for criminal offenders in lieu of jail or juvenile detention has become an increasingly common practice in law enforcement throughout the United States since the 1990s. Many possession-related offenders are assigned to court-mandated diversion programs such as drug courts, where they may be diagnosed by default as substance abusers. These policy trends have inflated recent estimates of marijuana "addiction," and by now, most marijuana abusers in treatment are criminal justice referrals (SAMHSA 2015).

According to a large survey released in 2015, the rate of reported marijuana use in the previous 12 months among adult Americans (18 or older) increased dramatically between 2002 and 2013, from 4.1 percent to 9.5 percent (Hasin et al. 2015). That study estimated the incidence of marijuana use disorder among the overall adult population to be 2.9 percent. Increased use rates may be in response to the expansion of legalization of cannabis for both medical and recreational uses and (relatedly) also to more tolerant attitudes toward marijuana among Americans. At the same time, however, the prevalence of marijuana use disorders among current users was estimated to be 11 percent in 2014, which represents a decrease from 14.8 percent in 2002 (Compton et al. 2016). Thus, the increasing trends in marijuana use were not associated with increases in cannabis use disorder diagnoses (see also Hasin et al. 2015).

Marijuana dependence has long been observed to co-occur with mental illness. U.S. adults with specific substance use disorders for nicotine, alcohol, cocaine, hallucinogens, inhalants, or psychotherapeutics are more likely to also show marijuana dependence, as are those who report major depressive episodes (Compton et al. 2016). Marijuana dependence is more often secondary in its co-occurrence with alcohol, opiate, or cocaine abuse than a stand-alone addiction, although a significant minority of those with co-occurring substance use disorders report marijuana as the primary substance abused (Degenhardt Hall, and Lynskey 2001). In large surveys of Americans, as many as 35.6 percent of all adults who reported having used marijuana in the past year reported at least one medical or psychological problem that they attribute to using it (Hasin et al. 2015). However, it has not been possible to establish a clear causal link to these problems because of the lack of control groups of nonusers in these studies (Earleywine 2002).

The incidence of marijuana dependence varies widely with age, sex, race, socioeconomic status, and other sociodemographic categories. For instance, there is evidence that smokers under the age of 18 have a larger risk of developing cannabis use disorder than adults (Winters and Lee 2008) and that more than 90 percent of U.S. cases of dependence arise between the ages of 15 and 35 (Anthony 2006). Age at first use is also associated with dependence and abuse. Among those who first tried marijuana at age 14 or younger, 11.5 percent were estimated to qualify as dependent or problem users (SAMHSA 2015). The risk of dependence was estimated in one longitudinal study to be one in six for those who were initiated into marijuana use in adolescence (Anthony, Warner, and Kessler 1994).

Overall, the prevalence of marijuana use disorders among U.S. users was recently estimated to be significantly higher in men than in women. Higher rates have also been found in non-Hispanic African Americans, Hispanics, non-Hispanic Asians, and non-Hispanic users of more than one race than among whites. Adults without a high school diploma have also been found to have a higher likelihood of a marijuana use disorder than those with higher education levels. People employed part-time, unable to work because of disability, or unemployed are at higher risk than those who are employed full time. Finally, data indicate that never-married adults are more likely to be classified as suffering from a marijuana use disorder than married ones (Compton et al. 2016). Adult residents of states that have legalized marijuana for nonmedical use (as of 2014) are more frequent users, but users in those states show no significant difference from other states in frequency of cannabis use disorder (Compton et al. 2016).

The risk of addiction to marijuana, along with its consequences, has historically been overstated by various government agencies and moral entrepreneurs in support of prohibition in the United States (Mosher and Akins 2013). However, while marijuana use disorder is now widely accepted as a real form of dependence, the definitions of what constitutes problematic or harmful use remain under debate (Temple, Brown, and Hine 2011).

Bienvenido Ruiz

See also: Dependence; Dependence, History of.

Further Reading

Anthony, James C. "The Epidemiology of Cannabis Dependence." In *Cannabis Dependence: Its Nature, Consequences and Treatment*, edited by Roger A. Roffman and Robert S. Stephens. Cambridge, MA: Cambridge University Press, 2006, 58–105.

Anthony, James C., Lynn A. Warner, and Ronald C. Kessler. "Comparative Epidemiology of Dependence on Tobacco, Alcohol, Controlled Substances, and Inhalants: Basic Findings from the National Comorbidity Survey." *Experimental and Clinical Psychopharmacology* 2 (1994): 244–268.

Asbridge, Mark, Cameron Duff, David C. Marsh, and Patricia G. Erickson. "Problems with the Identification of 'Problematic' Cannabis Use: Examining the Issues of Frequency, Quantity, and Drug Use Environment." *European Addiction Research* 20, no. 5 (2014): 254–267.

Compton, Wilson M., et al. "Marijuana Use and Use Disorders in Adults in the USA, 2002–14: Analysis of Annual Cross-Sectional Surveys." *The Lancet Psychiatry* 3, no. 10 (2016): 954–964.

Degenhardt, Louisa, Wayne Hall, and Michael Lynskey. "The Relationship Between Cannabis Use and Other Substance Use in the General Population." *Drug and Alcohol Dependence* 64, no. 3 (2001): 319–327.

Earleywine, Mitch. *Understanding Marijuana: A New Look at the Scientific Evidence.* Oxford, UK: Oxford University Press, 2002.

Hasin, Deborah S., et al. "Prevalence of Marijuana Use Disorders in the United States Between 2001–2002 and 2012–2013." *JAMA Psychiatry* 72, no. 12 (2015): 1235–1242.

Mosher, Clayton J., and Scott Akins. *Drugs and Drug Policy: The Control of Consciousness Alteration.* New York: Sage, 2013.

Smith, Charles H., and Kathi A. Borden. "Introduction to the Special Issue on Substance Use Disorders and Addictions." *Professional Psychology: Research and Practice* 51, no. 1 (2020): 1–4.

Substance Abuse and Mental Health Services Administration, Center for Behavioral Health Statistics and Quality. *Treatment Episode Data Set (TEDS): 2003–2013. National Admissions to Substance Abuse Treatment Services.* Rockville, MD: Substance Abuse and Mental Health Services Administration, 2015.

Substance Abuse and Mental Health Services Administration. *Key Substance Use and Mental Health Indicators in the United States: Results from the 2019 National Survey on Drug Use and Health.* Rockville, MD: Center for Behavioral Health Statistics and Quality, Substance Abuse and Mental Health Services Administration, 2020.

Temple, Elizabeth C., Rhonda F. Brown, and Donald W. Hine. "The 'Grass Ceiling': Limitations in the Literature Hinder Our Understanding of Cannabis Use and Its Consequences." *Addiction* 106, no. 2 (2011): 238–244.

Winters, Ken C., and Chih-Yuan S. Lee. "Likelihood of Developing an Alcohol and Cannabis Use Disorder during Youth: Association with Recent Use and Age." *Drug and Alcohol Dependence* 92, no. 1–3 (2008): 239–247.

Differential Association Theory/Social Learning Theory

Differential association theory, first formulated by criminologist Edwin Sutherland (1883–1950), attempted to show the process by which deviance from social norms and laws arises, including illegal marijuana use. Often misunderstood as a theory that asserts only that people are influenced by those around them, the theory actually has several components. Building on differential association theory and adding insights from psychological behaviorism, Ronald L. Akers (1939–) expanded the theory into what he termed social learning theory. While more often cited for his work on labeling theory, sociologist Howard S. Becker wrote an influential article *Becoming a Marihuana User* (1953) that is closely related to social learning theory. Taken together, differential association and social learning theory are widely supported as explanations for deviant social behavior in general and illegal marijuana use specifically.

Sutherland introduced differential association theory in his 1939 text *Principles of Criminology*. He continued to refine the theory until 1947. At his time of writing, marijuana use was heavily stigmatized as criminal deviance, making it a topic of interest to criminologists and sociologists. Sutherland's differential association theory attempted to explain how a person came to engage in deviant acts such as using marijuana. Social interaction was a key part of the process, and the key concept was that criminal behavior was learned, rather than innate or born of circumstance. It was learned by communicating with others within intimate personal groups. These groups could be families, or close-knit peer groups. It was in these groups, Sutherland said, that people become exposed to rationalizations for illegal activity, as well as practical tips for engaging in crimes (such as smoking pot) without getting caught. Values and ideas about what activities are and are not permissible played a role, modifying people's attitudes to be more or less favorable toward crime. In the process, people develop orientations to the law that predispose them to break it or honor it, though their involvement may be mediated by frequency, depth, and intensity of their criminal contacts and definitions of crime as favorable or unfavorable. In the context of marijuana deviance, the best-known demonstration of this kind of learning process is found in Howard S. Becker's *Becoming a Marihuana User* (1953), in which he describes how marijuana users have to learn how to ingest the drug, how to recognize the effects of the drug, how to enjoy the effects of the drug, and the subculture surrounding the drug.

Building on Sutherland's differential association theory, and adding insights from behaviorism in the field of psychology, Ronald L. Akers became known for social learning theory. The 1966 reformulation of differential association added the language of psychology to the theory, saying that criminal behavior is learned through operant conditioning. Operant conditioning refers to the process by which people who are motivated by the rewards of an activity to keep doing that activity, which becomes a learned habit. Not meant to supplant differential association theory, Aker's social learning theory was an expansion of it to account for the appearance, continuance, and cessation of deviant behaviors. For example, social learning theory takes into account the context in which norms and laws are broken. A marijuana user may have past (or present) associates who use the drug, may define the use of the drug in a way that encourages use, may receive positive reinforcement from peers when using the drug—or all of those factors may work in the opposite way, lessening the likelihood that someone will decide to use marijuana.

Akers' theory also provides explanations for why people who smoke marijuana continue to use it or give it up. The likelihood of continuing use is influenced by the social and nonsocial rewards (reinforcers) or punishments that occur. These not only affect the act of deviance itself but also the ideas that a person has about the deviance. If favorable ideas are weakened, cessation is more likely, and vice versa. Where there are no negative sanctions against the deviance, it is likely to continue. "Nonsocial" reinforcement or dissuasion from deviance involves the general reward system in society. It also includes the physical, emotional, and physiological effects of intoxication, which, if pleasant, are more likely to condition a person to seek those sensations out again and again. Social rewards can be symbolic, where a person seeks to amplify a social status, political identification, or prestige in society or in a subculture. Other rewards may be more interpersonal, like the satisfaction achieved in imitating a person held in high esteem who commits deviant acts.

Social learning theory delves into the process by which ideas favorable to or against deviance develop. One such process is "neutralizing definitions" by which people excuse their deviance. Examples include: "It's not hurting anybody" and "I can't help myself." Ideas favorable to or against deviance occur along a spectrum and might be more or less strongly held. The strength with which they are held predicts the likelihood of deviance or conformity to norms and laws.

Chelsea Starr

See also: Conflict and Labeling Theories; Social Bonding Theory/Social Control Theory; Theories of Use.

Further Reading

Akers, Ronald. *Social Learning and Social Structure: A General Theory of Crime and Deviance.* New York: Routledge, 2009.

Becker, Howard. "Becoming a Marihuana User." *American Journal of Sociology* 59 no. 3 (1953): 235–242.

Becker, Howard. *Outsiders: Studies in the Sociology of Deviance.* New York: Free Press, 1963.

Sutherland, Edwin, Donald Cressey, and David Luckenbill. *Principles of Criminology.* 11th ed. New York: Rowman & Littlefield, 1992.

Dispensaries

The term "dispensaries" can refer to any store that sells medications, but within the context of marijuana dispensaries, this typically refers to a government-regulated physical location where a person can legally purchase cannabis for medical or recreational purposes. Differing from the coffeeshops that emerged in Amsterdam in the 1970s, patrons of marijuana dispensaries are not permitted to smoke the product on the premises. Although medical marijuana dispensaries recognize state-issued medical marijuana permits and physician's recommendations, the federal ban on marijuana means that the cannabis products sold are not approved by the U.S. Food and Drug Administration (FDA) or legally registered with the federal government. Instead, medical and recreational marijuana states regulate dispensaries and the products they sell.

In 1992, the first public marijuana dispensary in the United States was opened in California following the success of Proposition P, a local provision to allow for medical marijuana. The San Francisco Cannabis Buyers Club was founded by the coauthors of Proposition 215, which passed in 1996. This statewide measure legalized medical marijuana, mostly for the treatment of those suffering from AIDS. This establishment became central to the medical marijuana debate and AIDS activism. The owners were subject to numerous arrests and raids by state agents (until the passage of Proposition 215) and federal agents in a long struggle to try and legitimize medical marijuana (Manta 2017).

As of 2019, in the 36 states that allow for medical marijuana dispensaries, the actual number of dispensaries in operation vary. The top five states with marijuana dispensaries have over 10 dispensaries per 100,000 residents (Wolinsky 2020). Oregon (16.5 per 100,000 residents) has the most, followed by Oklahoma (15.6 per 100,000 residents), Montana (15.1 per 100,000 residents), Colorado (14.1 per 100,000 residents), and Alaska (12.7 per 100,000 residents). The top five cities in terms of per capita dispensaries are Missoula, Montana; Medford, Oregon; Pueblo, Colorado; Eugene, Oregon; and Denver, Colorado (Wolinsky 2020).

Dispensaries differ from head shops that often sell marijuana paraphernalia and novel drugs such as synthetic cannabinoids (prior to the 2012 ban on synthetic cannabinoids such as Spice and K2; see Khey, Stogner, and Miller 2014) but are not permitted to legally sell marijuana. In some locations that permit recreational marijuana sales and use, lounges exist that allow patrons to legally consume marijuana. These establishments often differ from dispensaries, head shops, and Amsterdam's coffeeshops in that they allow users to "bring your own bud" (BYOBud), pay an entrance or membership fee, and use marijuana in the provided social space. For example, in Denver, Colorado, The Coffee Joint, located next to a dispensary, is the first legal lounge for consuming marijuana in the state, but patrons are not

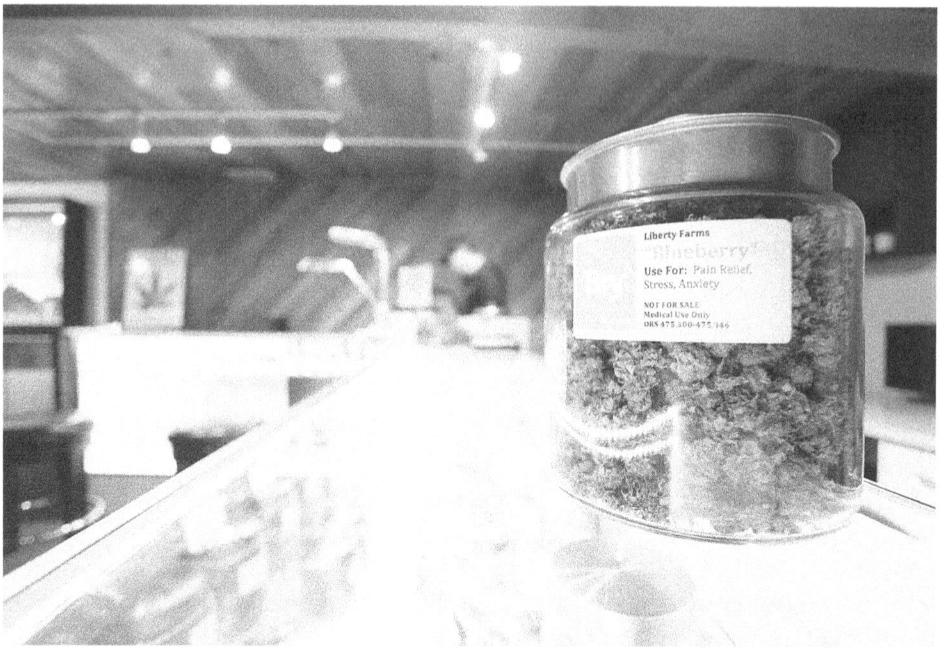

With the legalization of medical marijuana beginning with California in 1996, medical marijuana dispensaries have opened in many states. Patrons can legally purchase a variety of types of cannabis, including *Cannabis sativa* and *Cannabis indica*. (Peter Kim/ Dreamstime.com)

permitted to smoke, as smoking of any kind is still prohibited in public. As a result, only vaporizing and edibles are permitted. Some all-in-one shops have emerged. In California, the state is able to grant on-site consumption licenses. In San Francisco, for example, Moe Greens allows users to purchase products, including cannabis-infused beverages and cannabis concentrates, to consume in the different areas of the lounge. The Magnolia Dispensary, Vape Lounge, and Dab Bar in Oakland, California, permits patrons to bring their own cannabis products or purchase them at the on-site dispensary (Astorino 2019).

Regulations of dispensaries vary greatly across the states that permit medical or recreational marijuana, but all require some type of process to obtain a state license. A license can permit the sale of medical and/or recreational marijuana depending on state and local laws. The licensing process typically involves background checks and at least $5,000 worth of fees (Cohen 2018). Some states are more restrictive in the number of licenses that are permitted. For example, in Washington State the number of available state licenses is capped and can only be obtained by purchasing one from a current licensee or waiting in hopes that this number is expanded. Other challenges in obtaining a license include capital requirements indicating proof of adequate liquid assets and having a suitable location that follows state and city regulations not within close proximity to a school, church, park, arcade, and/or other location where children are frequently found (Cohen 2018).

Bryan Lee Miller

See also: Cannabis Drinks; Coffeeshops; Head Shops; Medical Uses.

Further Reading

Astorino, Dominiqu Michelle. "5 U.S. Lounges Where You Can Smoke Weed (Legally)." AFAR.com, August 16, 2019. https://www.afar.com/magazine/lounges-where-you-can-legally-smoke-weed-in-the-united-states

Cohen, Gary. "How Much Does It Actually Cost to Open a Dispensary?" National Cannabis Industry Association, September 25, 2018. https://thecannabisindustry.org/member-blog-how-much-does-it-actually-cost-to-open-a-dispensary/

Khey, David N., John Stogner, and Bryan Lee Miller. *Emerging Trends in Drug Use and Distribution*. Vol. 12. New York: Springer Science & Business Media, 2014.

Manta, Ashley. "Remembering the San Francisco Cannabis Buyers Club, the Nation's First Dispensary." *Leafly*, June 14, 2017. https://www.leafly.com/news/lifestyle/san-francisco-cannabis-buyers-club-nations-first-american-dispensary

Wolinsky, Jacob. "The Cities and States with Most Marijuana Dispensaries Per Capita." *Valuewalk*, January 24, 2020. https://www.valuewalk.com/2020/01/cities-states-most-marijuana-dispensaries/?fbclid=IwAR0_PUgE2q2ZdXWwDhh2tVRSVwBulZUtoQtpDYhlQ7r79OlP9nX_4IhWEgU

"Drug Abuse Message to Congress" (President Carter, 1977)

In 1977, President Jimmy Carter delivered a "Drug Abuse Message to Congress" in which he advocated repealing federal criminal statutes as they pertain to those apprehended for possession of an ounce or less of marijuana. Instead of criminal charges, he suggested instituting civil penalties for such infractions. Under federal criminal laws at the time of his address, a conviction for simple marijuana possession resulted in a $5,000 fine and the possibility of a short prison sentence; President Carter suggested a civil penalty consisting of a $100 fine (Walsh 1977). His views did not coincide with those of many members of Congress, however, most of whom remained supportive of the long-standing, punitive drug control policies held by the United States. As a result, his proposal to reform the nation's marijuana laws never gained much momentum, and within a matter of months, it had been largely forgotten.

The first attempt at cohesive drug enforcement came with the 1914 Federal Harrison Act. This legislation imposed taxes on specific drugs. It also required dispensaries to register with the government, and it mandated that they keep a detailed record of their pharmaceutical inventories (Musto 2002). The post-Harrison Act period was marked by an increase in illicit drug use by the general public and a subsequent large-scale shift toward anti-narcotic legislation. In concurrence with the prohibitive attitudes of lawmakers, Supreme Court decisions gradually increased penalties for possessing illicit substances from 1919 to 1925; by 1935, marijuana, cocaine, and heroin were heavily regulated, if not illegal, in all the states (White and Goreman 2000; Adrian 2015). The next couple of decades saw dramatic surges in property and violent crime that was attributed in some quarters to rising levels of drug abuse in American society. These trends prompted the Federal Bureau of Narcotics to petition Congress for tighter drug control legislation; the result was the Boggs Act of 1956, which increased the mandatory minimum sentence for the possession of narcotics (Musto 2002). Around the same period, the rise in crime influenced states to shift from flexible indeterminate sentencing to determinate sentencing practices, thus preventing inmates from exiting the correctional system early for good behavior. In 1971, mounting political pressures to address rising levels of illicit drug use and the proliferation of crime compelled the Nixon Administration (1969–1974) to declare a "War on Drugs." The war on drugs provided increases in funding and organizational support to law enforcement entities. The cumulative effect was that more individuals were incarcerated longer than they would have been in previous decades under more permissive laws.

A key concern driving Carter's address to Congress was that the existing laws and penalties regarding the possession of marijuana harmed the individual more so than the drug did. Operationally, his support for federal decriminalization would have little impact on reducing drug prosecutions since he did not direct individual states to adopt similar legislation and because few individuals were ever charged under the federal law to begin with. In other words, Carter's argument was more emblematic of a broader social movement than designed to meaningfully reduce incarceration for marijuana-related violations of the law—although decriminalizing the simple possession of marijuana would have the effect of encouraging federal law enforcement to focus on drug crimes that were more damaging to society (Hudak 2016).

In October of 1977, the Senate Judiciary Committee voted to pass President Carter's proposal, but it never garnered the collective approval of Congress. Carter never revisited this issue because his term in office became quickly consumed with other pressing domestic and international issues, including health care, fuel shortages, the Soviet Union's invasion of Afghanistan, and the Iranian Hostage Crisis. President Carter was defeated in his bid for reelection in November 1980, and any discussion of decriminalizing marijuana was quickly dismissed in the following decade due to cultural opposition to teen marijuana use.

Melody Hicks and Ben Stickle

See also: Anti-Drug Abuse Acts of 1986 and 1988; Comprehensive Drug Abuse Prevention and Control Act (1970); Marihuana Tax Act (1937); Nixon Administration "War on Drugs."

Further Reading

Adrian, Manuella. "What the History of Drugs Can Teach Us about the Current Cannabis Legalization Process: Unfinished Business." *Substance Use & Misuse 50*, no. 8–9 (2015): 990–1004.

Hudak, John. *Marijuana: A Short History.* Washington, DC: Brookings Institution Press, 2016.

Musto, David F. *Drugs in America: A Documentary History.* New York: New York University Press, 2002.

Walsh, Edward. "Carter Endorses Decriminalization of Marijuana." *Washington Post,* August 3, 1977. https://www.washingtonpost.com/archive/politics/1977/08/03/carter-endorses-decriminalization-of-marijuana/7e4b0e9a-90c9-4bdb-a49b-57290236a671/?noredirect=on&utm_term=.474d1bf31c99

White, Helene R., and Dennis M. Gorman. "Dynamics of the Drug-crime Relationship." *Criminal Justice* 1, no. 15 (2000): 1–218.

Drug Abuse Resistance Education (DARE)

The Drug Abuse Resistance Program, more commonly known as DARE, is an education-based program that seeks to prevent drug use, gang membership, and violence among adolescents. DARE was founded in Los Angeles, California, in

1983 as part of the broader War on Drugs campaign. Stemming from a collaboration between the Los Angeles County School District and the Los Angeles Police Department, DARE spread rapidly throughout the country. By 1994, DARE programs existed in all 50 states, as well as 6 other nations. DARE quickly became the most widely used school-based drug prevention program in the country (National Institute of Justice 2011).

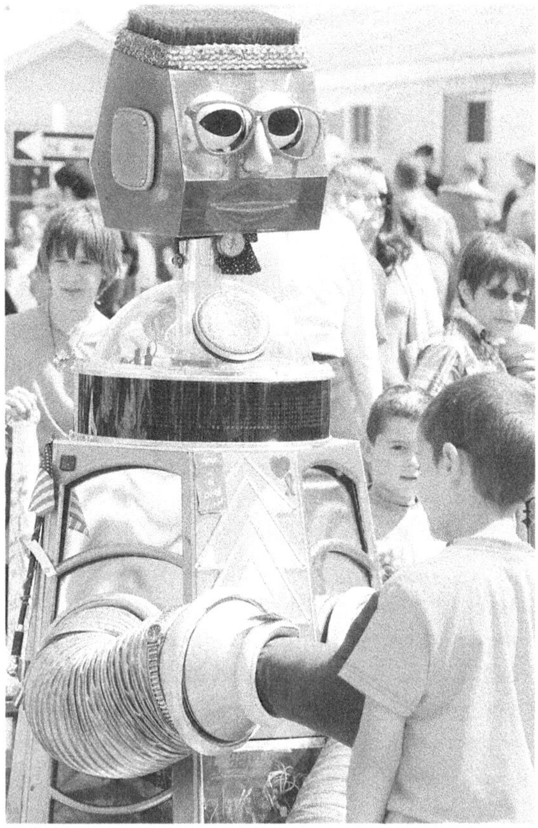

A DARE (Drug Abuse Resistance Education) robot talks to children at the 188th annual Great Geauga County Fair in Burton, Ohio, on September 5, 2010. DARE is a popular school-based drug use prevention program administered by specially trained law enforcement officers. Founded in 1983, it has been implemented in approximately 80% of school districts in the United States. (DARE America)

The DARE program curriculum has changed over time, in turn, so has the program's target population. Initially, DARE was developed for elementary-school children in the fifth and sixth grades because it was believed that preteens were most receptive to antidrug messaging and likely had not yet experimented—or been tempted to experiment—with drugs. DARE programs for children in middle school and high school were later introduced as well. Even so, the message remained largely the same; DARE sought to teach kids to resist the temptation of drugs and not fall prey to peer pressure to experiment with marijuana or other drugs. DARE was developed based on a psychological approach that stressed the role of social influence on delinquent behavior. To combat negative social influence, DARE attempted to strengthen the ability of adolescents to refuse negative situations and, more generally, build social competency and confidence (National Institute of Justice 2011).

DARE classes were held in classrooms by police officers who received 80 hours of training in areas related to teaching, classroom management, adolescent development, and drug competency. DARE programs consisted of 17 lessons provided on a weekly basis. The average lesson lasted 45 minutes to 1 hour and was primarily lecture based. Among other topics, these lessons instructed students in the areas of personal safety, the effects of drug use, resisting peer pressure, building self-esteem, stress management, decision-making, the influence of mass media, alternatives to drug use, drug-free role models, and gang pressures.

Several studies have sought to evaluate the effectiveness of DARE in achieving its intended goal—reducing adolescent drug use. Overall, the effect of DARE has been found to be negligible, if not counterproductive. For instance, one 1994 study examining 12 schools and 1,803 students found that attending the DARE program did not have a statistically significant effect on the reduction of students' initiation of alcohol use, cigarette smoking, or heavy drinking. Moreover, DARE did not affect the long-term attitudes of teens concerning drug use (Ennett 1994). Another study 2 years later examined 2,071 students across 31 elementary schools in Lexington, Kentucky, and found similar results. Students exposed to the DARE curriculum showed similar rates of alcohol, cigarette, and drug use, relative to students who did not participate in the DARE program. Similarly, attitudes toward drug use were not significantly impacted by attending the DARE program (Clayton, Cattarello, and Johnstone 1996).

In 2009, the DARE program was ended. However, DARE America, the nonprofit organization that administered DARE, developed a new program, keepin' it REAL, which was designed by prevention specialists. By promoting interactive lessons, as opposed to lengthy lectures, keepin' it REAL sought to more effectively engage with a new generation of students. Instead of teaching drug abstinence, keepin' it REAL taught students to be honest, responsible, and safe in an attempt to dissuade drug use. Instructors speak minimally in keepin' it REAL, allowing students more time to participate in activities designed to encourage healthy and responsible decision-making (Nordrum 2014). Numerous studies demonstrate that keepin' it REAL is more effective than DARE at keeping teens away from drugs, alcohol, and cigarettes (Hecht et al. 2003, 2008; Warren et al. 2006).

Matthew Costello

See also: Anti-Marijuana Campaigns in Popular Press; Differential Association Theory/Social Learning Theory; Gateway Drug Hypothesis; Law Enforcement Resources.

Further Reading

Clayton, Richard R., Anne M. Cattarello, and Bryan M. Johnstone. "The Effectiveness of Drug Abuse Resistance Education (Project DARE): 5-year Follow-up Results." *Preventive Medicine* 25, no. 3 (1996): 307–318.

Ennett, Susan T., et al. "Long-term Evaluation of Drug Abuse Resistance Education." *Addictive Behaviors* 19, no. 2 (1994): 113–125.

Hecht, Michael L., et al. "Culturally Grounded Substance Use Prevention: An Evaluation of the Keepin' It REAL Curriculum." *Prevention Science* 4, no. 4 (2003): 233–248.

Hecht, Michael L., et al. "Immediate and Short-Term Effects of the 5th Grade Version of the Keepin' It REAL Substance Use Prevention Intervention." *Journal of Drug Education* 38, no. 3 (2008): 225–251.

National Institute of Justice. "Program Profile: Drug Abuse Resistance Education (DARE) (1983–2009)." June 2, 2011. https://www.crimesolutions.gov/ProgramDetails.aspx?ID=99

Nordrum, Amy. "The New D.A.R.E. Program—This One Works." *Scientific American,* September 10, 2014. https://www.scientificamerican.com/article/the-new-d-a-r-e-program-this-one-works/

Warren, Jennifer R., et al. "Communicating Prevention: The Effects of the Keepin' It REAL Classroom Videotapes and Televised PSAs on Middle-school Students' Substance Use." *Journal of Applied Communication Research* 34, no. 2 (2006): 209–227.

Drug Cartels

Mexican drug cartels have a long history of supplying the United States with illicit substances. As early as the Prohibition era (1920–1933) in America, Mexico sent rum runners across the U.S. border to supply the American people with alcohol that they were unable to purchase legally. Today, Mexican cartels provide U.S. consumers with heroin, marijuana, methamphetamines, and other illicit substances. Mexican drug cartels have learned to maximize their advantage of sharing a border with one of the world's largest consumers of illicit substances. These cartels are run as profit-driven business organizations with the ability to change their spread and scope (based on consumer demand) to other sources to maximize profits. Once consisting of only four cartels, the current number of cartels and diversity of illicit products and services they provided has expanded to at least nine cartels, commonly referred to as drug trafficking organizations (DTOs) and transnational criminal organizations (TCOs). The nine major Mexican drug cartels are the Knights Templar, the Gulf Cartel, the Sinaloa Cartel, the Juarez/Carrillo Fuentes Organization, the Tijuana/Arellano Felix Organization (T/AFO), Los Zetas, the Beltran Leyva Organization (BLO), La Familia Michoacán (LFM), and the Cartel Jalisco New Generation (CJNG). These nine groups can be thought of as the parent organizations for numerous groups that have formed beneath them.

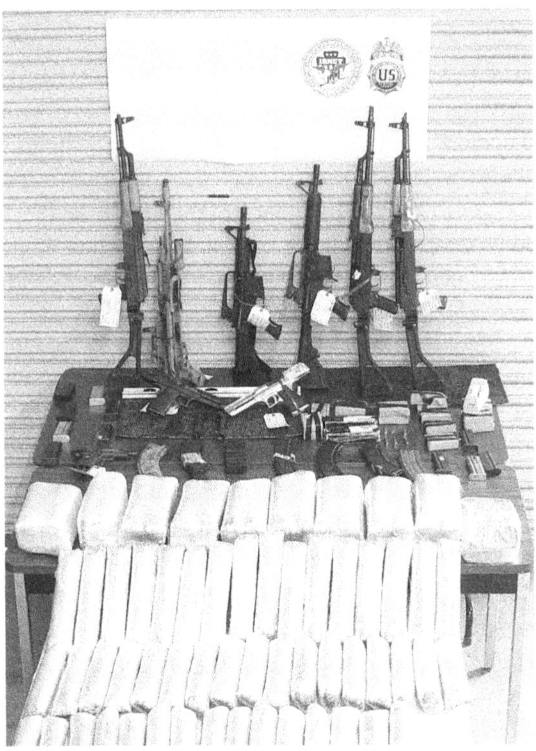

The War on Drugs has targeted drug trafficking both domestically and internationally. These operations have resulted in the seizure of drugs, weapons, and cash. Part of the seizure from one such operation is pictured here. "Project Coronado" resulted in 1,186 arrests and huge drug and money seizures against one of the world's most violent drug cartels, La Familia Michoacana, in 2009. (Drug Enforcement Administration)

The Gulf Cartel arose during the Prohibition era of the 1920s. It cooperated with other Central and South American organizations in the cocaine and marijuana trade and then later expanded operations to include methamphetamine and heroin. The oldest and most established cartel in Mexico is the Sinaloa Cartel, headed by Joaquin "El Chapo" Guzman (1957–). The Sinaloa Cartel gained its power and influence through the trafficking of South American cocaine, locally sourced methamphetamines, marijuana, and heroin to the U.S. market. The Congressional Research Service estimates that the Sinaloa Cartel accounts for 40–60 percent of the Mexican drug trade and brings in about $3 billion annually (Beittel 2015).

At one point in the 1980s and 1990s, the Juarez/Carrillo Fuentes Organization controlled nearly half of all narcotic trafficking between Ciudad Juarez and El Paso, Texas. The organization was once a prominent trafficker of marijuana and cocaine, but has recently become more involved in opium cultivation and heroin production and trafficking. The Tijuana/Arellano Felix Organization (T/AFO) is based in the border city of Tijuana and is responsible for a large proportion of the narcotics smuggled into Baja and Southern California. Los Zetas was originally the enforcement/assassination arm of the Gulf Cartel, and its leadership and members include a large number of former Mexican Special Forces and law enforcement officers. Los Zetas is considered one of the most aggressive cartels in Mexico. Much of its revenue comes from crime and violence (fuel theft, extortion, human smuggling, kidnapping, etc.).

The Beltran Leyva Organization (BLO) emerged as the result of a split from the Sinaloa Cartel. The BLO has splintered into at least five smaller groups. The BLO and its splinter groups have significant presence and influence in at least four Mexican states. La Familia Michoacán (LFM) was established in the 1980s and was originally based in the Mexican state of Michoacán. LFM has been known for providing social services to Mexican citizens in its territory. In 2010, LFM called for a truce with the Mexican government and now remains largely fragmented. The Knights Templar began as an offshoot of the LFM in 2011. According to the Congressional Research Service, LMF claims that its goal is to protect citizens of Michoacán from other criminal organizations. The Cartel Jalisco New Generation (CJNG) has been declared the most dangerous group by the Mexican government. The CJNG maintains an international presence, with operations throughout the Americas, Asia, and Europe. Present in 22 of the 32 Mexican states, this cartel controls many of Mexico's international ports, granting it ease of access to numerous smuggling enterprises.

Drug cartels remain a prominent threat for both the United States and Mexico. In the 2018 National Drug Threat Assessment, the U.S. Drug Enforcement Administration asserted that these groups represent the greatest threat to the United States in terms of public health, law enforcement, and national security (U.S. DOJ 2018). This threat led to a push by U.S. politicians to label drug trafficking organizations (DTOs) as foreign terrorist organizations (FTOs), but there is ongoing debate as to whether or not the levels of violence used by DTOs meet the U.S criteria for terrorist activity. Current political climates in both the United States and Mexico are calling for new solutions to these issues in order to reduce crime on both sides of the border.

Shelby I. Ingalls

See also: Drug Enforcement Administration (DEA); Street Crime.

Further Reading

Beittel, June S. "Mexico: Organized Crime and Drug Trafficking Organizations." *Washington: Congressional Research Service* 3 (2015). https://sgp.fas.org/crs/row/R41576.pdf

U.S. Department of Justice. "National Drug Threat Assessment." 2018. https://www.dea.gov/sites/default/files/2018-11/DIR-032-18%202018%20NDTA%20final%20low%20resolution.pdf

Drug Enforcement Administration (DEA)

The Drug Enforcement Administration, more commonly known as the DEA, is a U.S. federal agency tasked with enforcing "the controlled substances laws and regulations of the United States and bring to the criminal and civil justice system of the United States, or any other competent jurisdiction, those organizations and principal members of organizations, involved in the growing, manufacture, or distribution of controlled substances appearing in or destined for illicit traffic in the United States; and to recommend and support nonenforcement programs aimed at reducing the availability of illicit controlled substances on the domestic and international markets" (Drug Enforcement Administration n.d.-c, para. 1). The DEA incorporates various drug law enforcement efforts to combat drug law violations. The various efforts include crop eradication, asset forfeiture, and seizure; interagency coordination with other law enforcement agencies such as task forces both nationally and internationally; and drug interdiction (Drug Enforcement Administration n.d.-c). These are only a few of the many enforcement efforts utilized by the DEA to combat the rampant drug crime problem.

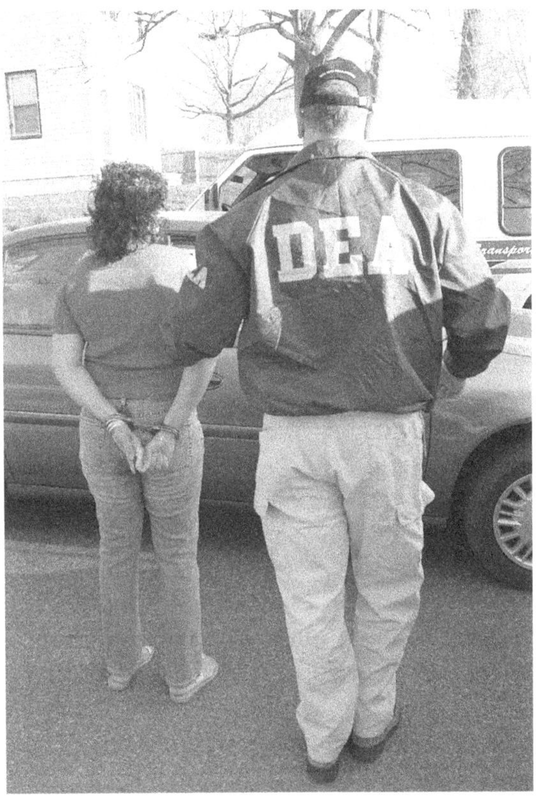

A Drug Enforcement Administration (DEA) officer arrests a suspected drug trafficker. Formed in 1973 with the merger of the Federal Bureau of Narcotics and Dangerous Drugs, the Office of Drug Abuse Law Enforcement, and agents from other federal agencies, the DEA is the nation's leading federal agency in charge of controlling illegal drugs. (Drug Enforcement Administration)

Crop eradication and substitution is a method used to limit drug supply, make drugs more expensive, and eventually decrease use (Bigwood and Phillip 2005). Researchers contend, though, that eradicating drug crops has had a nominal outcome on the cost or availability of illegal drugs such as cocaine in the United States. Critics also assert that the eradication programs have intensified human rights violations, reinforced undemocratic governments, and aided in shaping relationships between guerillas and peasant growers (Bigwood and Phillip 2005). Additionally, eradication can have a devastating impact on the environment through the utilization of toxic substances and fertilizers. According to the DEA, marijuana is the only popular illegal drug of abuse grown on U.S. soil. One of the DEA's primary anti-marijuana initiatives has been the Domestic Cannabis Eradication/Suppression Program (DCE/SP) to target drug trafficking organizations (DTO) engaged in marijuana cultivation (Drug Enforcement Administration n.d.-a). This program has had some success with eradicating marijuana plants, seizing assets, and arresting members of DTOs. In 2019, the DCE/SP, working in collaboration with 127 local and state law enforcement agencies, destroyed 3,232,722 cultivated outdoor cannabis plants and 770,472 indoor plants, thus eradicating more than 4 million marijuana plants overall.

Seizing and forfeiting the assets of those suspected of illegal drug trafficking is also done by the DEA, which uses this method to cripple the financial structure of drug trafficking groups globally. It uses this tool to target individuals as low in the drug trade hierarchy as couriers moving cash or drugs to the leadership of international drug cartels. The DEA reports that civil forfeiture is an effective weapon against profit-motivated drug crimes, but it is also one of the most controversial drug enforcement techniques undertaken by U.S. federal law enforcement agencies.

The DEA also employs task forces and others means of coordination with other international agencies such as Interpol and the United States. Task forces are arguably the most important means of interagency coordination utilized by the DEA. The DEA reports that interagency cooperation enables it to draw upon the expertise of law enforcement, share resources, and increase jurisdictions of state and local law enforcement officers by deputizing them as federal agents. Contributing agencies can obtain an equitable portion of forfeited drug profits, and the DEA may provide overtime pay and investigative expenditures for state and local agencies (Drug Enforcement Administration n.d.-d).

Drug interdiction is another method that is utilized by the DEA and international law enforcement agencies to stop illegal drugs from entering the United States. For example, the DEA's 2018 National Drug Threat Assessment reports several successful instances of drug interdiction (Drug Enforcement Administration 2018). One instance occurred in February 2018 when SEDENA (Mexico's Secretariat of National Defense) seized over 800 kilograms of cocaine, approximately 40 grams of fentanyl powder, about 4 grams of heroin, and around 5,000 pills containing fentanyl (Drug Enforcement Administration 2018).

These are only a few of the many enforcement efforts undertaken by the DEA to enforce U.S. drug laws and regulations and combat criminal drug enterprises such as cartels. Despite the controversies surrounding some of these different methods, such as asset forfeiture, the DEA continues to employ many of these methods in pursuit of their ultimate goal, reducing the use of drugs.

Lucas Maness

See also: Comprehensive Drug Abuse Prevention and Control Act (1970); Confidential Informants; Law Enforcement Efforts, Marijuana Control; Law Enforcement Resources.

Further Reading

Bigwood, Jeremy and Phillip Coffin. "Coca Eradication." *Institute for Policy Studies*, October 2005. https://ips-dc.org/coca_eradication/

Drug Enforcement Administration. "Cannabis Eradication." n.d.-a. Accessed August 23, 2021. https://www.dea.gov/cannabis-eradication

Drug Enforcement Administration. "DEA Asset Forfeiture." n.d.-b. Accessed August 23, 2021. https://www.dea.gov/dea-asset-forfeiture

Drug Enforcement Administration. "Mission: DEA Mission Statement." n.d.-c. Accessed August 23, 2021. https://www.dea.gov/mission

Drug Enforcement Administration. "Task Forces." n.d.-d. Accessed August 23, 2021. https://www.dea.gov/task-forces

Drug Enforcement Administration (DEA). "2018 National Drug Threat Assessment." 2018. https://www.dea.gov/sites/default/files/2018-11/DIR-032 18%202018%20 NDTA%20final%20low%20resolution.pdf

U.S. Department of State. Bureau of International Narcotics and Law Enforcement Affairs. "Eradication and Interdiction." 2019. https://www.state.gov/eradication-and-interdiction/

Warchol, Greg L., and Brian R. Johnson. "Guilty Property: A Quantitative Analysis of Civil Asset Forfeiture." *American Journal of Criminal Justice* 21, no. 1 (1996): 61–81.

Drug Policy Alliance (DPA)

The Drug Policy Alliance (DPA) is a multi-issue social movement organization that has used advocacy efforts to change laws and shift cultural norms around drug use and abuse. While the group has gained the most traction with respect to marijuana, they have been active on multiple interrelated fronts. For instance, DPA's work has also influenced criminal justice reform and harmed reduction efforts.

DPA was established in 2000 with the merger of two existing advocacy groups: The Drug Policy Foundation (established 1987) and The Lindesmith Center (established 1994). The organization has described itself as the "leading drug policy reform organization" and "the loyal opposition to the war on drugs." The organization partners with academic institutions and has received significant financial support from the George Soros' Open Society Foundations, as well as through collaborating with human rights groups (DPA 2019).

The organization played a financial and conceptual role in advancing a broad movement to end marijuana prohibition. Characterizing the war on drugs as both inefficient and racist, DPA has supported the decriminalization, medicalization, regulation, and legalization of marijuana in many states. DPA has also consulted with governmental and social movement activities around drug policy throughout the Americas, including Mexico, Guatemala, Colombia, and Uruguay. The group emphasizes its belief that racism is a primary motivation behind the war on drugs, including marijuana prohibition. It argues that law enforcement persistently targets people of color, disproportionately in Black and brown communities, for arrests and prosecutions of low-level drug offenses (Staggs 2019). However, rather than advance redistributive justice for those targeted by these efforts, their expertise and resources are directed toward opening new markets for legal and regulated use and sale of marijuana (DPA 2019).

These efforts reflect an upstream perspective that is reflected in DPA's work on reforming sentencing laws. For instance, California's Proposition 36 in 2000 established that statewide, first and second time "nonviolent drug offenders" could receive treatment instead of jail time. Nationally, DPA was involved in the

Obama-era Fair Sentencing Act (2010), reducing the disparity between punishment for convictions related to crack and powder cocaine.

DPA works in coalition with other groups such as the American Civil Liberties Union, National Cannabis Industry Association, Cannabis Trade Federation, and the National Association for the Advancement of Colored People (NAACP). Solidarities and spillover between such groups has illuminated the unequal growth of the marijuana industry through the partial repeals of prohibition. For instance, as people of color were disproportionately charged for marijuana-related offenses, these persistent criminal records create a barrier to entrance in the newly legalized industries, which grew out of their own efforts (Tolan 2019). Due to the slow pace of policy change, DPA and allied advocates direct many of their reform efforts to the grassroots and local levels.

In terms of harm reduction, DPA is working to shift the conversation about substance use toward a medical, evidence-based, and treatment-centered approach. As with marijuana law and criminal justice reform, DPA frames its work in terms of racial equity and justice by favoring a framework that emphasizes public health considerations over punishment and incarceration. Two examples of harm reduction are providing access to sterile syringes and creating pathways for individuals to receive medical attention to prevent overdose death without fear of criminal repercussions (DPA 2019).

Alex Espinoza-Kulick and Mario Alberto V. Espinoza-Kulick

See also: Drug Enforcement Administration (DEA); Medical Uses.

Further Reading

Drug Policy Alliance (DPA). *The Drug War, Mass Incarceration and Race.* New York: Drug Policy Alliance, 2016.

Drug Policy Alliance (DPA). *We Are the Drug Policy Alliance.* New York: Drug Policy Alliance, 2019.

Staggs, Brooke. "Los Angeles County Review of Pot Crimes Planned: Many Convictions May Be Cleared or Downgraded Under New Laws." *Daily News of Los Angeles*, April 1, 2019.

Tolan, Casey. "Harris Bill Would Decriminalize Marijuana at Federal Level: Former Federal Convicts Would See Convictions Expunged." *Monterey County Herald*, July 23, 2019.

E

Ecological Impacts

The ecological impacts of marijuana vary widely and depend upon numerous factors. These impacts can be categorized by the three primary ways cultivation and production of marijuana can adversely affect the environment: the *introduction of toxins into the environment*, the *depletion of scarce resources*, and the *disruption of ecosystems*.

While "meth labs" are notoriously hazardous, marijuana cultivation provides another example of how illegal drug production can introduce ecotoxins. Marijuana growers commonly use pesticides to protect their investments, and these highly toxic substances have been found in local water supplies (NDIC 2005). The toll is immense, as "the most toxic sites cost as much as $100,000 to clean up, leaving taxpayers with a bill that could reach $100 million or more in California alone" (Bernstein 2017). Moreover, the use of pesticides and rodenticides to protect young plants has proven lethal to numerous species, including mule deer, foxes, coyotes, northern spotted owls, ravens, and Coho salmon (Bauer et al. 2015; Helmer 2019). Indeed, one study found that 75 percent of dead fishers (an endangered mammal species) in California had been exposed to rodenticide (Gabriel 2012). In addition to pesticides, large quantities of synthetic fertilizers used to promote marijuana growth bring about yet more problems. These chemicals run off fields and enter water supplies, resulting in eutrophication, a form of water pollution that encourages algal growth that disrupts ecosystems and kills other aquatic life.

Outdoor cultivation also provides a telling example of how drug cultivation and the War on Drugs can alter ecosystems. While some experts estimate that 30 percent of Mexico's arable land is used for marijuana and opium poppy cultivation (Campbell 2010, 23), the recent tightening of the U.S./Mexico border has yielded numerous unintended consequences. One has been the creation of "super tunnels" to ferry drugs under the border (Reel 2015). Federal agents have found miles of long tunnels for such purposes, replete with rail lines and elevators. Such tunnels endanger the flora and fauna in the fragile desert landscape, while groundwater aquifers can be punctured and drained (Reel 2015). Another unintended outcome is increased cultivation on U.S. soil by Mexican drug cartels seeking to bypass the border altogether. These cartels have found the large expanses of unregulated national forest lands in the United States particularly suited for large-scale marijuana cultivation, with three major benefits: (1) access to large, unregulated expanses of remote land, (2) freedom from asset forfeiture laws, and (3) avoidance of border crossings. The majority of these operations are located in California, but Oregon; Washington; Hawaii; and even eastern states such as Tennessee, Kentucky, and West Virginia are now home to these clandestine plantations. Paradoxically, the number of such clandestine grow operations has increased since recreational marijuana has become legal in many states, most notably in California. Experts attribute this increase to the decreased severity of criminal punishment for marijuana-related offenses.

Despite its reputation as a weed, commercial-grade marijuana is actually a resource-intensive crop, and the ecological consequences are substantial. Marijuana cultivation has been linked to the loss of sensitive habitats because of illegal land clearing and logging. In addition, large-scale cultivation requires irrigation, and springs and streams are often diverted to water these plants (Helmer 2019). The removal of these water sources endangers the animals dependent on these drinking supplies while decimating aquatic systems and the organisms therein. Lethal effects related to marijuana cultivation have been documented for many species of fish and amphibians (Bauer et al. 2015). Less easily quantified are the impacts that occur when native species are replaced with the marijuana monocrop, which disrupts the complex interplays at work in the forest.

While most attention has been given to how outdoor marijuana cultivation impacts the environment, indoor production also has significant impacts. The shift to indoor, large-scale grow operations that has taken place since numerous states have legalized marijuana has placed a substantial burden on natural resources (Helmer 2019). Indoor producers consume considerable amounts of energy, with energy experts warning that heightened production could impose a large demand load on already burdened regional power grids. Indeed, the founder of the Resource Innovation Institute in Portland contends that legal indoor marijuana production in Colorado is responsible for 2 percent of the state's electrical load and 45 percent of all new demand, while electricity makes up 45 percent of the entire cost of running a marijuana grow operation (Crombie 2016). Additional research is needed to fully understand the environmental impacts of legal cultivation.

Robert Perdue and James Hawdon

See also: Drug Cartels; Law Enforcement Efforts, Marijuana Control; Online Marijuana Markets.

Further Reading

Bauer, Scott, et al. "Impacts of Surface Water Diversions for Marijuana Cultivation on Aquatic Habitat in Four Northwestern California Watersheds." *PloS one* 10, no. 3 (2015): e0120016.

Bernstein, Sharon. "Toxic Waste from U.S. Pot Farms Alarms Experts." *Reuters,* August 16 2017. https://www.reuters.com/article/us-usa-marijuana-environment/toxic-waste-from-u-s-pot-farms-alarms-experts-idUSKBN1AM0C3

Campbell, Howard. *Drug War Zone: Frontline Dispatches from the Streets of El Paso and Juárez*. Austin: University of Texas Press, 2010.

Crombie, Noelle. "Task Force Looks at Energy, Water Use Related to Marijuana Production." *The Oregonian*, June 8, 2016.

Gabriel, Mourad W. "Silent Forests: How Are Toxicants Associated with Marijuana Cultivation Impacting Wildlife on our Public and Tribal Lands?" California State University, 2012. https://scholarworks.calstate.edu/concern/publications/fq977x12c

Helmer, Jodi. "The Environmental Downside of Cannabis Cultivation." JSTOR Daily, 2019. https://daily.jstor.org/the-environmental-downside-of-cannabis-cultivation/

Miller, Char. "War in the Woods: Combating the Marijuana Cartels on America's Public Lands." *Journal of Forestry* 110, no. 2 (2012): 112.

National Drug Intelligence Center (NDIC). "Marijuana and Methamphetamine Trafficking on Federal Lands Threat Assessment." Last modified February, 2005. https://www.justice.gov/archive/ndic/pubs10/10402/back.htm

Reel, Monte. "Underworld: How the Sinaloa Drug Cartel Digs Its Tunnels." *New Yorker* 3 (2015): 22–28.

Edibles

Edibles are food products that contain cannabis. These products serve as an alternative to other forms of cannabis consumption, such as smoking and vaping. Popular examples of edibles include candies, gummies, and brownies. Oils, tinctures, and capsules are common edible alternatives in medical contexts. To create these homemade or commercially produced products, cannabinoids must be extracted from a cannabis plant through decarboxylation, a process that involves heating the cannabis flower in an oil-based liquid. During decarboxylation, which instantly occurs during smoking and vaping, tetrahydrocannabinolic acid (nonpsychoactive) is converted into tetrahydrocannabinol (THC), the prime psychoactive ingredient of cannabis. The THC dissolves into the oil-based liquid along with other cannabinoids, creating a cannabis-infused oil that can be added to medicinal products, food, or drinks to create edible cannabis products (Blake and Nahtigal 2019).

Edibles are increasingly formidable competition to traditional methods of consuming cannabis. Many reasons have been cited for their rise in popularity. Some users prefer edible consumption because the "high" can be long-lasting and less intense. Some reports suggest the effects of an edible peak around 2–4 hours after ingestion, while the effects of smoking or vaping peak around 20–30 minutes after ingestion. Health concerns related to smoking cannabis also contribute to the popularity of edible products. Specifically, there is a perception that edibles are a way to escape toxins present in cannabis smoke. Edibles are also lauded for their convenience and discreteness. These products lack smoke or smell and are often indistinguishable from nonpsychoactive food (Giombi et al. 2018).

Health concerns have been raised about edibles, though. A combination of inconsistent dosing and labeling, as well as the delayed onset of effects, can lead to over-ingestion and produce severe effects. Inconsistent dosing leads to variation in psychoactive effects, and many researchers have found that users often complain about the difficulty of controlling one's "high" during edible consumption. Unlike smoking and vaping, edible consumption has a delayed onset of psychoactive effects, which contributes to over-ingestion because users can consume a product and not feel "high" for 30–90 minutes. This long wait time may prompt uniformed users to consume more of an edible after not feeling a high, leading to intense effects. Accidental ingestion is another prominent concern. Adults, children, and pets are at risk of accidental ingestion due to how indistinguishable edible products can be from ordinary foods (Barrus et al. 2016).

The issues of over-ingestion and accidental ingestion have led to calls for increased regulation of labeling and dosing procedures. Supporters assert that

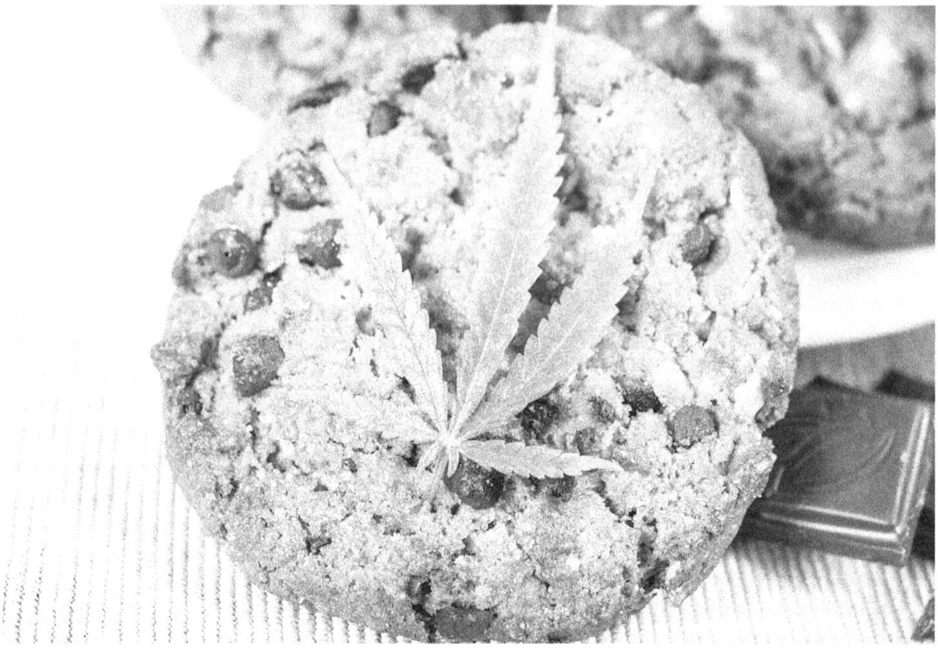

Marijuana can be consumed through edibles, which are food and beverages infused with cannabis. Rather than smoking or vaping, edibles are an alternative method of use, available in many forms such as this chocolate chip cookie containing marijuana. (Y991bh/Dreamstime.com)

such measures could better ensure that users follow dosing guidelines, improve dosing consistency, and make cannabis edibles more easily distinguishable from regular food. To minimize over-ingestion, some places in the United States where the retail sale of cannabis is legal require labeling that warns users of the delayed effects of edible consumption. Another effort for minimization of over-ingestion is the requirement for consistent distribution of THC throughout cannabis edibles. States have also taken action to combat accidental ingestion through manufacturing regulations. Some of these regulations include requiring child-proof packaging, restricting the manufacturing and packaging of products that may appeal to children, and requiring labeling that clearly indicates the presence of THC (Barrus et al. 2016).

Aubrey D. Johnson

See also: Cannabis Drinks; Cannabis Oils.

Further Reading

Barrus, Daniel G., et al. "Tasty THC: Promises and Challenges of Cannabis Edibles." *RTI Press* (2016): 1–17.

Blake, Alexia, and Istok Nahtigal. "The Evolving Landscape of Cannabis Edibles." *Current Opinion in Food Science* 28 (2019): 25–31.

Giombi, Kristen C., Katherine M. Kosa, Carrie Rains, and Sheryl C. Cates. "Consumers' Perceptions of Edible Marijuana Products for Recreational Use: Likes, Dislikes, and Reasons for Use." *Substance Use & Misuse* 53, no. 4 (2018): 541–547.

Europe

Europeans have relatively high use rates of several types of drugs, including marijuana, cocaine, and ecstasy. In fact, Europe has some of the highest rates of drug use in the world, and cannabis is among the most popular drugs in Europe. Based on data from the United Nations, approximately 5.1 percent of Europe's adult population (defined by the UN as people ages 15–64) use marijuana annually. This compares to the global average of 3.9 percent of the adult population (UNODC 2018).

Cannabis has a long history in Europe. Researchers have found indications of its use dating back to at least ancient Greece, when the cannabis plant was used medically. During the early Middle Ages, hemp cultivation was common, as the plant was used to make rope and cloth for sails. Although hemp was common in Europe during the Middle Ages, the recreational use of cannabis was limited, at least until the nineteenth century when French troops invaded Egypt and were introduced to hashish (Booth 2015).

Despite being criminalized in most European nations in the late nineteenth and early twentieth centuries, marijuana became increasingly popular in Europe in the 1960s and 1970s and has remained a popular recreational drug ever since (Hawdon 2005). Based on 2019 data from the United Nations (UNODC 2018) and the European Monitoring Centre for Drugs and Drug Addiction (EMCDDA 2019), an estimated 27.9 million Europeans use cannabis annually. Rates of marijuana use vary considerably across the continent, however. Western Europeans are almost three times as likely to use marijuana as are Eastern Europeans. While approximately 7.0 percent of the adult population of Western and Central Europe uses cannabis annually, only 2.4 percent of adults in Eastern Europe do (UNODC 2018).

MARIJUANA IN WESTERN EUROPE

Marijuana use in Europe is most associated with the coffeeshops of Netherlands, where cannabis is openly sold for personal consumption. Despite coffeeshops being a notorious feature of Dutch cities since the 1970s and the source of a thriving drug tourism industry, the Netherlands does not lead Europe in cannabis consumption rates. France and Spain report the highest rates of cannabis use in Europe, with approximately 11 percent of the adult population of both nations using the drug annually in the late 2010s. Similarly, Czechia, Italy, the Netherlands, and Switzerland all report relatively high rates of cannabis use, with rates in these nations ranging from approximately 8 percent to 10.2 percent of the adult population.

Despite these similar rates of use, the trends in consumption reported by these nations differ. For example, cannabis use increased by nearly 30 percent between 2010 and 2014 in France, and rates of use nearly tripled in Switzerland between 2008 and 2016. In contrast, rates have been relatively stable over this period in Spain and Czechia. Nations with rates of use ranging between 5 percent and 8 percent include Austria, Denmark, Estonia, Finland, Germany, Ireland, Norway,

Portugal, and the United Kingdom. The lowest rates of use in Western Europe are found in Belgium, Luxembourg, Poland, and Sweden, where rates of use range between 4 and 5 percent of the adult population (UNODC 2018; EMCDDA 2019).

MARIJUANA IN EASTERN EUROPE

By contrast, Croatia is the only Eastern European nation that reports rates of cannabis use above 7 percent of the adult population (7.9 percent). Albania (5.6 percent), Slovenia (4.4 percent), Slovakia (4.3 percent), Latvia (4.2 percent), and Bulgaria (4.2 percent) are the only other Eastern European nations that have higher use rates than the global average of 3.9 percent. The Russian Federation (3.4 percent), Romania (3.2 percent), Lithuania (2.7 percent), Ukraine (2.1 percent), Montenegro (1.8 percent), Bosnia and Herzegovina (1.5 percent), Hungary (1.5 percent), Belarus (1.1 percent), Turkey (1.1 percent), and Moldovia (0.7 percent) all report relatively low rates of marijuana use (EMCDDA 2019).

The fact that cannabis products are the most widely used illicit drugs in Europe is not surprising. As in other regions of the world, marijuana is the illicit drug of choice. However, Europe differs from many other regions in one important respect. While cannabis use is limited to adult males in some places around the world (Hawdon 2005), it is a habit of young people of both genders in Europe. Nearly 60 percent of young adults ages 15–34 in France have tried marijuana at least once in their lives. Similarly, nearly half of young adults in Denmark, Czechia, Spain, and Italy report having used cannabis at least once in their lifetimes.

Studies have also found relatively high rates of "regular" or monthly use in Europe. For example, between 20 and 25 percent of young adults in the United Kingdom are regular recreational cannabis users, and 35 percent of young Czechs used marijuana. In Spain, nearly 15 percent of 15- to 24-year-olds report using marijuana in the past month, and similar rates are seen in France, Italy, and the Netherlands. Throughout the European Union countries, more than one in 4 young Europeans have tried cannabis and more than 1 in 10 have used cannabis over the last month (EMCDDA 2019). In fact, the youthful recreational use of cannabis has become "normalized" in many Western European nations (Parker, Williams, and Aldridge 2002). The pattern of marijuana use being a youthful activity is also seen in Eastern Europe, although rates of use among youth are not as high as they are in many Western European nations.

CORRELATES OF MARIJUANA USE IN EUROPE

In both Western and Eastern Europe, cannabis use is more prevalent among males than females. For example, among young adults in EU countries, males are twice as likely to use cannabis regularly as are European females. Regular cannabis use is also correlated with occupational status, as managers are nearly twice as likely to use cannabis on a monthly basis as are manual workers. Urban young adults are slightly more likely to use cannabis on a monthly basis than are Europeans from rural communities, small towns, or medium-sized cities (Hawdon 2005). Thus, young professional males are the primary users of cannabis—the most widely used illicit substance in Europe. This is especially true in Western Europe. However, as in the United States and other developed nations, cannabis use is not limited to any particular group. It is relatively common in all social strata, at least among the young (Kraus et al. 2018).

THE LEGAL STATUS OF MARIJUANA IN EUROPE

Although Georgia is the only European nation—and one of four in the world—where recreational use of cannabis is legal, it is decriminalized in a number of countries. In these countries, possession is treated as a noncriminal offense, similar to a traffic violation. European nations that have decriminalized marijuana include Austria, Belgium, Estonia, Czechia, Italy, Portugal, Spain, Switzerland, and the Netherlands. Medical marijuana is legal in Croatia, Germany, Greece, Ireland, Italy, Lithuania, Luxembourg, Norway, the Netherlands, Portugal, Switzerland, and the United Kingdom. Complicating the use and legal control of cannabis in Europe are new high-potency strains of the plant, as the potency of both cannabis resin and herb has increased over the last decade. In addition, the introduction of new cannabis products such as edibles and concentrates is presenting a new challenge for European drug control efforts (EMCDDA 2019).

James Hawdon

See also: Africa; Central Asia; China and Southeast Asia; India and South Asia; Latin America; Middle East.

Further Reading

Booth, Martin. *Cannabis: A History*. New York: Macmillan, 2015.

European Monitoring Centre for Drugs and Drug Addiction (EMCDDA). *European Drug Report 2019: Trends and Developments*. Lisbon: EMCDDA, 2019.

Hawdon, James. *Drug and Alcohol Consumption as Functions of Social Structures: A Cross-Cultural Sociology*. No. 47. Lewistown, NY: Edwin Mellen Press, 2005.

Kraus, Ludwig, et al. "'Are the Times a-changin'? Trends in Adolescent Substance Use in Europe." *Addiction* 113, no. 7 (2018): 1317–1332.

Parker, Howard, Lisa Williams, and Judith Aldridge. 2002. "The Normalization of 'Sensible' Recreational Drug Use: Further Evidence from the North West England Longitudinal Study." *Sociology* 36: 941–965.

United Nations Office on Drugs and Crime (UNODC). *World Drug Report 2018*. Oxford, UK: Oxford University Press, 2018.

F

Family Life

Marijuana use interrelates with family relationships and processes. In particular, family lifestyle and dynamics have been associated with adolescents' and young adults' marijuana use, especially if their parents or siblings use marijuana. Parental use correlates with their children's marijuana use during adolescence and even has an association with the marijuana use of college students (Windle et al. 2017). Similarly, parental disapproval of marijuana use, which may be related to their own use or nonuse, is a deterrent for adolescents' marijuana use. Furthermore, older siblings' marijuana use is positively associated with younger siblings' use, especially if they have the same friends. Concordance between older siblings' and younger siblings' marijuana use is greater than it is for alcohol or cigarette use and generally decreases with age (Schuler et al. 2019).

Parenting styles and family relationships can also influence adolescents' and young adults' marijuana use. Parental monitoring and control is associated with reduced marijuana use among adolescents. Monitoring of behavior appears to be a stronger predictor of marijuana use during early adolescence, whereas family relationship quality is more important during middle and late adolescence. However, parental monitoring, even during the senior year of high school, is negatively associated with marijuana exposure opportunity in college (Pinchevsky et al. 2012). Feeling close to parents is associated with decreased marijuana use during adolescence, which is mediated through a sense of family belonging. Both a sense of family belonging and family attachment are associated with reduced odds of marijuana use for adolescents.

In addition, family processes influence adults' marijuana use. Partners in committed relationships tend to be concordant on marijuana use for both heterosexual and same-sex couples, which may be due to convergence effects (Derrick, Wittkower, and Pierce 2019). Research supports this contention, as a spouse's marijuana use prior to marriage is associated with an individual's increased risk of marijuana use during the first four years of marriage (Homish, Leonard, and Cornelius 2007). Relatedly, couples who are discordant on marijuana use have poorer relationship quality, including decreased relationship satisfaction for men and increased negative social exchanges for both men and women. At least some of partners' concordance on marijuana use is due to the fact that men who used marijuana prior to marriage tend to marry women who also used marijuana (Yamaguchi and Kandel 1997).

Adults who take on family roles including cohabiting, marital, and parental roles tend to have lower marijuana use. For instance, married and cohabiting couples tend to have lower marijuana use than those who are not dating, whereas daters and non-daters do not differ on marijuana use. Higher relationship quality is also associated with decreased marijuana use, but only for those whose partner does not use marijuana (Fleming, White, and Catalano 2010). Likewise, becoming a parent and being a primary caregiver reduces the odds of marijuana use during adulthood.

Lastly, marijuana use can influence family relationships and processes, although most of these associations are detrimental for the family. For instance, marijuana use is associated with more marital disruptions. Marijuana use is also correlated with intimate partner violence, although it is unclear whether this relationship is causal (Derrick et al. 2019). That is, marijuana use may only be a precipitating factor in intimate partner aggression for those who are already predisposed toward aggression (Derrick et al. 2019).

Anastasia S. Vogt Yuan

See also: Age; Gender; Theories of Use.

Further Reading

Derrick, Jaye L., L. David Wittkower, and Jace D. Pierce. "Committed Relationships and Substance Use: Recent Findings and Future Directions." *Current Opinion in Psychology* 30 (2019): 74–79.

Fleming, Charles B., Helene R. White, and Richard F. Catalano. "Romantic Relationships and Substance Use in Early Adulthood: An Examination of the Influences of Relationship Type, Partner Substance Use, and Relationship Quality." *Journal of Health and Social Behavior* 51, no. 2 (2010): 153–167.

Homish, Gregory G., Kenneth E. Leonard, and Jack R. Cornelius. "Predictors of Marijuana Use among Married Couples: The Influence of One's Spouse." *Drug and Alcohol Dependence* 91, no. 2–3 (2007): 121–128.

Pinchevsky, Gillian M., et al. "Marijuana Exposure Opportunity and Initiation During College: Parent and Peer Influences." *Prevention Science* 13, no. 1 (2012): 43–54.

Schuler, Megan S., Joan S. Tucker, Eric R. Pedersen, and Elizabeth J. D'Amico. "Relative Influence of Perceived Peer and Family Substance Use on Adolescent Alcohol, Cigarette, and Marijuana Use Across Middle and High School." *Addictive Behaviors* 88 (2019): 99–105.

Windle, Michael, et al. "Social Influences on College Student Use of Tobacco Products, Alcohol, and Marijuana." *Substance Use & Misuse* 52, no. 9 (2017): 1111–1119.

Yamaguchi, Kazuo, and Denise B. Kandel. "The Influence of Spouses' Behavior and Marital Dissolution on Marijuana Use: Causation or Selection." *Journal of Marriage and the Family* (1997): 22–36.

"420"

The term "420" (pronounced "four-twenty") is popular among marijuana users. While the precise definition of "420" is a bit ambiguous, broadly speaking, 420 simply refers to marijuana (Nguyen, Nguyen, et al. 2017). The term may trace its roots to a group of Northern California hippies in the early 1970s. Today, "420" is used to reference a variety of marijuana-related phenomena.

Some argue "420" was first coined by a group of five teenage boys—Steve Capper, Dave Reddix, Mark Gravitch, Larry Schwartz, and Jeff Noel—who attended

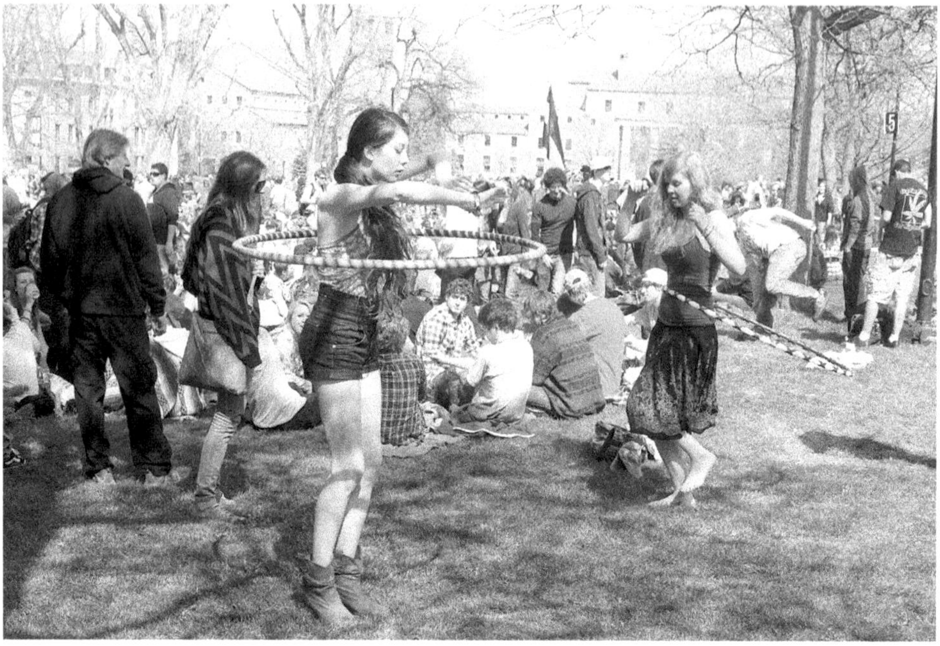

"420" is a symbol of the marijuana subculture. 420 day, celebrated here at University of Colorado, is one of the largest pro-marijuana rallies held annually on April 20 at 4:20 p.m. (James Insogna/Dreamstime.com)

a high school in San Rafael, California, in 1971. The group—known as "the Waldos"—had learned that a few members of the Coast Guard had been growing marijuana in a local forest, Point Reyes. Allegedly, the servicemen were weary of getting in trouble with their superiors, so at some point, they opted to abandon their crop. The Waldos decided to try to find the abandoned cannabis. The boys acquired a primitive map of Point Reyes made by one of the growers, outlining approximately where the abandoned weed could be found. After school, the group regularly met by a statue of Louis Pasteur outside of their high school to smoke marijuana and search for the deserted plants. Their meeting time was 4:20 p.m. On meeting days, they circulated a coded message throughout the school. The message simply read "420 Louis," referencing the time and place that they would meet to get high and prepare for their hunt. Eventually, the message was shortened to "420."

The Waldos had connections to the rock band, The Grateful Dead, which had formed in the San Francisco Bay area in 1965 and subsequently become one of the country's best-known bands. The boys introduced the term to the band members, who then began to use it in their performances. The phrase spread among the band's followers and gradually gained popularity among recreational marijuana users as well. A 1990 article in *High Times*, a magazine that caters to marijuana users, related the story of 420's origins and further spread its use among its readership.

Today, "420" is used in reference to a variety of marijuana-related phenomena. For instance, rental ads on Craigslist will commonly mention "420 Friendly" to indicate that marijuana users are welcome. "420" is also popular on social media.

There is a group on Facebook called "420 People," and "#420" is a common term on both Twitter and Instagram. There is even a subreddit (e.g., "r/420") for anything cannabis related. These social media groups provide an international, interactive, and educational platform for marijuana enthusiasts to communicate with one another. The term has even made its way into popular media, with references in the film *Pulp Fiction* and the television series *Rocko's Modern Life*. Additionally, many influential musicians, including Dr. Dre and Snoop Dogg, have referenced the term in their songs. Further, 4:20 p.m. is widely regarded as "marijuana happy hour"—the time of the day when users are encouraged to smoke pot.

Finally, April 20 (the twentieth day of the fourth month of the year) is recognized by many cannabis enthusiasts as International Pot-Smoking Day. This is a day when people are encouraged to come together and celebrate marijuana; it is a day when citizens in regions where marijuana use is prohibited gather in public and light up in an act of civil disobedience. In areas where recreational use has been legalized, users still gather and celebrate the drug, and many restaurants, including Pizza Hut and White Castle, advertise 420 deals. Large festival-like events have taken place on April 20 in various cities throughout the world, including New York City, Montreal, Sydney, and London. Arguably, one of the most popular of these festivals is the *Mile High 420 Festival* held in Denver, Colorado. The event includes musical performances and vendors selling all things related to marijuana.

Meghan Harrigan and Nathan E. Kruis

See also: Casual Users, Health Effects; *High Times*; Neurological Effects.

Further Reading

Nguyen, Anh, Long Nguyen, Dong Nguyen, Uyen Le, and Tuan Tran. "'420 Friendly': Revealing Marijuana Use via Craigslist Rental Ads." In *Workshops at the Thirty-First AAAI Conference on Artificial Intelligence*. 2017. https://arxiv.org/pdf/1612.07630.pdf

Nguyen, Anh, Hoang Pham, Dong Nguyen, and Tuan Tran. "Towards Monitoring Marijuana Activities via User-Generated Content Platforms and Social Networks." In *Public Health Intelligence and the Internet*, edited by Arash Shaban-Nejad, John S. Brownstein, and David L. Buckeridge. New York: Springer, 2017, 107–128.

G

Gaming

The video game industry is ever growing, becoming a leading form of entertainment for adults and children around the world. In 2020, there was an estimated 3.1 billion gamers globally, around 40 percent of the world's population. Given the popularity of video games, it is not surprising that the video gaming industry is now estimated to be worth more than $159 billion, making gaming the most lucrative entertainment industry, dwarfing both the movie and music industries. While video games are most popular in the Asia-Pacific region, globally, gaming industry revenue share is the second largest in the United States, trailing only China. In fact, in 2020 there were more than 214 million video game players in the United States. The average gamer in the United States is between the ages of 35 and 44 years old, although gaming is increasingly popular for all age demographics. Nearly two-thirds of U.S. adults and 70 percent of juveniles report playing video games regularly, and more than 75 percent of U.S. households have at least one member who plays video games. Most gamers play on consoles, but it is also common to play on smartphones, personal computers, handheld devices, and virtual reality devices.

Gamers commonly play video games for the sheer enjoyment of doing so. However, enjoyment is not the only benefit to playing that gamers cite. Some gamers cite the mental stimulation offered by video games, while others note that playing can sharpen their problem-solving skills (Bowen 2014). For other gamers, playing is a means to relax, unwind, and temporarily forget about daily stressors. Gaming can also serve as a social activity, allowing gamers to connect with acquaintances and strangers alike. Highlighting the increasingly communal nature of gaming, a recent report showed that around two-thirds of gamers typically play with others, either online or in person, and more than half of parents report playing video games with their children (Entertainment Software Association 2020).

Some gamers believe that marijuana intake enhances their experience, and perhaps their gaming acumen as well. Both marijuana and gaming are used by individuals to relax, and therefore, combining the two activities can enhance the feeling of relaxation. For other gamers, using marijuana while playing makes gaming more rewarding. Since tetrahydrocannabinol (THC), the main psychoactive compound in cannabis, releases dopamine and stimulates one's reward system, the sense of accomplishment felt by achieving a goal in a video game can be amplified by THC. Gamers also report enhanced enjoyment and sociability while using marijuana products. In other words, they feel happier and more apt to interact with other gamers when they are using marijuana (Cook 2018).

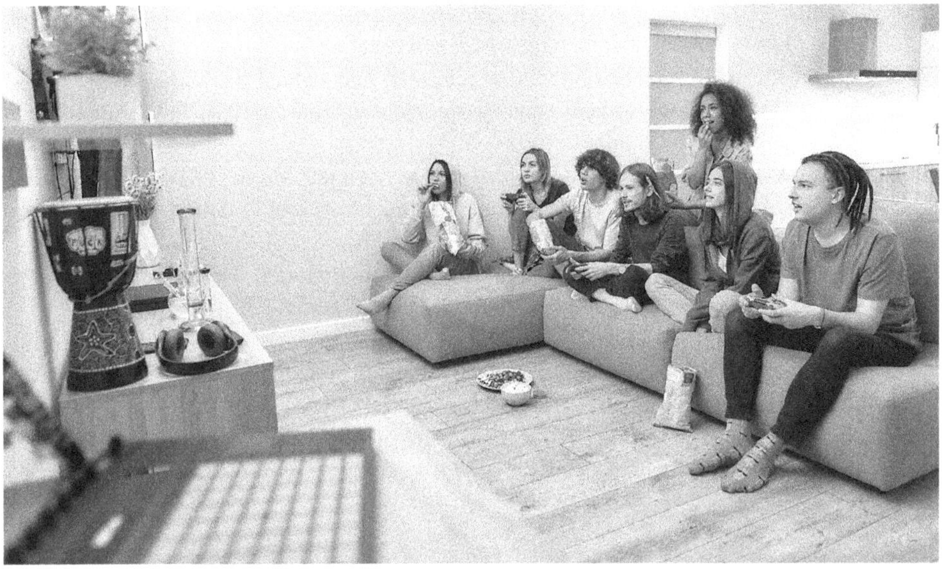

Young multicultural people eating snacks and playing video games after smoking marijuana from a bong. Some users claim marijuana enhances social experiences such as gaming. (Svitlana Ponurkina/Dreamstime.com)

The research on whether partaking in marijuana improves or hinders gaming proficiency is decidedly mixed. On the one hand, there is evidence that marijuana reduces motivation and impairs motor coordination, both essential to successful gaming (Sánchez Artiles et al. 2019). Similarly, marijuana can distort time perception (Sewell et al. 2013), slow reaction time, and reduce motor control (Kvålseth 1977). Again, in many video games, quick reactions and keen motor control are integral to success. Conversely, one study exploring memory retention found that a group of gamers given medical marijuana scored significantly higher on memory retention compared to the group that did not receive the treatment. Thus, for video games that require the retention of information, marijuana can bolster performance. Other work suggests that cannabis can improve focus and cognitive performance (Gruber et al. 2018), which are important factors in successful gaming. Additionally, long bouts of gaming, common in competitive gaming settings, can lead to pain and inflammation, which can be alleviated by cannabidiol (CBD), an active ingredient in cannabis. CBD can also have a calming effect on users, reducing stress and anxiety, and potentially improving the situational awareness and decision-making of gamers.

Matthew Costello

See also: Casual Users, Health Effects, Neurological Effects; Recreational Marijuana Laws; Sports.

Further Reading

Bowen, Lisa. "Video Game Play May Provide Learning, Health, Social Benefits, Review Finds." *Monitor on Psychology* 45, no. 2 (February 2014). http://www.apa.org/monitor/2014/02/video-game

Cook, Isabella. "Optimizing Your High Gaming Experience." *Cannabis Culture*, 2018. https://www.leafbuyer.com/blog/weed-video-games/

Entertainment Software Association. "2020 Essential Facts about the Video Game Industry." 2020. https://www.theesa.com/wp-content/uploads/2020/07/Final-Edited-2020-ESA_Essential_facts.pdf

Gruber, Staci A., et al. 2018. "The Grass Might Be Greener: Medical Marijuana Patients Exhibit Altered Brain Activity and Improved Executive Function after 3 Months of Treatment." *Frontiers in Pharmacology* 8: 983.

Kvålseth, Tarald O. "Effects of Marijuana on Human Reaction Time and Motor Control." *Perceptual and Motor Skills* 45, no. 3 (1977): 935–939.

Sánchez Artiles, Angel E., Areeba Awan, Mitchell Karl, and Antonello Santini. "Cardiovascular Effects of Cannabis (Marijuana): A Timely Update." *Phytotherapy Research* 33, no. 5 (2019): 1592–1594.

Sewell, R. Andrew, et al. "Acute Effects of THC on Time Perception in Frequent and Infrequent Cannabis Users." *Psychopharmacology* 226, no. 2 (2013): 401–413.

Garcia, Jerry (1942–1995)

Jerome John "Jerry" Garcia (August 1, 1942–August 9, 1995) was an American singer-songwriter, guitar player, ice cream flavor namesake, and founding member of the band the Grateful Dead. Garcia has been recognized as one of the top guitar players of all times by *Rolling Stone* magazine.

Garcia grew up in and around San Francisco, California. The son of a musician, he grew up playing piano and banjo. He went to live with his maternal grandparents as a child following his father's untimely death. At a young age, Garcia was introduced to contemporary guitarists such as John Lee Hooker, Hank Ballard, and B. B. King, by his older brother, Clifford. Inspired by their music, Garcia wished for an electric guitar and amplifier for his fifteenth birthday. When he instead received an accordion, he was able to convince his mother to exchange the accordion for a guitar at a local pawnshop.

Three years later, Garcia was forced to join the U.S. Army in 1960 as punishment for stealing his mother's car. However, by the end of the same year, he received a general discharge for excessive absence without leave by frequently missing roll call. The next year, Garcia survived a major car accident while out joyriding with friends. He viewed surviving as a wake-up call and began to take guitar playing seriously, joining several local bands in the early 1960s as a guitarist and vocalist. In 1965, Garcia joined several musicians from these earlier groups to assemble the band that would eventually come to be known as the Grateful Dead.

The Dead rose to prominence in the world of rock and roll quickly, in large part because they came to symbolize the 1960s counterculture era. They were known for their eclectic and psychedelic style, as well as being one of the first "jam bands," blending many genres including rock, blues, blue grass, country, and jazz. On stage, Garcia was known for his signature improvisation on guitar. As a result, it has been said that no two Grateful Dead shows were the same. From their formation in 1965 till 1995, when Garcia passed away, the Grateful Dead played 2,314 shows and

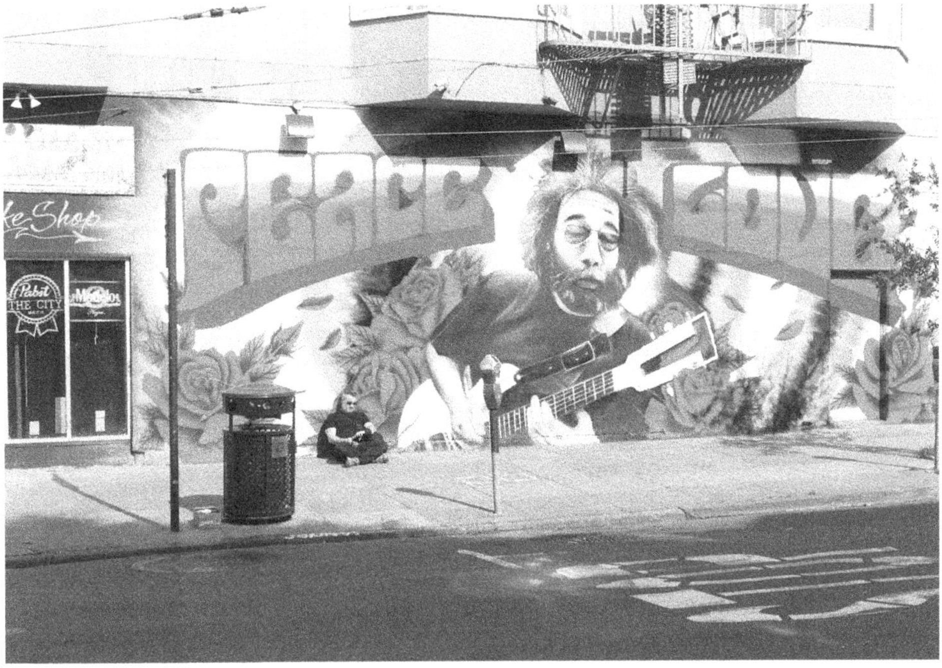

The Cole Street Mural, located on Cole and Haight in San Francisco, depicting guitarist and vocalist Jerry Garcia. Jerry Garcia (1942–1995) was the front man for the acid-rock band the Grateful Dead. The band was known for their live performances and was centered in the Haight-Ashbury district of San Francisco during the late 1960s and early 1970s. (Alexander Bernardo/Dreamstime.com)

earned a cult-like following from their fans—known as "Deadheads"—becoming a culture unto themselves. While they released 13 studio albums and had a number of hit songs, the band was best known for its live performances—recordings of which were freely made and traded by their Deadhead fans.

Although the band was most strongly associated with the psychedelic drug LSD (their sound engineer was Owsley Stanley who, in his spare time, produced massive quantities of the drug), drugs of all types could be found at Grateful Dead concerts.

Garcia himself was introduced to marijuana at the age of 15 and first began using LSD in 1964 at the age of 22. Throughout the 1970s, the band used cocaine in excess. Garcia began experimenting with heroin in 1975 and soon became dependent on both drugs to the point that he was spending an estimated $700 a day (equivalent to $1,900 in 2019) on drugs. Garcia was eventually confronted about his drug addiction in 1985 by his bandmates. By 1986, he was totally abstinent, but he relapsed several times over the next decade. Despite concerted efforts to remain clean and improve his lifestyle in the early 1990s, a history of obesity, smoking, and drug addiction caused his health to continue to decline. Garcia died from a heart attack while in drug rehab in 1995 at the age of 53. Since then, the remaining band members have reunited under the name "The Other Ones" for a number of tours. In 2019, it was announced that the Jerry Garcia estate would be launching a signature cannabis collection in 2020 in honor of Garcia.

John M. Eassey

See also: Beatles, The; Monkees, The; Nelson, Willie (1933–); Petty, Tom (1950–2017); Snoop Dogg (1971–); Woodstock.

Further Reading

Greenfield, Robert. *Bear: The Life and Times of Augustus Owsley Stanley III.* New York: St. Martin's Press, 2016.

Jackson, Blair, and David Gans. *This Is All a Dream We Dreamed: An Oral History of the Grateful Dead.* New York: Flatiron Books, 2015.

Kreutzmann, Bill, and Benjy Eisen. *Deal: My Three Decades of Drumming, Dreams, and Drugs with the Grateful Dead.* New York: St. Martin's Press, 2015.

Lesh, Phil. *Searching for the Sound: My Life with the Grateful Dead.* New York: Little, Brown and Co, 2005.

Scully, Rock, and David Dalton. *Living with the Dead: Twenty Years on the Bus with Garcia and the Grateful Dead.* New York: Little, Brown and Company, 1995.

Gateway Drug Hypothesis

The hypothesis that marijuana usage often becomes a "gateway" to "harder" drugs has been a reoccurring theory in the United States since the 1930s. The theory is that people progress through a sequence of drug usage beginning with legal and socially acceptable drugs (e.g., nicotine, alcohol), then to "soft" drugs (e.g., cannabis), and later to "harder" drugs (e.g., cocaine, heroin). This hypothesis has been repeatedly studied and is often used to support the criminalization of marijuana. However, despite the theory's wide popularity, the research on the relationship between marijuana usage and later use of illicit "hard" paints a mixed picture.

The theory of marijuana as a gateway drug dates back to the early 1930s, when Harry Anslinger (1892–1975) served as the first Commissioner of the U.S. Treasury's Federal Bureau of Narcotics between 1930 and 1962. Anslinger rose to particular prominence during the Boggs Act hearings (1951), when he claimed in testimony before Congress that over half of America's drug addicts "started on marijuana smoking. They started there and graduated to heroin; they took the needle when the thrill of marijuana was gone" (United States Congress 1975).

During the 1970s, the theory was often referred to as "progression theory" or "stepping-stone thesis." The hypothesis gained additional national prominence in 1970, when *Time* magazine published an article titled "Kids and Heroin: The Adolescent Epidemic." The article cited unnamed "experts," who claimed, "If a young person smokes marijuana on more than ten occasions, that chances are one in five that he will go on to more dangerous drugs" ("Nation: Kids and Heroin: The Adolescent Epidemic" 1970). Other news media sources began to cover the hypothesis, and public familiarity with the idea bloomed.

The concept gained further prominence in 1984 when Robert L. Dupont, director of the National Institute on Drug Abuse, first coined the term "gateway drug" in his book *Getting Tough on Gateway Drugs.* The gateway drug hypothesis became the focus of anti-marijuana rhetoric surrounding the "War on Drugs" campaign launched by President Ronald Reagan and his so-called "drug czar," Carlton Turner, during the 1980s. National antidrug programs such as Drug Abuse Resistance Education (DARE) emphasized the dangers of gateway drugs.

Supporters of the hypothesis point to several studies that lend support to the theory including Denise Kandel's pivotal *Stages in Adolescent Involvement in Drug Use*, which was published in 1975. Since then, numerous studies have purported to demonstrate a link between marijuana use and experimentation with and addiction to "harder" drugs. However, the theory came under heavy fire in the early 2000s in the wake of several studies that called into question the tenets of the theory and criticized the methods used by researchers who found grounds to support it.

Many researchers today do not put much stock in the "gateway theory," arguing that there is no scientific support for the hypothesis. One common objection to the theory is that correlation (i.e., marijuana usage and heroin usage) is not causation. In other words, while research may demonstrate a connection between marijuana usage and other drug usage, the studies cannot prove marijuana is what caused a person to use "harder" drugs. Others believe the theory fails to consider social status, education levels, psychological, racial, gender, and other essential differences among individuals or that the theory does not include substance use that is generally accepted by society, such as alcohol and caffeine. Still other critiques point out that the percentage of the American population that uses marijuana has changed over time, but that there has been no corresponding change in the number of "hard" drug users. Some researchers have even begun speculating that marijuana usage may provide a means for some people addicted to opioids and other drugs to wean themselves off those substances.

While the research to support the gateway drug hypothesis is declining, the failure to adequately "prove" the hypothesis has not stopped it from remaining a primary shaper of American drug policy, laws, and sentiments for nearly a century. Moreover, both proponents and critics of marijuana legalization agree that the hypothesis remains one of the most hotly debated elements of proposed legalization efforts.

Ben Stickle

See also: Anslinger, Harry (1892–1975); Drug Abuse Resistance Education (DARE); Reagan Administration "War on Drugs."

Further Reading

Calton, Chris. "The Gateway Drug Myth." Mises Institute, May 16, 2019. https://mises.org/wire/gateway-drug-myth

Drug Policy Alliance. "Debunking the 'Gateway' Myth." Drug Policy Alliance, February 12, 2017. http://www.drugpolicy.org/resource/debunking-gateway-myth

DuPont, Robert L. *Getting Tough on Gateway Drugs*. Washington, DC: American Psychiatric Press, 1984.

Kandel, Denise. "Stages in Adolescent Involvement in Drug Use." *Science* 190, no. 4217 (1975): 912–914.

"Nation: Kids and Heroin: The Adolescent Epidemic." *Time*, March 16, 1970. http://content.time.com/time/magazine/article/0,9171,909060,00.html

United States Congress. "Marijuana Decriminalization- Hearing before the Senate Subcommittee to Investigate Juvenile Delinquency." 94th Congress, 1st Session-Investigation of Juvenile Delinquency in the United States Senate, May 14, 1975. https://www.ojp.gov/pdffiles1/Digitization/45858NCJRS.pdf

Gender

Men are more likely than women to use marijuana in America. According to a 2017 survey, 13 percent of males identified as current marijuana users, while only 7 percent of women responded similarly (Statista Research Department 2019). Various studies likewise show higher rates of usage among males than females (Johnston et al. 2008; Substance Abuse and Mental Health Services Administration 2006). Additionally, the gap in usage rates between men and women appears to be increasing. While both men and women reported increased rates of marijuana usage between 2002 and 2014, men reported greater past-year usage rates than women, and since 2007, the rate of increase of marijuana usage is greater for men than women. During this time period, it is estimated that an additional six million men used marijuana in the past year, compared to four million additional women who reported using marijuana in the past year (Carliner et al. 2017). A recent study (Carliner et al. 2017) purports the widening gender gap in marijuana usage is largely driven by increases in usage by low-income men, especially during economic downturns as economic insecurity deepens.

The recent trends in marijuana usage by gender fit with a much longer pattern. Gender disparities in drug usage were the norm in premodern societies, in which drug use by women was generally discouraged, if not entirely disallowed. Modernization, however, has increased equitability in drug use between men and women. Drug use patterns are becoming more dependent on achieved statuses, or positions in society based on merit, rather than gender in modern societies.

Nevertheless, gender differences in marijuana usage still persist throughout much of the world. For instance, at least until the early 1980s, marijuana use was almost exclusively a male endeavor in Cambodia, West Africa, North Africa, Pakistan, and Brazil. Moreover, marijuana usage rates by men outpace female rates in places such as Rwanda, Jamaica, and China, while in much of the Middle East, women are forbidden by custom to partake in drug use (Hawdon 2005).

Interestingly, not only are men more likely than women to use marijuana in the United States, but a 2013 survey conducted by the Pew Research Center indicated they are similarly more likely to favor its legalization. This runs counter to the general trend of women staking more liberal positions than men on most social and criminal justice issues. Researchers believe that numerous factors contribute to the disparity in permissiveness. In part, they find that women report higher levels of religiosity than men, helping to explain the gap. However, more important is the simple fact that men partake in marijuana use more than women and are therefore more likely to support its legalization (Elder and Greene 2019).

There is also research suggesting that not only do men and women use marijuana at different rates but they often do so for different reasons. Notably, men are found to be more likely to try marijuana to satiate an urge for risk-taking, which has been linked to testosterone levels. On the other hand, women are more likely than men to use marijuana for functional reasons, such as coping with anxiety or physical ailments. Men and women even differ in how they often consume cannabis; women, for instance, are more likely than men to use topical cannabis products or cannabis products that appear unappealing to young children (Struik, Sanna, and Fattore 2018).

Matthew Costello

See also: Age; Race; Religion; Sexual Functioning; Sexual Orientation.

Further Reading

Carliner, Hannah, et al. "The Widening Gender Gap in Marijuana Use Prevalence in the US during a Period of Economic Change, 2002–2014." *Drug and Alcohol Dependence* 170 (2017): 51–58.

Elder, Laurel, and Steven Greene. "Gender and the Politics of Marijuana." *Social Science Quarterly* 100, no. 1 (2019): 109–122.

Hawdon, James. *Drug and Alcohol Consumption as Functions of Social Structures: A Cross-Cultural Sociology*. No. 47. Lewiston, NY: Edwin Mellen Press, 2005.

Johnston, Lloyd, Patrick M. O'Malley, and Jerald G. Bachman. *Monitoring the Future: National Survey Results on Drug Use, 1975–2003*. Vol. 1. Bethesda, MD: National Institute on Drug Abuse, US Department of Health and Human Services, National Institutes of Health, 2004.

Johnston, Lloyd, Patrick M. O'Malley, Jerald G. Bachman, J. G., and John E. Schulenberg. Monitoring the Future National Survey Results on Drug Use 1975–2007. Vol. I: Secondary School Students NIH Publication No. 08-6418A. Bethesda, MD: National Institute on Drug Abuse, U.S. Department of Health and Human Services, National Institutes of Health, 2008.

Statista Research Department. "Share of Consumers in the United States who Currently Smoke Marijuana as of July 2017, by Gender." S*tatista Research Department*, August 9, 2019. https://www.statista.com/statistics/737820/share-americans-gender-use-marijuana/

Struik, Dicky, Fabrizio Sanna, and Liana Fattore. "The Modulating Role of Sex and Anabolic-Androgenic Steroid Hormones in Cannabinoid Sensitivity." *Frontiers in Behavioral Neuroscience* 12 (2018): 249.

Substance Abuse and Mental Health Services Administration. "Results from the 2005 National Survey on Drug Use and Health: National Findings." SAMHSA, 2006. http://www. oas. samhsa. gov/nsduh/2k5nsduh/2k5Results. pdf

Gonzales v. Raich (2005)

Gonzales v. Raich (2005) is a landmark U.S. Supreme Court case that established federal preemption over state laws related to marijuana cultivation and use. Although some states have increasingly expanded medical marijuana laws and decriminalized and even legalized the recreational use of the drug, *Raich* established that pursuant to Congress's power under the Commerce Clause of the U.S. Constitution, the federal government can make illegal even the small-scale cultivation of marijuana for single use, which is otherwise legal under a state medical marijuana law. Since *Raich*, U.S. presidents have differed on their approaches to enforcing federal marijuana laws in the face of conflicting state laws, but the *Raich* case clearly establishes the power to enforce such federal laws at the executive's discretion.

Angel Raich and Diane Monson were Californians who used marijuana for medical purposes as permitted by California's Compassionate Use Act of 1996. Monson cultivated her own cannabis solely for medical use while Raich procured hers through caregivers who provided it to Raich without charge. Although her medical drug use was compliant with California law, Federal Drug Enforcement Administration agents raided Monson's home in 2002 and seized and destroyed six marijuana plants. The federal agents were enforcing the Controlled Substances Act (CSA) of 1970, which prohibits the manufacture, distribution, dispensing, or possession of any controlled substance, including marijuana, except in ways outlined in the CSA. The act classifies controlled substances into five schedules purportedly based on their accepted medical use, potential for abuse, and psychological and physical effects on the body. From inception, marijuana has been classified as a Schedule I drug, making manufacturing, distribution, dispensing, or possession of marijuana a federal criminal offense.

Raich and Monson brought a civil action against the federal government to resolve this conflict between state and federal law. Pursuant to the U.S. Constitution and the principles of American federalism, the power of the federal government is ostensibly limited: powers not delegated to the federal government are reserved for the states. Where power has been delegated to the federal government, the Constitution's Supremacy Clause and the related doctrine of preemption mean that any conflicting state laws must give way to the federal law.

As American history has progressed, much of the federal government's expanding reach has come, somewhat surprisingly, from the seemingly pedestrian Commerce Clause, which, in terse language, grants Congress the power to "regulate Commerce with foreign Nations, and among the several States, and with the Indian Tribes." Beginning with the New Deal, President Franklin D. Roosevelt's famous slate of laws and policies designed to lift the United States out of the Great Depression during the 1930s, the Commerce Clause became a potent source of expanding federal power as the Supreme Court adopted generous interpretations of what fell within the penumbra of "commerce."

Yet, the Court's ideological pendulum began to swing toward more conservative by the late 1990s. The case of *U.S. v. Lopez* (1995) marked a rare limitation on the federal commerce power and a potential signal of a resurgence of states' rights. The *Lopez* Court found Congress lacked the power under the Commerce Clause to create a federal criminal offense of possessing a firearm in a school zone. The Court reasoned that education was a quintessentially local activity and that irrespective of the merits or drawbacks of school gun zone laws any connection between gun violence, education, and commerce was too tenuous to support Congress's interloping in traditional state and local lawmaking territory. In the 2000 opinion of *U.S. v. Morrison*, the Court again found that Congress had surpassed its authority under the Commerce Clause in a provision in the Violence Against Women Act. Consequently, when the Court took up the *Raich* case it was unclear whether the justices would follow in the trend of *Lopez* and *Morrison* with the more conservative Court ruling against expansive federal power (and thus restoring some power to the states) or whether the Court would find the CSA a valid use of the power to regulate commerce.

AN HISTORIC—AND NARROW—DECISION

Justice John Paul Stevens authored the majority opinion in *Raich*, joined by Justices Anthony Kennedy, Ruth Bader Ginsburg, David Souter, and Stephen Breyer. The 5-4 majority held that the enforcement of the CSA in this instance did not violate the Commerce Clause; although the private cultivation and possession of marijuana were not themselves direct acts of interstate commerce, there was an "undisputed magnitude of the commercial market for marijuana," meaning because the available market for marijuana was so prevalent, it would be possible for individuals who claimed to privately cultivate and possess marijuana to enter that product into the commercial market. Therefore, the Court reasoned it was permissible for the federal government to regulate the private cultivation of marijuana for medical use under the Commerce Clause because it was necessary to prevent others from having access to the drug through the market.

The opinion relied on *Wickard v. Filburn* (1942) in which the Court had ruled the federal government could regulate wheat grown solely for private consumption if it proved that failure to do so would undercut the regulation of the interstate market for wheat. Applied to *Raich*, the Court reasoned a failure to regulate marijuana grown for private consumption could indeed undercut the government's ability to prevent marijuana from being traded via interstate commerce. The majority thus rejected the arguments based on *Lopez* and *Morrison*.

Justice Sandra Day O'Connor dissented in an opinion joined by Chief Justice William Rehnquist. She rejected the majority's view that the Commerce Clause should be applied in cases where marijuana is cultivated and possessed for personal medical use. Although she agreed that Congress could regulate in areas that substantially affected interstate commerce as outlined in *Wickard*, Justice O'Connor argued there was insufficient proof in *Raich* of the specific ramifications of homegrown medical marijuana on interstate commerce. In *Wickard*, the government provided real numbers demonstrating the impact of homegrown wheat on interstate commerce. In *Raich*, the government provided no real numbers regarding the exact impact. The dissent claimed that without clear evidence, a power could not arbitrarily be taken away from the states and given to the federal government. Therefore, O'Connor followed the lead of *Lopez* and *Morrison* and found the CSA to be beyond the "outer limits" of Commerce Clause authority. By ruling in favor of broader federal government power, the dissent claimed the Court was undercutting the chief virtues of federalism, which should allow the states to act as "laboratories of democracy," empowered to try new policies and foster innovation without risk to the rest of the country.

Justice Clarence Thomas also dissented from the majority opinion in a separate opinion. He argued that if Congress could regulate "a half-dozen cannabis plants for personal consumption," then Congressional power had "no meaningful limits." Based on the majority's reasoning, he argued that Congress could now regulate "quilting bees, clothes drives, and potluck suppers."

Since the *Raich* opinion in 2005—and despite its holding—the number of states passing medical marijuana laws has increased. Moreover, beginning with Colorado and Washington in 2012, an increasing number of states have legalized or decriminalized the use of marijuana for recreational purposes. These developments mean that increasingly in those states, individuals may use marijuana without the threat of state-level criminal liability. However, the federal government is an independent jurisdiction that continues to list marijuana as a Schedule 1 illicit drug under the CSA of 1970. Accordingly, an individual in a recreational marijuana state may be lawfully (under state law) celebrating April 20 by consuming marijuana, or may be using cannabis for medical purposes pursuant to a doctor's prescription, and yet still be in violation of federal law, just as the Court found Angel Raich and Diane Monson to be. The reference to celebrating April 20 refers to the rise of "420" as drug use argot for consuming marijuana, sometimes translated to a time of day, 4:20, or the twentieth date of the year's fourth month. For example, the phrase "It's 420!" would signal an indication that "It's time to smoke marijuana!" and given the prevalence of the euphemism (the origins of which are unclear), April 20 has become a celebrated day among marijuana enthusiasts.

The extent to which the federal government enforces its marijuana prohibition, however, is a separate issue and depends upon the particular executive administration in power. (The uncertainty of federal enforcement has caused various issues in the emerging legal state marijuana markets, for example, those related to concerns over whether federally backed banking institutions should be used for business that is legal under state law but illicit under federal law.) Under President Barack Obama's administration, for example, the Department of Justice adopted a hands-off approach, effectively deferring to state marijuana laws. The Trump administration reversed course, however, with Attorney General Jeff Sessions issuing a memorandum to U.S. attorneys citing marijuana as a "dangerous drug" and its production, sale, or use "a serious crime" and rescinding the Obama-era hands-off policies (Marijuana Enforcement Memorandum, Office of the Attorney General Jeff Sessions, 2018). Since then, an expanding number of states have continued to adopt more liberal policies toward marijuana use, even as the Trump administration has sought to enforce federal criminal laws related to marijuana, as permitted by *Gonzales v. Raich*. Under such a policy, enforcement depends on the discretion of prosecutors and law enforcement in the given jurisdiction and is subject to traditional discretionary considerations over how finite criminal justice resources should be allocated. Ultimately, federal enforcement of marijuana laws is far from certain, but per *Raich*, it's certainly permissible.

Rhys Hester and Paige Kennett

See also: Drug Enforcement Administration (DEA); Law Enforcement Efforts, Marijuana Control.

Further Reading

Gonzales v. Raich (2005), 545 U.S. 1.

Marijuana Enforcement Memorandum, Office of the Attorney General Jeff Sessions, January 4, 2018. https://www.justice.gov/opa/pr/justice-department-issues-memo-marijuana-enforcement

Ramsey, Michael D. "American Federalism and the Tragedy of Gonzales v. Raich." *University of Queensland Law Journal* 31, no. 2 (2012): 203–232.

Rivikin, David B., and Elizabeth Price Foley. "Federal Antidrug Law Goes Up in Smoke." *Wall Street Journal*, December 28, 2014.

Young, Earnest A. "Just Blowing Smoke? Politics, Doctrine, and the Federalist Revival after Gonzales v. Raich." *The Supreme Court Review* 1 (2005): 1–50.

Gravity Bongs

A gravity bong is an apparatus used to consume cannabis using a system of air pressure and water to extract smoke from a small bowl of lit cannabis. It can be created using a variety of materials such as buckets, plastic bottles, or even glass. While some methods of cannabis consumption are labeled based on the apparatus itself, a gravity bong is named as a result of the physics utilized by the bong, or what is colloquially known as a rig. Gravity bongs use the negative pressure created by water leaving the bong's chamber through a small hole (or holes) in the bottom of the chamber. This pulls air through the burning cannabis at the top of the bong and fills the chamber with smoke. The lit cannabis exists within a small lid or "bowl" on top of the bong and is removed in order to consume the smoke. The amount of smoke created is dependent on the size of the chamber, the amount of marijuana used, and the materials used to create the bong.

There are two commonly known types of gravity bongs, distinguished by their use of water within the rig. The water either leaves one smaller chamber to enter another larger one below (i.e., a traditional gravity bong) or leaves the rig entirely (i.e., a "waterfall" gravity bong). The traditional system encourages the user to push the smoke-filled chamber back into the water, which then forcefully pushes the smoke through the hole as water fills the chamber through the holes in the bottom. "Waterfall" gravity bongs do not have this option because the water is not collected after leaving the first chamber, so the user just inhales the smoke from the top of the bong using their own lung power.

It is believed that these methods of cannabis consumption are more effective at achieving a "high" than other smoking techniques due to the forceful method in which the smoke is inhaled and the sheer amount of smoke taken in each hit. In fact, several veteran cannabis users have stated warnings about the intensity of gravity bongs and encourage new smokers to avoid them. However, there is no scientific evidence thus far supporting or contradicting this assumption.

Gravity bongs have no official origin date but seemed to have gained popularity in the late 1990s across the United States. The materials required to create these bongs are commonly found in most households, thus making them one of the most accessible and affordable pieces of paraphernalia available. It wasn't until the early 2000s that gravity bongs were commercialized and sold. In 2004, David Daily began to sell a glass gravity bong known as the "Gravitron." This was the first gravity bong made entirely of glass, which was chosen to reduce potential hazards of using plastic and aluminum pieces. In 2017, "The Stundenglass," made with aircraft-grade aluminum and surgical grade steel, joined the market. The continuing development of these types of bongs exhibits their growing popularity and alludes to an increase in economic demand.

Gabrielle L. Lory

See also: Blunts; Bongs and Water Pipes; Dabbing.

Further Reading

Khey, David N., John Stogner, and Bryan Lee Miller. *Emerging Trends in Drug Use and Distribution.* Vol. 12. New York: Springer Science & Business Media, 2013.

Miller, Bryan Lee, John M. Stogner, and J. Mitchell Miller. "Exploring Butane Hash Oil Use: A Research Note." *Journal of Psychoactive Drugs* 48, no. 1 (2016): 44–49.

H

Hashish

Hashish, hash, or hash oil refers to a psychoactive substance made from the resin of the cannabis plant. Both ancient and more modern processes for the growth, collection, and purification of cannabis resin glands are used to form this cannabis concentrate. Depending on the process used and temperature, the product can either be a solid form (pressed) or paste-like substance (bubble hash). Hashish typically has a higher level of tetrahydrocannabinol (THC) than herbal forms of cannabis and can be consumed as an edible product, vaporized, or mixed with herbal products and smoked.

Hashish is one of the oldest forms of marijuana consumption, with the first written references to hashish dating back to northern India in the twelfth century. The Hindu term "charas" references hashish, and the drug plays an important role in the culture and rituals of the Hindu religion, especially among the Shaiva sect. Prior to the sixteenth century, hashish was exclusively used as an edible, as early written references frequently mention the "hashish-eaters" (Booth 2015). Smoking hashish was not common until the introduction of tobacco. Since hashish itself is not combustible, it was mixed with tobacco in order to be smoked.

Modern hashish users still consume it as an edible, but the product is also used in a variety of devices similar to those used for other marijuana concentrates such as vaporizers and bongs. It can also be mixed with herbal (plant) parts of marijuana and consumed in joints, pipes, and other smoking devices. In the United States, hashish has a history of being less popular than herbal marijuana, whereas European consumption of hashish has historically remained higher (Sznitman, Olsson, and Room 2008). Currently, hashish is more common than herbal marijuana in Europe, although since the early 2010s other forms of cannabis concentrates have been growing in popularity in the United States, especially butane hash oil (BHO).

Although there is some debate over the exact terminology, hashish generally refers to the natural extraction of resin from cannabis (without the use of chemicals). Other cannabis concentrates, such as those that utilize a chemical separation agent such as ethanol or butane, are considered different from traditional hashish. Hashish is manufactured by a process that collects resin from fresh female cannabis plants. In traditional methods, the flowering plants are pressed or rubbed with two hands in order to create a small ball of sticky resin. In mechanical separation methods, dried plant material is sifted through screens that produce a powder known as "kief," which can be pressed into blocks of hashish through the application of heat. Another mechanical method of separation involves using ice water and processes of agitation and separation to extract a purified form of hashish sometimes referred to as bubble hash (Rosenthal 2014).

Bryan Lee Miller

See also: Ancient Religions; Butane Hash Oil; Central Asia; Edibles; Europe; India and South Asia; Religion; Tetrahydrocannabinol (THC).

Further Reading

Booth, Martin. *Cannabis: A History*. New York: Macmillan, 2015.

Rosenthal, Ed. *Beyond Buds: Marijuana Extracts—Hash, Vaping, Dabbing, Edibles and Medicines*. Piedmont, CA: Quick Trading Company, 2014.

Schaffer Library of Drug Policy. "Guide to the Different Types of Hashish." n.d. Accessed August 20, 2021. http://druglibrary.org/MedicalMj/hash/guide_to_the_different_types_of_.htm

Sznitman, Sharon Rödner, Börje Olsson, and Robin Room. "EMCDDA Monographs." *EMCDDA Monographs* (2008). http://www.chanvre-info.ch/info/ru/IMG/pdf/att_53355_EN_emcdda-cannabis-mon-full-2vols-web-3.pdf

Head Shops

During the 1960s, numerous storefronts opened in American cities championing counterculture ideals, selling marijuana paraphernalia, and creating a safe space for those looking to surround themselves with like-minded individuals. Though the framework and look of a modern head shop is not that different from those of decades ago, their role within society has somewhat changed from a bastion that was disenfranchised politically and socially to a more traditional capitalist enterprise. Regardless, for half a century head shops have served individuals interested in exploring psychoactive substances using the guise that their products are intended to be used with tobacco rather than any illicit substance.

The term "head shop" has become less common in today's world. Perhaps, owners and patrons wanted to distance themselves from drug user labels and terms associated with illicit substances. Regardless, shops of this variety operate today in the United States under labels such as "smoke shop," "vape shop," or something of that ilk. There are approximately 10,591 vape stores in the United States identified by the "Yelp" website's database (Galstyan, Galimov, and Sussman 2019, 119). The origins of the head shop label are intriguing; at the time, "head" was used as a derogatory term for substance users by those opposing psychoactive drug use (likely as an abbreviated version of "pothead"), yet counterculturalists accepted the "head" label as a badge of honor. They had long referred to one another as "heads" and saw it as a label that reflected their choice to get "turned on and tuned in"—altered their state of consciousness with drugs to achieve a higher level of harmony with the wider world. "Feed your head" was even a line repeated at the end of a 1967 Jefferson Airplane song, "White Rabbit," which served as an anthem of the late 1960s' counterculture. Some have described "head" as originating as an acronym for "he eats acid daily" since "acid head" also became a common colloquial term, but as "head" was used prior to LSD's introduction, this explanation for the term, and ultimately the "head shop" label, seems unlikely.

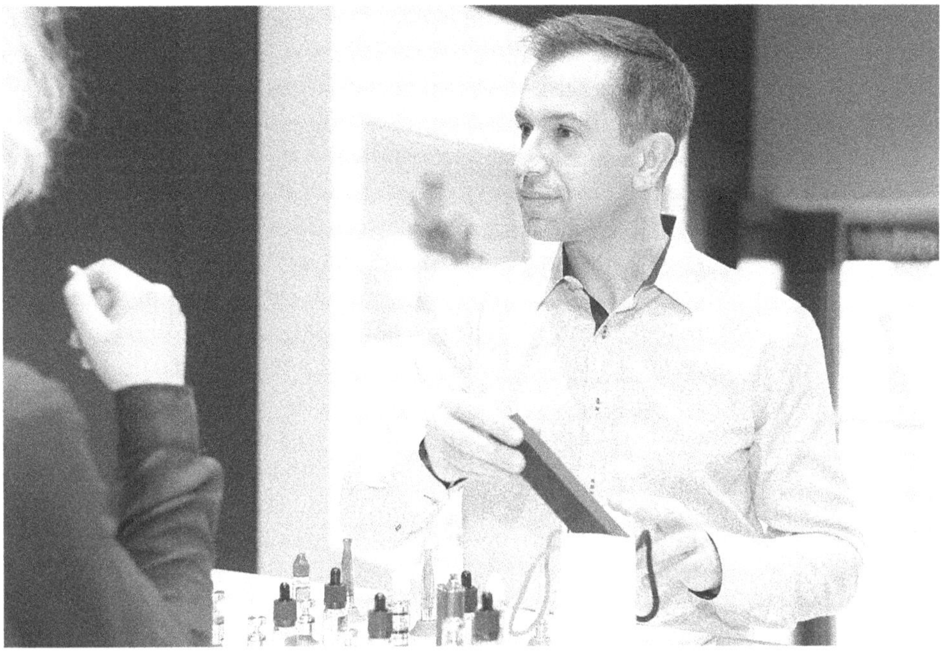

A man makes a purchases in a head shop. Head shops are stores that sell drug-related paraphernalia such as rolling papers, vaporizers, pipes, waterpipes, and bongs. (Auremar/Dreamstime.com)

Initially, head shops served as what we would now label a "safe space" for hippies and activists who were harassed and degraded by other members of society. They provided a meeting place for those looking to explore policy and societal reform. The open forum and accepting culture were primary concerns; profitability was secondary (Glickman 1970, 34). These stores, however, were profitable. A significant demand existed for rolling papers, marijuana paraphernalia, and items for enhancing interactions with a variety of illicit drugs (Davis 2015, 39); "hip capitalists" were rewarded for creating this niche industry (Davis 2015, 27). Yet, some of the profits generated were returned to the counterculture that sustained them in the form of flyers promoting drug policy reform, support for decriminalization campaigns, and the like.

The thinly veiled guise of selling products for tobacco use has been effective in sidestepping legal restrictions. Clerks are trained to discuss how the products might be used with tobacco and avoid using language that violates the law. Customers asking about illicit products or using paraphernalia with illicit substances are turned away to avoid risks to the business. Some head shops have violated laws and endured law enforcement raids, but the industry's long-standing awareness of policy has enabled cautious storefronts to remain in operation. Concerned parents' groups and the "War on Drugs," more generally, forced some stores to rebrand themselves and/or retreat politically to continue to serve their clientele.

In addition to paraphernalia, items associated with the substance use experience are traditionally sold at head shops. Originally, this inventory would have included posters, incense, Eastern religious texts, and music that was thought to improve a high or trip. Today's head shops continue to sell these items but have expanded to include clothing, newer smoking devices, and items related to hobbies associated with marijuana use. For example, frisbees and disc golf supplies are prevalent at head shops in the Southeastern United States. Some shops are now profiting on the sale and use of e-cigarettes; at these shops, customers may be given the chance to try flavors and learn about different hardware (Allem et al. 2015, 794). Head shops also have profited extensively from the novel psychoactive drug (NPD) or "legal high" industry in the last 15 years.

Novel psychoactive drugs (NPDs) generally mimic the actions of commonly abused drugs such as marijuana, stimulants, hallucinogens, and opiates. These drugs are formulated, marketed, and used to sidestep legal restrictions (Khey, Stogner, and Miller 2014). In addition to synthetics developed to mimic existing psychoactives (e.g., synthetic cannabinoids such as "spice" and synthetic cathinones such as "bath salts"), the NPD term also encompasses ethnobotanicals in recently fortified or strengthened forms (e.g., kratom, *Salvia divinorum*; Khey et al. 2014). These products often exist in a legal gray area for a limited window of time. Due to issues with the language of the Federal Analogue Act of 1986, they may be sold and marketed as "not for human consumption" prior to scheduling even though many chemically qualify as an analogue of a scheduled substance. Head shops sales facilitated the popularity of synthetic cannabinoids referred to as "spice," but their use has significantly dropped since federal regulation clarified their status and led to their removal from shelves in 2012. Head shops still sell a number of novel psychoactives that are not regulated in their jurisdiction. Locally, ethnobotanicals are more common on store shelves than synthetics; head shops toured by the author currently sell an array of kratom products (teas, resins, or capsules made from leaves of the *Mitragyna speciosa* tree) as well as for those looking to manage pain or deal with opioid withdrawal. Products made from *Salvia divinorum*, a plant native to the Oaxaca region of Mexico, sit on the shelves of head shops in neighboring states. The sales of NPDs is perhaps the biggest issue with modern head shops.

Despite attacks on the head shop industry as enterprises that depend on the illicit behavior of others for their existence, defenders contend that these outlets serve a vital, positive role in society. They still offer a respite to the disenfranchised substance users. They offer products and paraphernalia in a regulated environment that may increase safety. In recreational and marijuana states, they offer equipment that facilitates use of marijuana in an established manner. They even provide a safe space for communication between substance users in marijuana prohibition states (so long as the customer refers to tobacco use as opposed to marijuana).

John Stogner and Lucas Maness

See also: Coffeeshops; Recreational Marijuana Laws.

Further Reading

Allem, J. P., et al. "Tobacco Attitudes and Behaviors of Vape Shop Retailers in Los Angeles." *American Journal of Health Behavior* 39, no. 6 (October 2015): 794–798. https://doi.org/10.5993/AJHB.39.6.7

Davis, Joshua Clark. "The Business of Getting High: Head Shops, Countercultural Capitalism, and the Marijuana Legalization Movement." *The Sixties: A Journal of History, Politics, and Culture* 8, no. 1 (June 2015): 27–49. https://doi.org/10.1080/17541328.2015.1058480

Farber, David. "Building the Counterculture, Creating Right Livelihoods: The Counterculture at Work." *The Sixties: A Journal of History, Politics, and Culture* 6, no. 1 (May 2013): 1–24. https://doi.org/10.1080/17541328.2013.778706

Galstyan, Ellen, Arthur Galimov, and Steve Sussman. "Commentary: The Emergence of Pod Mods." *Evaluation & the Health Professions* 42, no. 1 (March 2019): 118–124. https://doi.org/10.1177/0163278718812976

Glickman, Art. "The Corner Store: Mod Boutiques in Lansing Turns Tidy Profit by Offering Clients a Feeling of Freedom." *Wall Street Journal*, September 17, 1970: 34.

Khey, D. N., J. Stogner, and B. L. Miller. *Emerging Trends in Drug Use and Distribution.* Cham, Switzerland: Springer International Publishing. 2014.

Hemp

Hemp is a variety of the *Cannabis sativa* plant. It is often referred to as industrial hemp, and it has been cultivated by humans for centuries. Hemp has been used in religious rituals and as a source of food, medicine, paper, and fiber, and it may be one of the earliest plants ever to be cultivated by humans. The production of hemp has evolved into the manufacturing of a variety of products, including health foods, organic products, clothing, construction materials, biofuels, and plastics (Yonavjak 2013).

Although derived from the same species, hemp and marijuana are distinct strains of the *C. sativa* plant. Hemp contains very low concentrations of tetrahydrocannabinol (THC) and grows taller and denser than marijuana, which is grown for its budding flowers and intoxicating effects. In the United States, hemp products have enjoyed market growth in recent years, with retail sales exceeding $500 million annually in the early 2010s, yet major companies must import hemp seeds, oil, and fibers for their products (Yonavjak 2013). Decriminalization of cannabis, which reflects a shift in public perception of marijuana, has also been seen by hemp enthusiasts as boosting the prospects for their industry.

Hemp production and use in the United States predates the nation, as the earliest European colonists planted and cultivated it. Hemp was even legal tender in a number of colonies, including Virginia, Maryland, and Pennsylvania (PBS 2016). In the early days of the United States, hemp farming was mandatory in several states, and it was a staple of the early nation's agricultural economy. Indeed, even the Declaration of Independence was written on hemp paper (Yonavjak 2013). In the early eighteenth century, hemp production continued to thrive, and the American government encouraged the cultivation of hemp for items such as rope, ship sails, and clothing. As time passed, however, hemp began to be supplanted by cotton, timber, and other materials, and production of the substance steadily declined. The hemp industry was already a shadow of its onetime self in 1937 when the passage of the Marijuana Tax Act delivered a crushing blow. The act levied a tax on anyone who dealt commercially in cannabis, hemp, or marijuana, and its passage virtually destroyed what remained of the

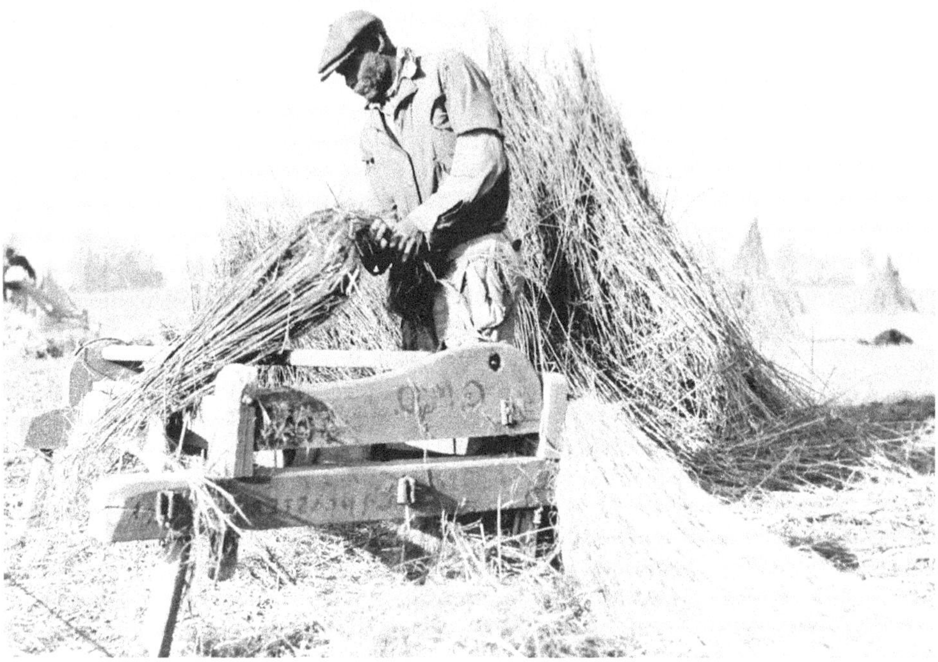

A worker processes hemp in Kentucky. Hemp was first introduced to Kentucky in 1775, and it was an important part of the state's economy during the centuries that followed. In the 1930s, the distinction between industrial hemp and the drug marijuana blurred, and hemp crops were eventually outlawed in the United States. The potential economic impact of hemp crops on Kentucky led to a widespread legalization movement in the 1980s and 1990s. (Public Records Division, Kentucky Department for Libraries and Archives)

U.S. hemp industry. However, during World War II after the Philippines fell to the Japanese in 1942, the Department of Agriculture introduced the "Hemp for Victory" campaign, a video that encouraged U.S. farmers to plant hemp in response to reduced imports of Filipino hemp and Indian jute (Anderson 2011). In response, U.S. production of hemp jumped 20 times higher in 1942 than in 1941 (Anderson 2011). During the war years, hemp was used to make uniforms, canvas, and rope.

While hemp production decreased substantially in the postwar years, by the turn of the twenty-first century, strong support for local industries and sustainable ecology prompted legislation to encourage hemp cultivation and new industry research. Widely used in the production of raw materials, major U.S. companies were forced to import hemp to make a variety of products, estimating the U.S. hemp industry to be valued at $500 million (USD) in 2012 (Yonavjak 2013). Congress acknowledged the importance of the commodity with the passing of a 2014 farm bill that allowed universities and state departments of agriculture to cultivate industrial hemp for limited purposes. By the mid-2010s, 30 states had adopted similar policies (National Conference of State Legislatures 2016), and the hemp industry gathered fresh momentum. The U.S. industrial hemp market, in fact, was valued at approximately $1 billion in 2019, while the total value of the global industrial market was an estimated $4.71 billion. This surging market is being driven by an increased demand for hemp oil and fibers for personal care, as well as demand for hemp in the automotive, food, construction, and textile industries (Grand View Research 2020).

Craig A. Depken, II and Shanyn Viars

See also: *Cannabis indica*; *Cannabis sativa*.

Further Reading

Anderson, Brian. 2011. "Hemp against Hitler: How Cannabis Helped America Win World War II." *Vice*, August 19, 2011. https://www.vice.com/en_us/article/533qed/hemp

Grand View Research. "Industrial Hemp Market Size, Share & Trends Analysis Report by Product." *Market Analysis Report*. Report ID: GVR 2-68038-389-8, 2020. https://www.pbs.org/wgbh/pages/frontline/shows/dope/etc/cron.html

National Conference of State Legislatures. *State Industrial Hemp Statutes*. Chicago: National Conference of State Legislatures, 2016.

PBS. "Marijuana Timeline." PBS.org, 2016. https://www.pbs.org/wgbh/pages/frontline/shows/dope/etc/cron.html

Siff, Stephen. "The Illegalization of Marijuana: A Brief History." *Origins: Current Events in Historical Perspective* 7, no. 8 (2014): 1–3.

Yonavjak, Logan. "Industrial Hemp: A Win-win for the Economy and the Environment." *Forbes.Com*, March 29, 2013. https://www.forbes.com/sites/ashoka/2013/05/29/industrial-hemp-a-win-win-for-the-economy-and-the-environment/?sh=336dcd9d289b

High Times

High Times is a cannabis-oriented publication that made its debut in 1974. Founded by the late Tom Forçade (1945–1978), the magazine comprised journalists and activists who often critiqued the federal government's War on Drugs, advocated for the end of cannabis prohibition, and celebrated the pleasures of marijuana consumption (every issue's "centerfold" photo spread featured marijuana or cannabis-inspired art). The magazine was a counterculture staple, in part due to its features of pro-pot celebrities; countercultural figures; and activists such as Tommy Chong, Bob Marley, Cher, Andy Warhol, Susan Sontag, and Noam Chomsky. Today, *High Times* features reports on the cannabis legalization movement, cannabis cultivation, relevant entertainment and culture stories, and critiques of federal marijuana policies.

High Times debuted when founder Tom Forçade rented a space at the National Boutique Show, an annual trade convention. The National Boutique Show, held in New York City, attracted countercultural business owners who sold drug paraphernalia. At the convention, Forçade's team made industry connections and spread the word about *High Times* with a promotional flyer that featured article ideas. Following their success at the event, Forçade and colleagues went on to produce *High Times*' first issue in 1974. The issue, of which only 10,000 copies were printed, sold out quickly. By its fifth issue in 1975, *High Times* had increased printing more than tenfold, and by 1977, 400,000 copies of every issue were being printed. As a result, the magazine's advertising strength grew. *High Times* offered a space for head shops and paraphernalia producers to advertise their businesses at a time when marketing opportunities for such endeavors were scarce. Because of this, *High Times* has been recognized as influential in the expansion of the head shop and cannabis paraphernalia industry, increasing both consumer choice and the reach of producers (Davis 2015). Though the 1970s were a time of growth for the nascent publication, Forçade, the man at the center of *High Times*, committed suicide at the age of 33 in 1978.

Forçade's suicide did not stop *High Times*' growth, however. Indeed, the magazine continued to expand after his death. In 1988, *High Times* produced its signature event, the Cannabis Cup, a convention where cannabis cultivators and consumers come together to appreciate cannabis and recognize the best of the cannabis industry. The Cannabis Cup has expanded and become a multinational event where producers can compete in categories such as "Best Seed Company," "Best Indica Flower," and "Best Vaporizer."

High Times also has an online presence. The website HighTimes.com features reports on topics relevant to cannabis culture, and the magazine's newsletter keeps subscribers informed on these topics as well. E-commerce is another part of *High Times*' online presence. Visitors can purchase apparel, magazine subscriptions and back issues, how-to books and DVDs, and *High Times*–branded accessories. In response to the censorship of cannabis-related content, *High Times* launched High Times Television (HTTV). This streaming channel is home to interviews, documentaries, how-to videos, entertainment videos, original series, and news reporting (Gold 2018).

Aubrey D. Johnson

See also: Cheech and Chong; Marley, Bob (1945–1981); Moral Panics; Nelson, Willie (1933–); Snoop Dogg (1971–); Woodstock.

Further Reading

"About High Times." *High Times*, March 15, 2020. https://hightimes.com/about/

Davis, Joshua Clark. "The Business of Getting High: Head Shops, Countercultural Capitalism, and the Marijuana Legalization Movement." *The Sixties* 8, no. 1 (2015): 27–49.

Garner, Dwight. "4 Decades of Inhaling Deeply: A History of 'High Times'." *New York Times*, October 21, 2014. https://www.nytimes.com/2014/10/22/books/high-times-a-40-year-history-of-the-magazine.html/

Gold, Chloé Harper. "High Times Announces Launch of High Times TV." *High Times*, August 9, 2018. https://hightimes.com/news/high-times-announces-launch-high-times-tv/

"High Times Greats: The Life and High Times of Tom Forçade." *High Times*, September 11, 2019. https://hightimes.com/culture/high-times-greats-life-high-times-tom-forcade/

Hippies

Modern-day "hippies" are commonly known as a coalition of social actors who are strong advocates for environmental justice and notoriously affiliated with the recreational and medicinal use of marijuana. While they are most strongly related to marijuana advocacy, they have also been in conversation, coalition, and tension with groups interested in drug use, rural farming, and Indigenous sovereignty. While hippies are often characterized by the popular media as grungy individuals

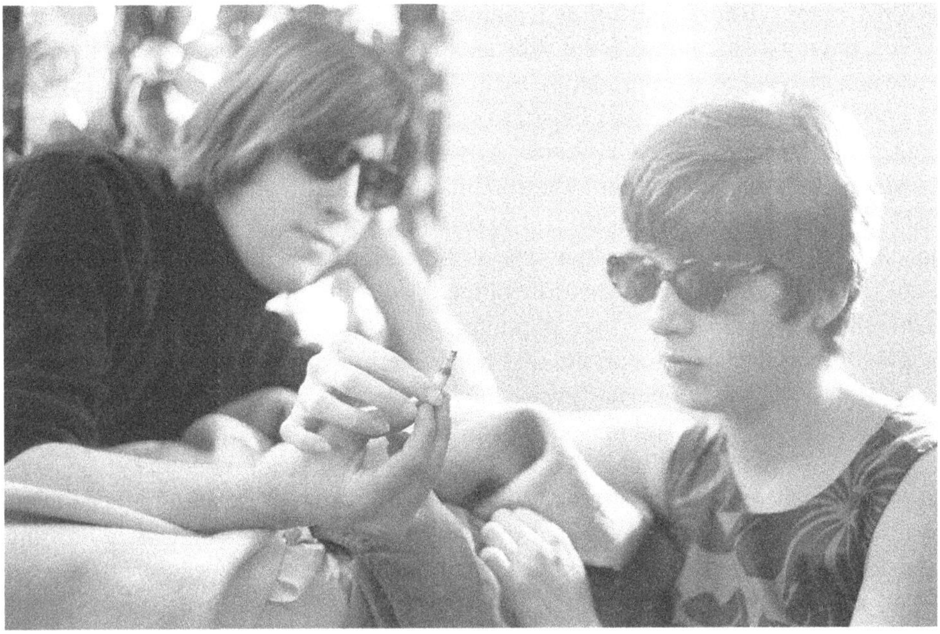

Hippies were members of the drug counterculture in the 1960s largely drawn from the middle classes. Known for their drug use and open sexuality, the Hippies were critical of dominant institutions such as capitalism and organized religion. They were also outspoken advocates for Civil Rights, ending the war in Vietnam, and legalizing marijuana and other drugs. (Library of Congress)

wearing open-toed shoes, floral or tie-dye shirts, baggy canvas pants, circular tinted-bifocals, and headbands, they play an important role in the history of marijuana and American social life broadly, especially through resistance to American imperialism and the war on drugs.

Hippies were related to the larger countercultural and subcultural movements that have come to define the 1960s, including ethnic power movements, sexual and gender liberation struggles, and anti-war campaigns. Through direct contact, cultural appropriation, and spillover between movements, revolutionary ideas and social tensions were front and center in many communities at the time. In particular, in large urban centers (e.g., New York, San Francisco, Los Angeles), a stock of affordable housing drew in diverse populations of immigrants, communities of color, and white individuals who demonstrated harmonious ethnic and cultural diversity that has inspired progressive social movements. However, hippies were unlike other constituencies because they were mostly white and largely middle class or well off. As a result, their defining connection to the struggle tended to be ideological (such as high levels of concern about civil rights, civil liberties, and environment protection). Thus, while hippies sought to distinguish themselves from their peers and parents through dress, attitude, action, and lifestyle, they usually had the education and family standing to access a comfortable, mainstream life (Issitt 2009).

Growing and smoking marijuana is a common practice among hippies, and one way of bringing individuals together in a shared identity. Because hippies stood against many cultural norms and mainstream practices during the 1960s and 1970s, having a shared preferred substance like marijuana operated as a signal of cohesion, as well as distinguishing them from the dominant systems they sought to upend and replace. Hippies began to cultivate marijuana from naturally occurring plants in places like California, as well as those brought from other established farms and distribution systems. Individuals cultivated plants for personal use, and later sale (Rendon 2012). Importantly, while drug use, including marijuana, has come to define a major aspect of the hippy subculture, there were some within the community who turned against drugs completely as a distinct way of achieving freedom. Rather than pursuing a substance-fueled high, these hippies aligned themselves with churches and religious institutions as a radically chosen, individualized path to liberty (Shires 2007).

At first, hippies smoked marijuana leaves, which have relatively lower concentrations of THC than the buds that became more popular for medicinal and recreational usage. Still, getting high provided an intellectual dividing line for hippies, whose choice of drug also reflected the value they placed on small-scale farming and locally oriented, organic culture. Many at the time were swept up in what some call the "back-to-the-land" movement among American urbanites in the 1960s and 1970s. Although many hippies romanticized agricultural life as being freer than their urban dwellings, after acting on these ideas, they were met with the harsh realities of rural life. The continuous demanding physical labor of living close to the land defied the idea of a slow-paced or simple lifestyle. Further, the actions of local governments to enforce building codes defied naive ideas about the ability to live freely off the land. In this context, broad-scale production and sale of marijuana was an appealing opportunity to increase one's economic standing while also maintaining a physical and symbolic connection to the countercultural foundations of hippy life (Rendon 2012).

The naive perspective of hippies toward rural life extended into both symbolic and direct violence against Native American communities. While many middle-class white Americans viewed the rural countryside as an open space in which to advance their own interests, tribal governments and nations had rights to these lands, including specific sacred sites. While hippies were quick to adopt what they saw as the dress and spiritual demeanor of Native Americans, this was typically in direct conflict with actual American Indians living on reservations and in cities. For instance, hippies attempted to impose their practices and ideas about drug use and nudity as the pinnacle of freedom, in defiance of the laws, ceremony, and norms of existing communities. In response to continuous disrespect and law-breaking, Pueblo, Hopi, and Navajo leadership declared hippy visitors unwelcome on tribal lands (Smith 2012).

Although the issues championed by hippy movements have shifted and developed over the years, the mark they have made on public discourse is undeniable. In addition to the mainstreaming of marijuana use, hippies have shaped the formation and endurance of environmental social movements, multicultural and racial justice efforts, public perception of land use and rights, and even religious doctrines.

Mario Alberto V. Espinoza-Kulick and Alex Espinoza-Kulick

See also: Beat Generation Writers; Garcia, Jerry (1942–1995); Nelson, Willie (1933–); Woodstock.

Further Reading

Hawdon, James. *Drug and Alcohol Consumption as Functions of Social Structures: A Cross-cultural Sociology*. No. 47. New York: Edwin Mellen Press, 2005.

Issitt, Micah. *Hippies: A Guide to an American Subculture*. Santa Barbara, CA: ABC-CLIO, 2009.

Rendon, Jim. *Super-charged: How Outlaws, Hippies, and Scientists Reinvented Marijuana*. Portland, OR: Timber Press, 2012.

Shires, Preston. *Hippies of the Religious Right*. Waco, TX: Baylor University Press, 2007.

Smith, Sherry L. *Hippies, Indians, and the Fight for Red Power*. New York: Oxford University Press, 2012.

"Howl"

"Howl (for Carl Solomon)" is a 1955 poem written by the American Beat poet Allen Ginsburg. The poem, considered by some as one of the greatest works of American literature, critiques American society and openly discusses drug use and sex. "Howl" was first read at Six Gallery in San Francisco in front of, among others, fellow Beat writer Jack Kerouac and City Lights bookstore owner Lawrence Ferlinghetti. After seeing Ginsberg read, Ferlinghetti offered to publish the work. To avoid the censorship he knew would come from the U.S. government, Ferlinghetti had the poem published in England in October 1956 as *Howl and Other Poems*. As expected, the book of poems faced immediate calls for censorship from U.S. officials due to the open and graphic discussion of drug use and both heterosexual and homosexual sex.

In 1957, 520 copies of the book were seized on the way into the country by U.S. custom officials. Ferlinghetti and City Lights manager Shigeyoshi Murao were both charged with the distribution of obscene material. A lengthy trial ensued, and Ferlinghetti and Murao, with the help of the American Civil Liberties Union, were found not guilty. After nine literary experts testified in defense of the literary merits of "Howl," Judge Clayton Horn determined that the poem was not obscene and had "redeeming social importance." He wrote, "An author should be real in treating his subject and be allowed to express his thoughts and ideas in his own words" (Morgan and Peters 2006; The Allen Ginsberg Project 2017). The publicity brought about by the trial made *Howl* a surprising commercial success, and by 1967, there were 146,000 copies of the book in print (Ramazani, Ellman, and O'Clair 2003, 336)—an astounding number for a contemporary book of poetry. By the early 2000s, *Howl and Other Poems* had sold more than 1 million copies worldwide and been translated into 24 languages (Block 2006).

The poem itself is written in three sections (with some considering the poem "Footnote to Howl" an unofficial fourth section). Judge Horn, in his ruling on the obscenity case, provided a surprisingly apt synopses of the three parts:

> The first part of "Howl" presents a picture of a nightmare world; the second part is an indictment of those elements in modern society destructive of the best qualities

> of human nature; such elements are predominantly identified as materialism, conformity, and mechanization leading toward war. The third part presents a picture of an individual who is a specific representation of what the author conceives as a general condition. (Morgan and Peters 2006; The Allen Ginsberg Project 2017)

Drug use is a central theme of "Howl." While marijuana is mentioned and alluded to several times, Ginsberg's verses about the effects of peyote and other hallucinogens, as well as heroin, contributed more to the overall atmosphere of the poem. In fact, Part II of the poem was written while Ginsburg was under the influence of peyote. The poem does little to sensationalize these more potent drugs. Instead, it focuses on their deleterious effects on habitual users. This perspective is clear from the very first line of the poem: "I saw the best minds of my generation destroyed by madness, starving hysterical naked, dragging themselves through the negro streets at dawn looking for an angry fix" (Ginsberg 1956, 9). Ginsberg's poem uses a barrage of language to viscerally re-create a schizophrenic, often nauseating atmosphere of drug users' experiences. However, while much of "Howl" seems to emphasize Ginsberg's concern around the negative impacts of drug use, his comments in a number of interviews suggest that he viewed marijuana as a mind-expanding, beneficial drug. As he tells the story, there was a time when he first started using marijuana, "smoking grass once or twice a week on elegant and selected special occasions," and his new experiences with the drug "made the whole universe swing." He was studying the work of French artist Paul Cézanne at the time, and Ginsberg had arranged to see some of the artist's watercolors at the Museum of Modern Art. According to Ginsberg, he smoked some marijuana in the garden before the show, and he explained what he saw in Cézanne's work by stating, "I discerned his use of space, understanding his use of hot colors advancing and cold colors receding. 'Eyeball kicks' I called it in "Howl"—optical consciousness" (Sloman and Barkin 1982).

The book *Howl and Other Poems* contains six additional poems, several of which also mention marijuana—some more explicitly than does "Howl." Most notable, perhaps, is the overtly political poem, "America," which makes several positive references to marijuana consumption. Ginsberg's words even playfully imply that his use of marijuana is as much a part of his identity as is his nationality.

The cultural influence of *Howl and Other Poems,* both in 1956 and today, is hard to overstate. Along with Jack Kerouac's *On the Road* and *Naked Lunch* by William S. Burroughs, it is one of the touchstones of the continuing legacy of Beat culture.

Steve Trost

See also: Beat Generation Writers.

Further Reading

The Allen Ginsberg Project. "60th Anniversary of the Howl Verdict." 2017. https://allenginsberg.org/2017/10/t-o-3-60th-anniversary-howl-verdict/

Block, Melissa. "After 50 Years, Ginsberg's Howl Still Resonates." *All Things Considered,* NPR, October 27, 2006. https://www.npr.org/transcripts/6393328

Ginsberg, Allen. *Howl and Other Poems*. San Francisco, CA: City Lights Books, 1956.

Morgan, Bill, and Nancy J. Peters. *Howl on Trial*. San Francisco, CA. City Lights Publishers, 2006.

Ramazani, Jahan, Richard Ellman, and Robert O'Clair. *The Norton Anthology of Modern and Contemporary Poetry. Vol. 2: Contemporary Poetry*. New York: W. W. Norton and Company, Inc., 2003.

Sloman, Larry, and George Barkin, "Interview: Allen Ginsber." *High Times*, #86, October 1, 1982: 33. https://hightimes.com/culture/high-times-greats-allen-ginsberg/

Hydroponics

Hydroponics is a method of plant growing without the utilization of soil. Water containing mineral nutrients is utilized during the plant growth, exposing the plants roots directly to the liquid. Marijuana, like other plants such as tomatoes, peppers, cucumbers, lettuce, and various flower types, can thrive in hydroponic systems. In fact, skillful use of hydroponics can produce bigger, better, and higher-quality varieties of all these plants. In addition to larger, healthier, and greater yielding plants, hydroponic marijuana can have higher levels of tetrahydrocannabinol (THC) and can be cultivated every three to four months, faster than the three- to six-month range for soil-planted cannabis (La Barge and Noakes 2005).

Hydroponic growing of marijuana largely developed as a response to increased legal pressure and stigma surrounding the domestic production of marijuana during the 1990s and early 2000s. Domestic cannabis cultivation largely moved to more clandestine locations to avoid law enforcement detection. Hydroponic

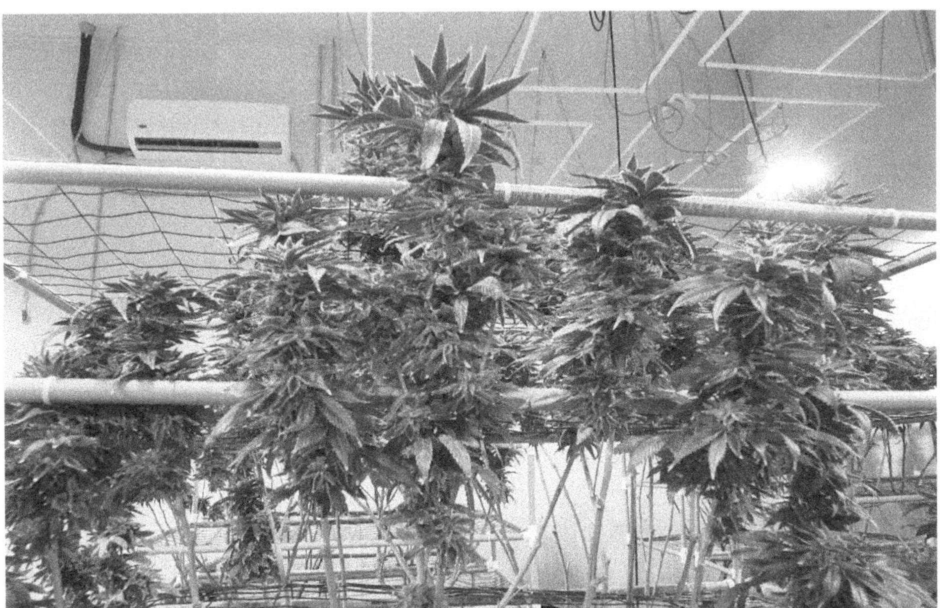

Cannabis leaves and stems are grown hydroponically in a garden. Hydroponics is a horticultural technique that uses a mineral-nutrient solution in water instead of soil. It is a technique most commonly used in indoor marijuana grow shops. (Luyag2/Dreamstime.com)

systems allow for marijuana to be cultivated in hidden locations with size limitations (such as basements) and produce crops in a controlled environment (Easley 2016).

Larger indoor hydroponic operations can be costly, with initial start-up costs of over $25,000 for equipment and supplies along with increased electricity consumption to control lighting systems. This has even led to electricity theft for illegal indoor growers, utilizing over $1,000 of electricity per month (Dadgari 2018; La Barge and Noakes 2005). Indoor growers utilizing an entire bedroom, basement, or garage are able to produce between 10 and 20 plants with yields of up to a couple of hundred thousand dollars per year (Boylstein and Maggard 2013). Small-scale operations for personal use and hobbyists that utilize a closet or small space for 2–4 full-sized plants can produce $20,000–$30,000 of marijuana per year. In a study of illicit hydroponic growers in northern Florida, the interview participants downplayed the profitability of the practice, but instead described their passion for caring for the plants (Boylstein and Maggard 2013). Among marijuana growing enthusiasts, hydroponics provides both a challenging and rewarding method of cultivating marijuana.

The legalization of the medical and recreational marijuana in some states has led to the expansion of the commercial cannabis industry. Many commercial growers have utilized advanced hydroponic systems to produce a controlled environment for consistent and larger yields of high THC marijuana (Easley 2016). Additionally, in states that permit the growing marijuana for personal use, hydroponic growing systems remain popular.

Bryan Lee Miller

See also: Tetrahydrocannabinol (THC).

Further Reading

Boylstein, Craig, and Scott R. Maggard. "Small-Scale Marijuana Growing: Deviant Careers as Serious Leisure." *Humboldt Journal of Social Relations* 35, no. 1 (2013): 52–70.

Dadgari, Ryan. "Powering Mary Jane: Marijuana and Electric Public Utilities." *Golden Gate University Environmental Law Journal* 10 (2018): 55.

Easley, Nic. "Hydroponics or Soil?: How to Choose the Right Growing Method for Cultivation Operation." *Cannabis Business Times*, December 5, 2016.

La Barge, Armand P., and Karen Noakes. "Indoor Marijuana Growing Operations." *The Police Chief* 72, no. 3 (2005): 28–31.

I

Impaired Driving

In 2018, there were over 33,654 fatal traffic accidents in the United States, and driving under the influence of drugs significantly contributes to that total. During the same year, the Substance Abuse and Mental Health Services administration estimated that 43.5 million Americans age 12 or older used marijuana. While alcohol is related to the most drugged-driving fatalities, the National Highway Traffic Safety Administration (NHTSA) identified cannabis as the most prevalent nonalcohol drug found in drivers. In 2018, approximately 12 million U.S. residents age 16 years and older—4.7 percent of the nation's total 16 and older population—reported driving under the influence of cannabis (Azofeifa et al. 2019).

Indeed, a commonly referenced concern raised against cannabis legalization is the impairing effects of the drug and the impact these effects may have on driving-related behaviors and crash risk. Due to the nature of cannabis (e.g., fat soluble) and potentially confounding factors (e.g., experience, use behavior, consumption type, user body type), there is no clear narrative about the relationship between cannabis and driving impairment or crash risk.

To assess the effects of cannabis on crash risk, it is important to explore the synthesis of multiple studies. For instance, a 2012 synthesis of nine studies found a significant correlation between acute cannabis consumption and fatal crash risk. In contrast, a 2018 meta-analysis of 24 relevant studies was unable to confirm a significant relationship between cannabis-impaired driving and traffic collisions, injuries, or death. The analysis concluded that fitness to drive cannot be determined by cannabis's presence alone (Hostiuc et al. 2018).

As the authors of these syntheses also note, there are important limitations to gaining consensus on the topic including methodological flaws such as biased sampling, inappropriate analyses, or unreliable data (e.g., self-report); inconsistent measurement of "cannabis use" or "cannabis impairment"; time between incident and bodily fluid testing; test cutoffs; and publication and interpretational bias (Hostiuc et al. 2018; Rogeberg 2019).

Furthermore, researchers commonly rely upon large traffic databases, such as the NHTSA's Fatality Analysis Reporting System (FARS), to assess crash risk in the United States. However, limitations of FARS nonalcohol drug data make it impossible to accurately infer lessons about nonalcohol drug impairment, crash causation, or comparisons to alcohol (Berning and Smithers 2014). Many of these limitations are present in state and local databases as well.

Cannabis use has been correlated with an increase in the distance that drivers maintain between themselves and the vehicle ahead, increased lane weaving, and a greater likelihood of driving below the speed limit (Hartman et al. 2016).

Studies also indicate with relative consistency that the combination of alcohol and cannabis results in impairing effects greater than either drug on its own. Some research works suggest chronic users develop a tolerance to some of the impairing effects of cannabis (Colizzi and Bhattacharyya 2018), while other research works have suggested chronic use leads to impairments that remain even after extended cessation of use (Busardò et al. 2017).

Understanding the relationship between cannabis and impairment is challenging due to the complex nature of the drug's chemistry. As cannabinoids are fat soluble, the relationship between the presence of tetrahydrocannabinol (THC, and other cannabinoids) in bodily fluids (such as saliva, blood, and urine) and behavioral or cognitive impairment is difficult to understand. Additionally, many consumer-related variables must be considered, including the body mass index (BMI); experience with cannabis and driving, separately and together; frequency of cannabis use; method of consumption (e.g., inhaled, ingested) and, if ingested, stomach contents when ingested; and amount used in a session. The chemical composition of the drug itself is also a factor. As of 2019, however, no relationship has been established between THC concentration in bodily fluids and behavioral or cognitive impairment (Chow et al. 2019).

C. Cozette Comer

See also: Casual Users, Health Effects; Law Enforcement Efforts, Marijuana Control; Neurological Effects.

Further Reading

Azofeifa, Alejandro, et al. "Driving under the Influence of Marijuana and Illicit Drugs among Persons Aged ≥16 Years—United States, 2018." *MMWR Morbidity and Mortality Weekly Report* 68, no. 50 (2019): 1153–1157. https://doi.org/10.15585/mmwr.mm6850a1

Berning, Amy, and Dereece D. Smither. *Understanding the Limitations of Drug Test Information, Reporting, and Testing Practices in Fatal Crashes.* No. DOT HS 812 072. United States. Department of Transportation. National Highway Traffic Safety Administration, 2014. https://crashstats.nhtsa.dot.gov/Api/Public/ViewPublication/812072

Busardò, Francesco P., et al. "Neurocognitive Correlates in Driving under the Influence of Cannabis." *CNS & Neurological Disorders - Drug Targets* 16, no. 5 (August 9, 2017). https://doi.org/10.2174/1871527316666170424115455

Chow, Robert M., et al. "Driving under the Influence of Cannabis: A Framework for Future Policy." *Anesthesia & Analgesia* 128, no. 6 (2019): 1300–1308.

Colizzi, Marco, and Sagnik Bhattacharyya. "Cannabis Use and the Development of Tolerance: A Systematic Review of Human Evidence." *Neuroscience & Biobehavioral Reviews* 93 (2018): 1–25.

Hartman, Rebecca L., et al. "Cannabis Effects on Driving Longitudinal Control with and Without Alcohol." *Journal of Applied Toxicology* 36, no. 11 (2016): 1418–1429. https://doi.org/10.1002/jat.3295

Hostiuc, Sorin, et al. "The Association of Unfavorable Traffic Events and Cannabis Usage: A Meta-Analysis." *Frontiers in Pharmacology* 9 (2018): 99.

Rogeberg, Ole. "A Meta-Analysis of the Crash Risk of Cannabis-Positive Drivers in Culpability Studies—Avoiding Interpretational Bias." *Accident Analysis & Prevention* 123 (2019): 69–78.

Substance Abuse and Mental Health Services Administration. 2019. *Key Substance Use and Mental Health Indicators in the United States.* Rockville, MD: Center for Behavioral Health Statistics and Quality, Substance Abuse and Mental Health Services Administration.

Incarceration for Marijuana Offenses

The criminalization of marijuana during the so-called War on Drugs campaign that began in the 1970s and peaked in the 1980s resulted in increased arrest and incarceration rates for marijuana-related offenses. During this time, racial disparities in how the American justice system adjudicated marijuana offenses were stark (Reinarman 2015, 15; Maurer and King 2007, 3). Starting in the 2000s, momentum for the decriminalization and legalization of marijuana has grown so strong that many states have legalized pot for medicinal and even recreational use. However, marijuana remains illegal according to federal law, so vulnerability to potential legal consequences for growing, selling, possessing, or using marijuana remains, even in states that have legalized pot.

A major shift in the criminalization of marijuana began in the 1970s with the enforcement of the Controlled Substances Act, a law passed in 1970 that categorized marijuana as a schedule I illicit drug subject to felony charges. Shortly after the classification of marijuana as an illicit drug, Richard Nixon declared a "War on Drugs" in 1971. This "get tough movement" was built on the belief that establishing and enforcing harsher penalties on illegal drug production, distribution, and use would incapacitate current offenders, deter future potential offenders, and reduce the crime rate (Latessa, Johnson, and Koetzle 2020; Clear 2009). The Carter administration took a different stance on pot, announcing its support for marijuana legalization in 1977. But little came of this initiative, and when Republican Ronald Reagan became president in January 1981, the War on Drugs—and marijuana—resumed. In the early 1980s, law enforcement agencies saw a dramatic increase in drug arrests, with three-fourths of those arrests attributed to marijuana (Mauer and King 2006). The biggest spike in incarceration rates came between 1990 and 2002, a period in which 700,000 Americans were being charged with marijuana possession charges annually. These trends dramatically increased U.S. incarceration rates compared to other nations (Reinarman 2015, 15).

The high arrest and incarceration rates for marijuana offenses had a detrimental effect on the African American community (as did a simultaneous crackdown on crack cocaine, which was more prevalent in Black communities than powder cocaine, which was much more likely to be used by whites). African Americans only made up 14 percent of the marijuana user population but made up 30 percent of arrests for marijuana violations (King and Mauer 2006, 3). In 2000, 51 percent of the convictions for the possession of marijuana and 63 percent of convictions of trafficking marijuana led to incarceration (Mauer and King 2006, 12). Additionally, in the same year, at the state level, offenders convicted of a marijuana felony had an average sentence period of 28 months while incarcerated and 40 months for probation (Mauer and King 2006, 12–13). Incarcerated marijuana offenders were responsible for 59 percent of trafficking offenses, 23 percent of possession offenses, and 15 percent of possession with the intent to distribute offenses in that same year (Mauer and King 2006, 14). Based on the patterns of sentencing in 2000, hypotheses conclude that the prison population approximately included 68,000 individuals incarcerated within state and federal facilities for a marijuana offense (Mauer and King 2006, 14). Presently, the effects of the War on Drugs are still apparent. Data collected by the Federal Bureau of Investigation (FBI) using the Crime Reporting Program concluded that a total of 1.6 million arrests were made in 2018. Of those arrests made, 37 percent were for marijuana possession and 3 percent were for selling or distributing marijuana (James and Sacco 2020, 2). In the same year, the Drug Enforcement Agency (DEA) arrested over 5,000 individuals for marijuana offenses and arrested an additional 4,000 individuals for the same offense in 2019 (James and Sacco 2020, 2).

California was the first state to legalize the use of medical marijuana with the enactment of Proposition 215 in 1996. However as of November 2020, a total of 36 states as well as the District of Columbia, Guam, Puerto Rico, and the U.S. Virgin Islands have passed similar legislature. In addition, 15 states have enacted or passed laws legalizing recreational use of marijuana. Of those 15 states, 13 have legalized recreational pot use through ballot referendums that put the question of legalization directly to voters rather than state legislatures. The legalization of recreational marijuana engenders questions about future sentencing policies. Currently, penalties and sentencing vary significantly across states. Oregon passed a couple of legislative measures that focus on the reduction of marijuana as a felony conviction and distinguishing penalties based on weight. Oregon also modified sentences for felony marijuana offenses. Following Oregon, Montana created a sweeping bill (HB 133) that modified and reduced penalties for marijuana possession to a misdemeanor with little to no time in jail (McInes 2019). Literature on the effects of criminalization and legalization on incarceration rates is scarce, but states that have decriminalized marijuana use have experienced a monumental drop in low-level marijuana arrests. In fact, one year after decriminalizing marijuana possession, arrest rates declined 86 percent in California, 67 percent in Connecticut, and 90 percent in Massachusetts (Neill Harris 2019, 7). Although reductions in arrest rates have been observed overall, the racial disparity in arrest and sentencing rates is still present at both the state and federal level. Missouri, for example, decriminalized marijuana in 2014. Since then, African Americans in the state have been 2.6 times more likely to be arrested on marijuana charges compared to other offenders by race (ACLU Missouri 2020). In an analysis of 2017 drug offenders at the federal level, results revealed that Black drug offenders had longer sentences of up to 20 months more when compared to other drug offenders of different racial origin (Testa 2020, 13).

In addition to reduced penalties for marijuana, talk about the possibility of expungement for marijuana-related convictions has also intensified. In Illinois, for example, some individuals can receive clemency for their convictions of possession up to 30 grams of marijuana due to the Cannabis Regulation and Tax Act (McInes 2019). The state of Delaware, meanwhile, provided direct expungement for conviction and arrest records for individuals who were either convicted or charged of particular offenses regarding marijuana (McInes 2019). As of 2020, however, federal legislation still finds marijuana possession, distribution, and use to be illegal and thus a federal crime (Davidson 2016, 2154). Currently, new bills are being proposed at the federal level to remove marijuana as a federal drug such as the Marijuana Justice Act of 2019 introduced by Senator Cory A. Booker. In addition to the Marijuana Justice Act of 2019, movement to expunge marijuana offenses at the federal level has also been advocated with the Marijuana Opportunity and Reinvestment and Expungement (MORE) Act of 2019, a bill introduced by Democratic Senator Kamala Harris (CA), which seeks to reduce the effects of mass incarceration from the War on Drugs by decriminalizing marijuana at the federal level and expunging the sentences of offenders convicted of marijuana-related offenses. Although the momentum for reform of federal marijuana laws seems to be on the rise, the MORE Act did not come up for a vote in the Republican-controlled Senate.

Olivia P. Shaw

See also: Drug Enforcement Administration (DEA); Incarceration Rates; Incarceration, Use during.

Further Reading

ACLU Missouri. "New ACLU Report: Black People Still 2.6 Times More Likely to Get Arrested for Marijuana in Missouri." April 23, 2020. https://www.aclu-mo.org/en/news/new-aclu-report-black-people-still-26-times-more-likely-get-arrested-marijuana-missouri

Clear, Todd R. *Imprisoning Communities: How Mass Incarceration Makes Disadvantaged Neighborhoods Worse*. New York: Oxford University Press, 2009.

Clear, Todd R., Patricia M. Harris, and S. Christopher Baird. "Probationer Violations and Officer Response." *Journal of Criminal Justice* 20, no. 1 (1992): 1–12.

Davidson, Adam. "Learning from History in Changing Times: Taking Account of Evolving Marijuana Laws in Federal Sentencing." *The University of Chicago Law Review* 83 (2016): 2105–2161.

Hanson, Karmen, and Alise Garcia. "State Medical Marijuana Laws." October 12, 2020. https://www.ncsl.org/research/health/state-medical-marijuana-laws.aspx

Hudak, John. *Marijuana: A Short History*. Washington, DC: Brookings Institution Press, 2016.

James, Nathan, and Lisa N. Sacco. "Criminal Records Expungement and the Marijuana Opportunity Reinvestment and Expungement (MORE) Act of 2019." *HeinOnline* (2020): 1–4. https://www.everycrsreport.com/reports/IN11506.html

King, Ryan S., and Marc Mauer. "The War on Marijuana: The Transformation of the War on Drugs in the 1990s." *Harm Reduction Journal* 3, no. 1 (2006): 6.

Latessa, Edward J., Shelley L. Johnson, and Deborah Koetzle. *What Works (and Doesn't) in Reducing Recidivism*. Abington, UK: Routledge, 2020.

Maurer, M., and R. S. King. *The 25-year Quagmire: The War on Drugs and Its Impact on American Society*. Washington, DC: The Sentencing Project, 2007. https://www.sentencingproject.org/publications/a-25-year-quagmire-the-war-on-drugs-and-its-impact-on-american-society/

Musto, David F. "Opium, Cocaine and Marijuana in American History." *Scientific American* 265, no. 1 (1991): 40–47.

Neill Harris, Katherine, and William Martin. "The Case for Marijuana Decriminalization." Rice University Baker Institute for Public Policy, April 16, 2019. https://

www.bakerinstitute.org/media/files/files/b4b661ec/bi-report-041619-drug-mjdecrim.pdf

Reinarman, Craig. "Prohibition and Its Discontents: Understanding People in Their Social Worlds Understanding People in Their Social Worlds." *Contexts* 14, nos. 4, 11 (2015): 15–16.

Svrakic, Dragan M., Patrick J. Lustman, Ashok Mallya, Taylor Andrea Lynn, Rhonda Finney, and Neda M. Svrakic. "Legalization, Decriminalization & Medicinal Use of Cannabis: A Scientific and Public Health Perspective." *Missouri Medicine* 109, no. 2 (2012): 90.

Teigen, Anne, and Karen McInnes. "Legalization." Marijuana Overview, October 17, 2019. https://www.ncsl.org/research/civil-and-criminal-justice/marijuana-overview.aspx#Expungement

Testa, Alexander, and Jacqueline G. Lee. "Trends in Sentencing of Federal Drug Offenders: Findings from U.S. District Courts 2002–2017." *Journal of Drug Issues*, September 2020. https://doi.org/10.1177/0022042620959071

Incarceration Rates

The impact of marijuana on the incarceration rate is a contentious point of debate in the United States, on both the federal and state levels. The United States has the highest incarceration rate in the world, and in 2018, it is estimated that 40 percent of arrests were for marijuana-based offenses (FBI 2018). While several states are experimenting with legalization or have decriminalized of marijuana, it was still considered a Schedule 1 Drug under federal law in 2020.

Criminal charges related to possession and use of marijuana require significant resources of the American criminal justice system, affecting police, courts, and corrections. In 2010, approximately 52 percent of all drug arrests were marijuana based, according to the American Civil Liberties Union. There were 8.2 million people arrested for marijuana-related crimes between 2001 and 2010, with 88 percent of individuals charged for possession of small amounts. With this volume of arrests, the costs associated with policing services, judicial hearings, and temporary housing in jails create a significant expense for taxpayers. Unfortunately, the costs continue to rise when the arrest moves to prosecution and potential incarceration. An estimated $3.6 billion is spent every year on the enforcement of state laws related to marijuana (American Civil Liberties Union 2013).

An examination into marijuana and incarceration found that in 2001 alone, $2.1 billion of all funds distributed to law enforcement in the United States was used on enforcing marijuana laws (Beckett and Herbert 2009). Of that, over 80 percent was explicitly used for possession alone. The study further found there were around 28,000 prisoners in state and federal prisons incarcerated for marijuana. The average annual cost for housing a prisoner in the United States in 2016 was $34,704, which means marijuana offenders may cost American taxpayers as much as $600 billion annually. Although marijuana offenders may seem to be a small percentage of the incarcerated population, the amount of money required to house low-level offenders is significant.

When viewing marijuana through the lens of prosecution, it is essential to note that every state has different laws pertaining to its legality. States such as California and Colorado have legalized marijuana for recreational use while others, such as

Arkansas and Florida, are known to heavily fine and even imprison people for pot possession. Most states that enforce marijuana laws label possession of a small amount as a misdemeanor, with the penalty being jail sentences of less than one year. These penalties have resulted in a heavy flow of people convicted of marijuana-related crimes moving in and out of the U.S. corrections system. In general, however, these offenders influence the overall prison population little compared to those sentenced on felony charges requiring more than a year in prison.

Federal laws related to marijuana, meanwhile, have remained largely unchanged for a half century. Before the 1970s and President Richard Nixon's "War on Drugs," law enforcement had less focus on investigating illegal substances. However, the focus shifted when Congress passed the Comprehensive Drug Abuse Prevention and Control Act of 1970. The act provided the federal government with resources to prosecute marijuana offenders and increased minimum sentences significantly beyond penalties imposed by state governments. Further, the act classified marijuana as a Schedule 1 Narcotic (i.e., high abuse potential and no medical use) and funded the creation of the Drug Enforcement Administration (DEA). This was a substantial expansion in the federal government's judiciary process, and drug cases entering the system increased by over 1,000 percent. Many of the standards, laws, and organizations created or funded in the 1970s remain in effect today (Newbern 2000).

Continuing into the 1980s, the War on Drugs expanded with the Anti-Drug Abuse Act of 1986, which gave U.S. attorneys the ability to impose mandatory minimum sentences for criminals convicted on drug charges. Offenders convicted and sentenced to federal prison for marijuana possession, for example, are required to serve a minimum of 85 percent of the sentence. Someone possessing 1 kilogram of marijuana can receive 6–12 months in prison if convicted, while 2–3 kilograms can lead to several years behind bars. Further, possession of 100 marijuana plants requires a minimum sentence of 5 years, and possession of 1,000 plants requires a minimum of 10 years. These long sentences are the minimum requirement, and federal judges may—and often do—levy even longer sentences. The threat of extended sentences may be why 98 percent of defendants take the option of pleading guilty (Pew Research Center 2019) and accepting a reduced sentence every year rather than risk a mandatory minimum sentence.

Many groups have emerged to oppose the "War on Drugs" and mandatory minimum sentences, including Families Against Mandatory Minimums (FAMM), Coalition for Public Safety, and Law Enforcement Against Prohibition (LEAP) (Criminal Justice Policy Foundation 2019). These groups oppose the federal statutes related to strict prison sentences for most drugs and argue that these harsh penalties are to blame for a significant increase in the prison population since the 1970s. These organizations work to influence lawmakers and build public support for sentencing reforms at the federal level.

Many people believe that marijuana contributes significantly to mass incarceration. According to a special report conducted by the U.S. Department of Justice in October 2015 that examined all drug offenders in federal prison at the end of the 2012 fiscal year, marijuana offenders received an average sentence of 88 months. This length is the shortest, in prison terms, for all types of drug offenders convicted of federal crimes (crack cocaine offenders received the longest sentences with an average of 170 months). Marijuana offenders accounted for 11,517 of the 94,215 drug offenders incarcerated in federal prisons. Moreover, 51 percent of marijuana offenders received between 1 and 5 years in prison for their crime, and 25.8 percent received 5 and 10 years, with only 1 percent sentenced to less than a year in prison (Taxy, Samuels, and Adams 2015).

It is quite possible the reason that about one-fourth of inmates convicted of marijuana-related offenses under federal law fall between five and ten years is because of federally mandated minimum sentencing. However, despite the set punishments initiated by the federal government, those who are convicted because of marijuana are among the least prominent types of convicts, in terms of numbers. According to the Prison Policy Initiative, there were 225,000 people held in federal prisons or jails in 2018, with 100,000 of these individuals incarcerated on some drug violation (Wagner and Sawyer 2018). While this may indicate that drug offenses have a substantial impact on the mass incarceration of individuals in federal prisons, the trend for marijuana appears to remain stable. Only a small portion of the drug offender population in federal prisons is made up of marijuana-based crime, and it leads to the shortest sentences.

David Boaz, the executive vice president of the libertarian Cato Institute, suggests lesser sentences in marijuana cases could have a positive impact on the nation's economy. Like many other critics, he asserts that the cost of keeping marijuana offenders incarcerated is a financial burden on the government. If marijuana users were legally employed, he argues, they would be contributing to society. Furthermore, he believes longer sentences in marijuana cases increase "black-market crime." He says, "It seems clear that rising penalties, while they may deter some drug use, also increase the price of illegal drugs," and contends that America would "be better served by keeping violent criminals in prison longer by freeing up beds now used by marijuana offenders" (Boaz 2019).

Ben Stickle and Ezekiel Hall

See also: Bush (George H.W.) Administration "War on Drugs"; Bush (George W.) Administration "War on Drugs"; Comprehensive Drug Abuse Prevention and Control Act (1970); Drug Enforcement Administration (DEA); Incarceration for Marijuana Offenses; Incarceration, Use during; Law Enforcement Action Partnership (LEAP); Nixon Administration "War on Drugs"; Reagan Administration "War on Drugs."

Further Reading

American Civil Liberties Union. "Marijuana Arrests by the Numbers." 2013. https://www.aclu.org/gallery/marijuana-arrests-numbers

Beckett, Katherine, and Steve Herbert. "The Consequence and Costs of Marijuana Prohibition." 2009. https://faculty.washington.edu/kbeckett/The%20Consequences%20and%20Costs%20of%20Marijuana%20Prohibition.pdf

Boaz, David. "Marijuana Sentencing Guidelines." 2019. https://www.cato.org/publications/congressional-testimony/marijuana-sentencing-guidelines

Criminal Justice Policy Foundation "Mandatory Minimums and Sentencing Reform." 2019. https://www.cjpf.org/mandatory-minimums

Federal Bureau of Investigation (FBI). "2018 Crime in the United States." 2018. https://ucr.fbi.gov/crime-in-the-u.s/2018/crime-in-the-u.s.-2018/topic-pages/persons-arrested

Newbern, Alistair E. "Good Cop, Bad Cop: Federal Prosecution of State-legalized Medical Marijuana Use after United States v. Lopez." *California Law Review* 88 (2000): 1575.

New York Times Editorial Board. "Outrageous Sentences for Marijuana." *New York Times,* April 14, 2016. https://www.nytimes.com/2016/04/14/opinion/outrageous-sentences-for-marijuana.html

Pew Research Center. "Only 2% of Federal Criminal Defendants Go to Trail, and Most Who Do Are Found Guilty." 2019. https://www.pewresearch.org/fact-tank/2019/06/11/only-2-of-federal-criminal-defendants-go-to-trial-and-most-who-do-are-found-guilty/

Taxy, Sam, Julie Samuels, and William Adams. *Drug Offenders in Federal Prison: Estimates of Characteristics Based on Linked Data.* Washington, DC: US Department of Justice, Office of Justice Programs, Bureau of Justice Statistics, 2015.

Wagner, P., and W. Sawyer. "Mass Incarceration: The Whole Pie." Prison Policy Initiative, 2018. https://www.prisonpolicy.org/reports/pie2018.html

Incarceration, Use during

The prison population of the United States is one of the largest in the world. As of late 2018, almost one and a half million Americans were incarcerated in both state and federal prisons (Carson 2020). Given the easy access to marijuana that prevails across much of the United States, problems with marijuana distribution and use among the prison population have plagued some of these correctional institutions.

The issue of contraband has been a lasting issue among correctional administrators. Previous research has noted the various ways in which prisoners obtain and store contraband, including marijuana, within correctional facilities. Namely, the use of books, envelopes, and other common items often hold items illegal within these settings (Kalinich and Stojkovic 1985, 1987). The use of these various items, most notably the use of books from the prison library, allows prisoners to hide the substance from other inmates and guards, thus avoiding confiscation (Bouchard and Winnicki 2000). Within the various black markets of prison, legal items such as cigarettes can oftentimes be traded in exchange for marijuana (Lankenau 2001).

In terms of the prevalence of the use of marijuana within correctional facilities, research is inconclusive. Research has noted individuals entering prison often display signs of either drug dependence or abuse. According to the Bureau of Justice Statistics, 58 percent of state prisoners met the criteria for drug dependence or abuse upon beginning their sentences (Bronson and Stroop 2017). Additionally, the use of marijuana was the highest reported substance ever used by prisoners in their lifetime, with 80 percent of state prisoners reporting previous use (Bronson and Stroop 2017). As of 2018, over 78 percent of individuals on parole or supervised release reported using illegal marijuana during their life (National Center for Drug Abuse Statistics 2019).

Although marijuana is an evident item of contraband within correctional facilities, marijuana is also an illegal substance in many states within the United States. Thus, legality issues can arise as marijuana is both an external contraband (i.e., illegal to possess within the free world) and an internal contraband (i.e., illegal to possess within correctional facilities). Prisoners who face issues related to the possession of marijuana as external contraband could potentially be held liable for additional criminal charges.

Many other states, however, have legalized marijuana for medical and/or recreational use. One state that has legalized both uses is California, where in 2019, a state appeals court overturned a decision to charge five inmates with felony possession of marijuana within a California Department of Correction and Rehabilitation (CDCR) facility. The court ruled that Proposition 64, the 2016 voter initiative that legalized marijuana in the state, did not classify the possession of less than an ounce of cannabis in prison as a felony within the state. The court did note that the possession may be against CDCR policies but was not in fact a violation of state law.

Marc D. Glidden

See also: Decriminalization; Incarceration for Marijuana Offenses.

Further Reading

Bouchard, Joseph, and Amanda Winnicki. "You Found What in a Book?" Contraband Control in the Prison Library." *Library and Archival Security* 16 no. 1 (2000): 47–61.

Bronson, Jennifer, and Jessica Stroop. *Drug Use, Dependence, and Abuse among State Prisoners and Inmates, 2007–2009*. Washington, DC: Bureau of Justice Statistics. 2017.

Carson, Ann E. *Prisoners in 2018*. Washington, DC: Bureau of Justice Statistics. 2020.

Hill, Michael O. "Permanent Confiscation of Prison Contraband: The Fifth Amendment Behind Bars." *The Yale Law Journal* 93, no. 5 (1984): 901–917.

Kalinich, David B., and Stan Stojkovic. "Contraband: The Basis of Legitimate Power in a Prison Social System." *Criminal Justice and Behavior* 12, no. 4 (1985): 435–451.

Kalinich, David B., and Stan Stojkovic. "Prison Contraband System: Implications for Prison Management." *Journal of Crime and Justice* 10, no. 1 (1987): 1–21.

Lankenau, Stephen E. "Smoke'em If You Got'em: Cigarette Black Markets in US Prisons and Jails." *The Prison Journal* 81, no. 2 (2001): 142–161.

National Center for Drug Abuse Statistics. "Marijuana Incarceration Statistics." 2019. https://drugabusestatistics.org/

India and South Asia

Despite the long history of drug use in the region—as well as the region's notoriety as a major global center for the production of illegal drugs—Asia has the lowest rate of illegal drug use among the major regions of the world. This is true despite the fact that nearly 30 percent of the world's cannabis users live in Asia. Thus, while millions of Asians use illegal drugs such as marijuana, rates of use, as a percentage of the total population, are relatively low throughout the region. Not surprisingly, the most commonly used illicit drug in Asia is marijuana. An estimated 56.6 million Asians use marijuana, according to the United Nations (UNODC 2018). Although this figure represents approximately 29 percent of the world's marijuana users, it is only 1.9 percent of the region's adult population, which the UN defines as 15–64. This is the lowest rate of use among the major regions of the world and significantly below the 2018 report's global estimate that 3.9 percent of the adult population use marijuana annually.

Within Asia, South Asia has the second highest rate of marijuana use in Asia, at least based on data reported to the United Nations. The average use rate in South Asia is approximately 2.6 percent of the adult population (UNODC 2004). Bhutan reports the highest rate of use in the region, with approximately 4.2 percent of the adult population believed to use cannabis annually. Bangladesh, Nepal, and India all have use rates ranging from 2.5 percent to approximately 3.5 percent of the adult population. The island nation of Maldives, meanwhile, has average use rates for the region at 2.5 percent of the adult population (UNODC 2018). Sri Lanka has rates of marijuana use that are slightly below the subregion's average. In Sri Lanka, where rates appear to be stable, 1.4 percent of the adult population uses marijuana (UNODC 2018).

MARIJUANA USE IN INDIA

The use of marijuana on the Indian subcontinent is ancient and deeply rooted in the region's culture. Marijuana was probably first used as an intoxicant in India around 1000 BC and soon thereafter became an integral part of Hindu culture. Cannabis is used in three different preparations in India. *Bhang* is made from the leaves and stems of uncultivated plants and blended into a liquid drink. *Ganja* is the flowering tops of cultivated plants and is smoked. *Charas* is similar to hashish and is obtained by scraping and pressing the resin from the leaves of the cultivated plants. It is also smoked. Even today, marijuana is used as a food, as medicine, for recreation, as an aphrodisiac, and for religious purposes (Courtwright 2001). While high-caste Hindus are not permitted to use alcohol, bhang is used at religious ceremonies and during marriage ceremonies and family festivals. Some Hindus devoted to Shiva smoke marijuana as an offering during the annual Maha Shivaratri festival, which is in remembrance of overcoming darkness and ignorance and involves prayers, fasting, and meditating. During the Holi, which is the festival of spring, bhang drinks are consumed.

Laborers in India use bhang in much the same way as Americans use alcohol. Older, male, rural farmers use ganja during "smoke breaks" (Hawdon 2005). In the urban areas, marijuana use is more common among the wealthier youth and the "lower and criminal classes" (Courtwright 2001, 40). The pattern is similar in Nepal, where cannabis grows wild and is cultivated in the mid-lands. Nepal, in fact, is a leading source for the transnational marijuana trade, but the percentage of people using it for recreation is relatively small. Users tend to be male and older, although urban youth have increasingly used marijuana since the 1970s. A pattern found throughout the region is that among school-age children, the stronger the child's Western cultural orientation, the greater her or his use of cannabis (Emdad-ul Haq 2000).

THE LEGAL STATUS OF MARIJUANA IN SOUTH ASIA

Cannabis use and possession is illegal throughout South Asia. It has been illegal in India, for example, since the passage of the Narcotic Drugs and Psychotropic

Substance Act in 1985. The cultivation, production, possession, and transportation of marijuana is met with punishments ranging from 6 months in prison and a fine for possession of small quantities to 10–20 years in prison for those caught with large quantities of cannabis. More recently, there has been increased interest among Indian politicians to legalize medical marijuana, and even some prominent politicians have called for the legalization and regulation of recreational cannabis use (Tharoor and Tharoor 2018). During the annual Maha Shivaratri festival, Nepal suspends its prohibition on cannabis use, and although not everyone participating in the festival uses it, thousands of those who attend honor Shiva by smoking marijuana to aid in their meditation (McLaren 2019).

James Hawdon

See also: Africa; Central Asia; China and Southeast Asia; Europe; Hashish; Latin America; Middle East.

Further Reading

Courtwright, David T. *Forces of Habit*. Cambridge, MA: Harvard University Press, 2001.

Emdad-ul Haq, M. *Drugs in South Asia: From the Opium Trade to the Present Day*. London, UK: MacMillan Press, 2000.

Hawdon, James. *Drug and Alcohol Consumption as Functions of Social Structures: A Cross-Cultural Sociology*. No. 47. Lewistown, NY: Edwin Mellen Press, 2005.

McLaren, Eirk. "How Hinduism's Cannabis God Fuels India's Weed-Loving Culture." *Herb*, August 14, 2019. https://herb.co/news/culture/shiva-india-ganja-culture/

Tharoor, Shashi, and Avinash Tharoor. "High Time India, the Land of Bhang, Legalises Marijuana." *The Print,* October 18, 2018. https://theprint.in/opinion/when-india-legalises-weed/66245/

United Nations Office on Drugs and Crime (UNODC). *World Drug Report 2004*. Oxford, UK: Oxford University Press, 2004.

UNODC. *World Drug Report 2018*. Oxford, UK: Oxford University Press, 2018.

J

Joints

Joints are dried cannabis flower rolled in cigarette rolling papers and smoked like a cigarette. The use of joints is so common within the cannabis community that the image of a marijuana cigarette is synonymous with that subculture in the United States and around much of the world. Marijuana cigarettes are known by many other names as well, depending on the nation and culture. For example, in the United States, the term "spliff" is used when the cannabis flower is mixed with tobacco. But in Europe and the Caribbean, they refer to a marijuana cigarette without tobacco as a spliff (Canna Connection 2020), whereas the term "blowtjie" is used when referring to cannabis mixed with tobacco (Sifaneck et al. 2003). There are many more terms for a marijuana cigarette that can be listed here, but some of the more common terms include J, bone, dutch/dutchy, doobie/dooby, tube, and cone. Some variation on terms relates to the style that the joint is rolled in; for example, a cone is a joint rolled with the lighting end larger than the inhalation end, and it often features a cardboard filter or crutch to keep the dried flower out of one's mouth.

To understand the origins of smoking marijuana in this manner, one must look first to the origin of rolling papers used for tobacco. Once tobacco was brought back to Europe from the new world, cigars quickly became very popular with the upper classes. While the lower classes could not afford cigars, they gathered the discarded butts of these cigars and rerolled the remaining tobacco in scraps of newspaper. As this behavior caught on around Europe, paper makers in Spain saw an opportunity and started to produce small thin papers specifically for rolling tobacco (Canna Connection 2020). The first record of people using cigarette papers for rolling cannabis was from Mexico in the 1850s (Desiree 2020), although the practice was likely in use for some time prior. This use was recorded by a pharmacist from University of Guadalajara while observing field laborers smoking a mix of cannabis and tobacco. By 1870, marijuana cigarettes were being marketed in the United States as a treatment for asthma and other respiratory issues, under the name Griimault's Indian Cigarettes (Desiree 2020).

The popularity of cannabis, and joints in particular, can largely be traced to the Jazz music scene and the banning of alcohol by the Eighteenth Amendment. While there is disagreement over the origins of the term joint being used for a marijuana cigarette, some trace it to this era as it was also a common reference to a seedy or disreputable place of accommodation or entertainment—an apt description of the speakeasies in which jazz music was commonly performed. Cannabis was very popular among musicians of this scene, as it was viewed as a method of intoxication that enhanced creativity without the loss of motor control that came with consuming

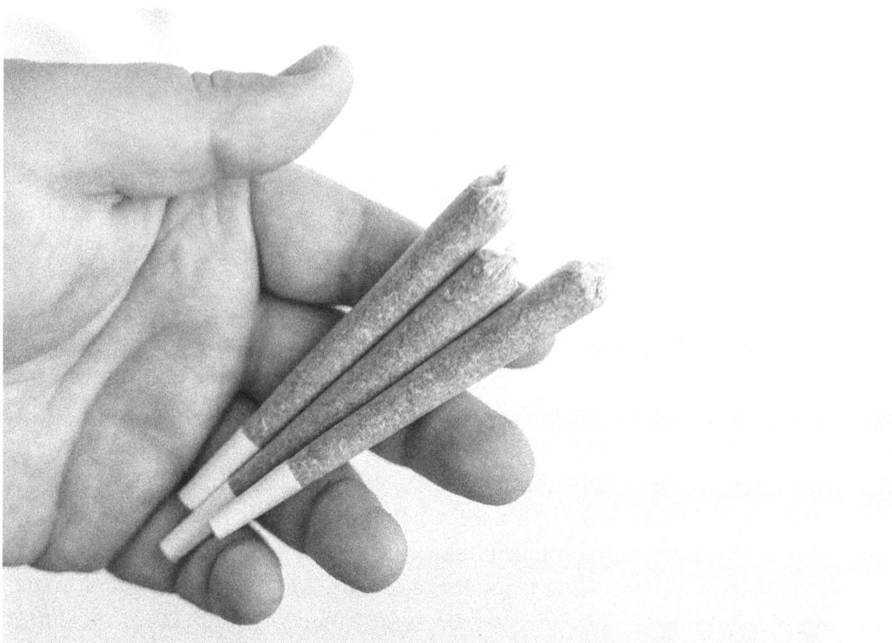

Joints are rolled marijuana cigarettes. Joints are a common method of smoking marijuana in many cultures, including among American youth. Other methods of use include smoking pipes, vaping, or ingesting edibles. (Ded Mityay/Dreamstime.com)

alcohol. As prohibition pushed alcohol sales underground, jazz musicians began to tour the country to play at these establishments and brought their "jazz cigarettes" with them, exposing other parts of the nation to this method of consuming marijuana (Desiree 2020). This exposure boomed into full-blown counterculture acceptance in the 1960s with the emergence of the hippie movement.

Even as it remained underground and subject to legal prosecution, cannabis began to develop as a counterculture of its own. A multitude of new brands of rolling papers specifically designed for cannabis, rather than tobacco, hit the market. These were often larger and thicker than traditional cigarette papers (Desiree 2020). More recently, this proliferation has only magnified. One can now purchase rolling papers in a huge variety of sizes, materials, and even flavors.

The emergence of the legal market for cannabis in 1999 (medical) and 2014 (recreational) in some American states has also had a major impact on cannabis generally and joints specifically. For the first time, pre-rolled joints featuring a variety of cannabis strains were made available for legal purchase. Joint rolling has also become viewed as an art form in itself, with many books providing guidance on how to roll a mind-boggling variety of joint styles and even official joint rolling competitions being held. While legalization has provided a plethora of alternatives to smoking cannabis flower, with vaping quickly gaining popularity, joints are still a mainstay of cannabis smoking. This is especially true for older generations that initiated cannabis use before many of these alternatives were accessible (Murphy et al. 2015).

Jebadiha E. Potterf

See also: Blunts; Bongs and Water Pipes; Gravity Bongs; Dabbing.

Further Reading

Canna Connection. "The History of Cannabis Joints." Updated February 7, 2020. https://www.cannaconnection.com/blog/19229-the-history-of-cannabis-joints

Desiree, Serene. "Cannabis in History: The Journey of the Joint." Leafly, 2020. https://www.leafly.com/news/cannabis-101/cannabis-history-journey-joint

Murphy, Fiona, et al. "Baby Boomers and Cannabis Delivery Systems." *Journal of Drug Issues* 45, no. 3 (2015): 293–313.

Sifaneck, Stephen J., Charles D. Kaplan, Eloise Dunlap, and Bruce D. Johnson. "Blunts and Blowtjes: Cannabis Use Practices in Two Cultural Settings and Their Implications for Secondary Prevention." *Free Inquiry in Creative Sociology* 31, no. 1 (2003): 3–14.

L

Latin America

Even though pre-Columbian civilizations in Latin America and the Caribbean already used a wide variety of drugs (such as peyote in Mesoamerica and the coca leaf in the Andean region) for medical and ceremonial purposes before the arrival of the Spaniards in the continent, it was not until the establishment of the Spanish colonial system that cannabis first appeared and started to be produced and commercialized in the region. There is historiographical evidence that it was Christopher Columbus and his hemp-roped fleet who brought the first cannabis seeds to Latin America in 1492. The first use of marijuana in Latin America was by early African slaves toiling in Brazil in the mid-1500s. The lives of these slaves were miserable, but they were allowed to both grow and smoke marijuana. While there are some other records of recreational consumption of cannabis leaves during the seventeenth and eighteenth centuries in some Spanish colonies, it was mostly used for medical and manufacturing purposes during this period.

Throughout the nineteenth century, and especially after most Latin American and Caribbean countries became independent from Spain between 1810 and 1830, the recreational consumption of marijuana started to increase gradually. Most postcolonial legal systems did not prohibit its use, and the effects and risks associated with it were largely unknown or regarded as inconsequential. By the beginning of the twentieth century, the recreational consumption of marijuana was a popular activity, to the point that in many Latin American and Caribbean countries marijuana cigarettes were produced and distributed in legal markets. During the Mexican Revolution (1910–1920), for example, the consumption of marijuana was very popular among the troops; several cultural products from the period, including popular songs, novels, and poems, make reference to the recreational consumption of marijuana.

After the United States passed the Marijuana Tax Act of 1937, most Latin American and Caribbean countries aligned their drug policies with the new American one and prohibited or taxed the production, commercialization, and consumption of marijuana. These policies predominated in the region until the 2010s, when some Latin American countries started decriminalizing the production and/or possession of marijuana for personal consumption with considerable limitations (e.g., Argentina and Mexico in 2009). However, in 2013, the Senate of Uruguay passed a law that fully legalized the production, distribution, and consumption of marijuana for recreational purposes—similar to the ones that the states of California (Amendment 64) and Washington (Initiative 502) were proposing at the time. This made Uruguay the first Latin American country to approve and implement a policy of this nature.

Currently, as a potential measure to mitigate the drug trafficking and violence crises that many Latin American and Caribbean countries are going through, and in the wake of recent pro-marijuana policies implemented in several American states and countries such as Canada, many governments in the region are debating the possible legalization of certain narcotics—starting with marijuana—just as in the Uruguayan case.

Antonio Paniagua Guzmán

See also: Ancient Religions; California; Colonial America; Drug Cartels; Hemp; Marihuana Tax Act (1937); Trafficking; Washington State.

Further Reading

Bagley, Bruce M., and Jonathan D. Rosen. *Drug Trafficking, Organized Crime, and Violence in the Americas Today*. Gainesville: University Press of Florida, 2015.

Campos, Isaac. *Home Grown: Marijuana and the Origins of Mexico's War on Drugs*. Chapel Hill: University of North Carolina Press. 2012.

Courtwright, David T. *Forces of Habit: Drugs and the Making of the Modern World*. Cambridge, MA: Harvard University Press, 2009.

Pardo, Bryce. "Cannabis Policy Reforms in the Americas: A Comparative Analysis of Colorado, Washington, and Uruguay." *International Journal of Drug Policy* 25, no. 4 (2014): 727–735.

Walker, William O. *Drug Control in the Americas*. Albuquerque: University of New Mexico Press, 1981.

Watt, Peter, and Roberto Martínez. *Drug War Mexico: Politics, Neoliberalism and Violence in the New Narcoeconomy*. London, UK and New York: Zed Books. 2012.

Youngers, Coletta, and Eileen Rosin. *Drugs and Democracy in Latin America: The Impact of U.S. Policy*. Boulder, CO: L. Rienner. 2005.

Law Enforcement Action Partnership (LEAP)

Law Enforcement Action Partnership (LEAP), formerly Law Enforcement Against Prohibition, is a 501(c)(3) nonprofit made up of criminal justice practitioners and stakeholders that advocate for criminal justice and drug policy reforms ("Who We Are" 2019). The nonprofit was founded in 2002 by five police officers with a focus primarily on drug policy reform but has since branched out to address police-community relations, harm reduction, incarceration, and global issues ("Who We Are" 2019). Harm reduction involves policies and programs aimed at reducing the consequences associated with drug use. This typically focuses on consequences to one's health by advocating for things such as methadone therapy, needle and syringe disposal, and safer drug use practices (Andersen and Järvinen 2007; Kammersgaard 2019; Riley et al. 1999). LEAP represents one of the only criminal justice organizations against drug prohibition ("Drug Policy" 2019). LEAP's position on marijuana is guided by a medical model of drug abuse, which calls for treatment for drug users instead of incarceration (Mason, Lusk, and Gintzler 1992) and by calling attention to the harms to communities wreaked by the War on Drugs ("Drug Policy" 2019). To achieve its goal, LEAP relies on speaking engagements, media appearances, testimony, and support of allied efforts ("2018 Annual Report" 2019;

"Who We Are" 2019). Further, its activities are not confined to the United States, as it also advocates internationally ("Global Issues" 2019).

LEAP's stance toward marijuana is guided by its principles about illicit drugs as a whole. Specifically, LEAP views drug abuse as a public health problem that should be regulated to protect public health. LEAP thus advocates against drug prohibition and that law enforcement action should only be taken against anyone creating harm while under the influence ("Drug Policy" 2019).

To ensure a medical approach is taken, LEAP suggests that those seeking help from drug addiction should receive support and treatment. LEAP argues that support and treatment can be financed from cost savings resulting from ending drug prohibition ("Drug Policy" 2019). Their medical approach also views the government as being obligated to determine and convey to the public the public health risk of each illicit drug ("Drug Policy" 2019). To help regulate drug use, LEAP advocates for a balanced approach incorporating public, private, and medical input tailored to each drug ("Drug Policy" 2019). As part of drug prohibition, LEAP advocates for expungement of drug records, release of drug offenders, and restoration of voting rights ("Drug Policy" 2019). Taking a global stance, LEAP points to the harms caused by the War on Drugs as an issue involving the United States, Mexico, Afghanistan, and most of Central America ("Global Issues" 2019). To reach global success, LEAP cites examples of drug policy reform in places like Portugal, where the use of all drugs has been decriminalized, and Switzerland, where robust nationwide drug treatment is offered ("Global Issues" 2019).

LEAP's advocacy at the federal and state level and beyond speaks to the range of their marijuana reform efforts. In 2019, LEAP representatives testified before the United States House Financial Services Committee in support of the Secure and Fair Enforcement (SAFE) Banking Act, which they testified would protect legitimate, tax-paying marijuana businesses and their employees from victimization by allowing them access to financial services ("LEAP Quarterly Winter 2018" 2019). Principally, they argued that the traditional cash-only system for marijuana businesses made them targets for theft ("LEAP Quarterly Winter 2018" 2019). At the state level, LEAP has expressed written support of issues such as decriminalization of marijuana and expungement of marijuana convictions ("2018 Annual Report" 2019). The group has also advocated for medical marijuana and has called for clear medical marijuana legislation that would allow police officers to more easily identify medical marijuana users ("2018 Annual Report" 2019; "LEAP Quarterly Fall 2018" 2019; "LEAP Quarterly Winter 2018" 2019). Their law enforcement representatives have commented in support of marijuana legalization in Connecticut, Delaware, Florida, Maryland, Michigan, New Hampshire, New Jersey, North Dakota, New York, and in Washington D.C. ("2018 Annual Report" 2019; "LEAP Quarterly Fall 2018" 2019; "LEAP Quarterly Winter 2018" 2019). Finally, LEAP provided testimony to legalize marijuana in the Northern Mariana Islands ("LEAP Quarterly Fall 2018" 2019).

Jose Torres

See also: Law Enforcement Efforts, Marijuana Control; Law Enforcement Resources; Medical Marijuana and the Law.

Further Reading

Andersen, Ditte, and Margaretha Järvinen. "Harm Reduction–Ideals and Paradoxes." *Nordic Studies on Alcohol and Drugs* 24, no. 3 (2007): 235–252.

"Drug Policy." Law Enforcement Action Partnership, 2019. https://lawenforcementactionpartnership.org/our-issues/drug-policy/

"Global Issues." Law Enforcement Action Partnership, 2019. https://lawenforcementactionpartnership.org/our-issues/global-issues/

Gray, James. *Why Our Drug Laws Have Failed and What We Can Do about It: A Judicial Indictment of the War on Drugs*. Philadelphia, PA: Temple University Pres, 2001.

Kammersgaard, Tobias. "Harm Reduction Policing: From Drug Law Enforcement to Protection." *Contemporary Drug Problems* 46, no. 4 (2019): 345–362.

"LEAP Quarterly Fall 2018." Law Enforcement Action Partnership, 2019. https://lawenforcementactionpartnership.org/fall2018/

"LEAP Quarterly Winter 2018." Law Enforcement Action Partnership, 2019. https://lawenforcementactionpartnership.org/winter2019/

Mason, Derek T., Mark W. Lusk, and Michael Gintzler. "Beyond Ideology in Drug Policy: The Primary Prevention Model." *Journal of Drug Issues* 22, no. 4 (1992): 959–976.

Rahtz, Howard. *Drugs, Crime and Violence: From Trafficking to Treatment*. Falls Village, CT: Hamilton Books, 2012.

Riley, Diane, Ed Sawka, Peter Conley, David Hewitt, Wayne Mitic, Christiane Poulin, Robin Room, Eric Single, and John Topp. "Harm Reduction: Concepts and Practice. A Policy Discussion Paper." *Substance Use & Misuse* 34, no. 1 (1999): 9–24.

"2018 Annual Report." Law Enforcement Action Partnership, 2019. https://lawenforcementactionpartnership.org/wp-content/uploads/2019/07/LEAP-Annual-Report-2018-online.pdf

"Who We Are." Law Enforcement Action Partnership, 2019. https://lawenforcementactionpartnership.org/about-us/who-we-are/

Woods, Neil, and Drug Wars: *The Terrifying inside Story of Britain's Drug Trade*. London, UK: Ebury Press, 2018.

Law Enforcement Efforts, Marijuana Control

With roughly 18,000 local and state police departments covering 50 states and the District of Columbia, it is unsurprising that a wide range of law enforcement responses to marijuana can be found across the United States. The vagaries of law enforcement's response to marijuana are compounded by the variations in state marijuana laws, as well as local prosecutorial emphasis. In short, there are likely as many legal approaches to marijuana as there are police agencies in the United States. In general, however, law enforcement efforts against marijuana that are being carried out today necessarily focus on one of three aspects: growing marijuana, transporting marijuana to markets, and sale and possession of marijuana.

Law enforcement has targeted marijuana production as one prong of its effort to control distribution. Marijuana can be grown inside a properly equipped building or grown outside in a favorable environment. Eradication of marijuana, while generally used in reference to removing outside plants, can be applied to dismantling inside operations as well. The goal of eradication is to prevent the plants from growing to maturity and harvested for sale. Indoor marijuana operations can be more difficult for growers to conceal. Not only must the grower worry about the odor, but the grower must also account for the large amounts of water and electricity required to grow marijuana indoors. Because the growing lights used in indoor operations generate plant-killing heat, venting heat from the structure is critical for the grower. However, growing indoors brings the potential for significant profits, as the growing environment can be strictly controlled and optimized.

Law enforcement uses a number of investigative techniques to detect indoor marijuana operations. In addition to traditional investigative techniques, a number of counterdrug teams utilized thermal imaging equipment to help identify building heat signatures, which might be indicative of a marijuana grow. The imaging scans were normally done after investigators developed other probable cause supporting the marijuana operation; the thermal scans were final steps before completing the search warrant affidavit. Throughout the 1990s, thermal imaging could be done without a warrant, as it is nonintrusive and does not require the police officer to be within the curtilage of the structure. In 2001, the Supreme Court ended warrantless use of thermal imaging in the United States in *Kyllo v. United States*. Canada's Supreme Court reached the opposite conclusion three years later, holding in *Her Majesty the Queen v. Tessling* (2004) that search warrants are unnecessary for thermal imaging scans performed outside of the curtilage (yard) of a private home.

Marijuana growers also utilize remote areas of national forests or other sparsely populated areas for their operations. In some states, local and state law enforcement use their own airborne assets to locate marijuana plots. In other states, law enforcement agencies partner with the National Guard to utilize military assets to locate and eradicate marijuana grow operations in outdoor settings, including public lands. Some researchers have argued eradication efforts are misplaced and ineffective, especially with the steady rise in states that have legalized marijuana for medical or recreational purposes. However, eradication undoubtedly has an impact: in 2017, the Commonwealth of Kentucky located and destroyed over 465,000 marijuana plants removed from outdoor plots (Justice and Public Safety Cabinet 2018). Outdoor marijuana eradication brings unique hazards to law enforcement and the public, as growers have been known to set booby traps around marijuana plots to protect their crops from poachers and law enforcement.

Law enforcement also targets transportation of marijuana through various interdiction efforts. Some interdiction happens at the national borders and entry ports of the United States through a combination of federal, state, and local efforts. However, much of the interdiction occurs on the nation's highways, well within the national borders. Take Kansas, for example. Kansas borders Colorado, which has legalized recreational marijuana. Interstate 70 runs the length of Kansas, connecting Denver to Kansas City, St. Louis, and beyond. In a 2015 report, the Kansas Highway Patrol noted 11 major interdiction seizures. Eight of the 11 seizures involved marijuana, and all of them on Interstate 70. KHP reported over 3,700 pounds of marijuana seized, almost all of it on Interstate 70 (Kansas Highway Patrol 2015). KHP lists criminal interdiction as one of its primary duties, even having a dedicated "Domestic Highway Enforcement Team" (which KHP designates as Troop N).

Law enforcement officers can attend any number of interdiction training courses. KHP offers courses, as does the Ohio State Highway Patrol. Private training exists as well. Desert Snow is considered one of the founding programs, developed by a former California Highway Patrol officer. All of these programs emphasize driving and behavior recognition, interview techniques, and search techniques. Interdiction efforts focus on private vehicles as well as commercial vehicles and tend to be most common from state police agencies (including highway patrols). The heavy involvement of state police in interdiction efforts is likely a result of two factors. First, state police and highway patrol agencies emphasize highway safety; it is their primary jurisdiction. Frequently, these agencies are also responsible for commercial vehicle inspection, so state troopers are more likely to have the necessary training to inspect commercial vehicles. Second, interdiction techniques are problematic in urban areas. Troopers stopping motorists for minor violations on the highway is an inconvenience, which affects motorists potentially from different states and cities. Local police stopping motorists for minor violations in a neighborhood creates a feeling of harassment in the neighborhood. With a significant portion of street-level drug crime centered in predominantly minority neighborhoods, harassing traffic stops potentially damage an already frayed community relationship with local police.

Law enforcement efforts toward the sale and possession of marijuana vary significantly by jurisdiction. Some agencies may face legal hurdles, such as laws making small amounts of marijuana either legal or not a criminal offense. Other agencies may face prosecutorial or local cultural hurdles, where local expectations place weight limits for prosecution. However, targeting the sale of marijuana is important, especially to local law enforcement. While the exact details frequently remain out of the public domain, home invasions (or residential robberies) are commonly tied to drug trafficking. Public perception of such lawbreaking is that it typically involves junkies breaking into homes to support their meth or heroin habits, but marijuana can be a driving force behind these criminal activities as well. Residential robbers, for example, often look to steal marijuana product or cash generated by marijuana sales from known dealers. Home invasions generate significant risks to all involved. The robbers forcing entry are sometimes armed with guns, bringing all the hazards associated with firearms. The robbers could mistakenly invade the wrong apartment, or the targeted drug dealer may have recently moved. Residents, especially if they are dealing with drugs and are armed to protect themselves, may react to the home invasion by using firearms to defend themselves. Home invasions can generate public fear, as the public usually learns only of the home invasion and rarely of the drug-related nature.

Jonathan F. Bastian

See also: Impaired Driving; Law Enforcement Action Partnership (LEAP); Law Enforcement Resources.

Further Reading

Justice and Public Safety Cabinet. *2017 Combined Annual Report Kentucky Office of Drug Control Policy and Kentucky Agency for Substance Abuse Policy*, 2018. https://odcp.ky.gov/Reports/2017%20Final%20KYODCP-KYASAP%20Annual%20Report.pdf

Kansas Highway Patrol. *Reversing the Trend of the Disappearing Trooper*, 2015. http://kslegislature.org/li_2016/b2015_16/committees/ctte_h_trnsprt_1/documents/testimony/20160128_06.pdf

Kyllo v. United States, 533 U.S. 27 (U.S. Supreme Court 2001).

Pollack, Harold A, and Peter Reuter. "Does Tougher Enforcement Make Drugs More Expensive?" *Addiction* 109, no. 12 (2014): 1959–1966. https://doi.org/10.1111/add.12497

Potter, G., L. Gaines, and B. Holbrook. "Blowing Smoke: An Evaluation of Marijuana Eradication in Kentucky." *American Journal of Police* 9, no. 1 (1990): 97–116.

Shepard, E.M., and Paul R. Blackley. "The Impact of Marijuana Law Enforcement in an Economic Model of Crime." *Journal of Drug Issues* 37, no. 2 (2007): 403–424. https://doi.org/10.1177/002204260703700209

Wilkins, Chris, Krishna Bhatta, and Sally Casswell. "The Effectiveness of Cannabis Crop Eradication Operations in New Zealand." *Drug and Alcohol Review* 21, no. 4 (2002): 369–374.

Law Enforcement Resources

Law enforcement agencies throughout the United States have a multitude of resources at their disposal to aid in the enforcement of marijuana-related laws. The most common of these resources comes in the form of officer training and education at local and regional training academies. In addition, drug prevention programs like DARE (Drug Abuse Resistance Education) are commonly found in schools and communities throughout the nation. Task forces also have emerged over past several decades, which focus on drug use and trafficking. Federal law enforcement agencies like the Drug Enforcement Agency (DEA) also conduct large-scale investigations into drug trafficking that extend well beyond the scope or capacity of local law enforcement. Finally, case law has extended probable cause to police officers, giving them the discretion to conduct warrantless searches of individuals based on the detection of marijuana odor. However, with recent legalization efforts of some forms of marijuana at the state level, this standard of probable cause is under further scrutiny.

TRAINING AND EDUCATION

Police academies and training centers across the country have increased training for recruits on how to investigate and carry out drug investigations. Several public websites belonging to police training facilities describe a variety of courses intended to certify law enforcement specific skills. For instance, the Midwest Counterdrug Training Center offers classes pertaining to roadside interdiction, developing drug informants, undercover investigations, gang investigations, and a multitude of other related topics. Another online resource, policeone.com, provides free articles and advertises online training as well as promotions for training academies across the country. Training focusing on specific illicit substances, including marijuana, is offered through many of these training academies, which also provide instruction on drug laws, trafficking trends, and other factors that pertain to the illegal drug industry in general.

Many of the discussed police trainings are focused on individual officers hoping to interdict drug offenses in the occurrence of daily patrols. An increasingly popular tactic among law enforcement agencies nationwide, however, is the development of drug-specific investigation units. These are commonly identified as Vice Narcotics units. Many of these detective-led investigative teams are found in large metropolitan areas. Such investigatory teams have historically developed in response to high rates of drug use and abuse in the urban setting. However, smaller police departments have also turned to these types of units to combat drug use in their communities. A commonly used approach is for several smaller departments to form a joint task force. Such joint task forces help to alleviate the financial burden of member departments because each participating department dedicates only one or two members to the task force.

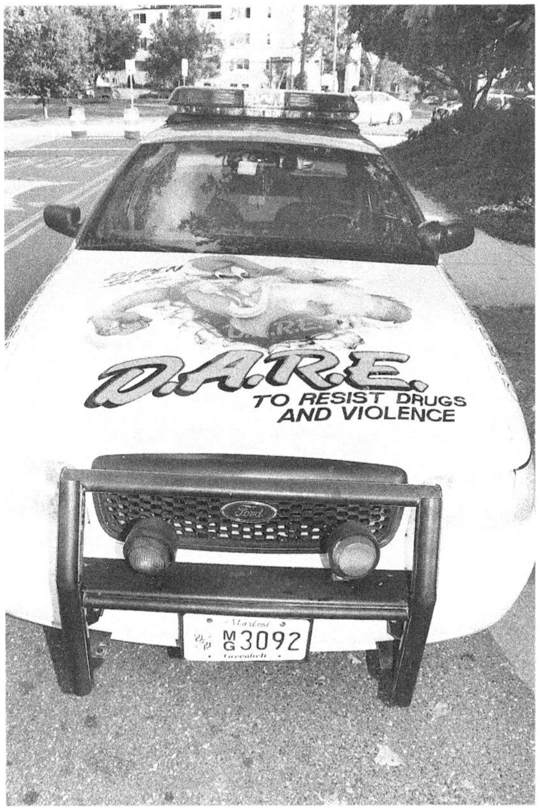

A police car has an anti-drug message on its hood. (Thomas Carter/Dreamstime.com)

Typically, these task forces operate in geographic regions of neighboring jurisdictions. The mantra that "crime knows no borders" is used literally to develop investigative teams with members from each participating jurisdiction to ensure that investigations don't stall when an offender crosses jurisdictional lines. The most common of these joint task forces is a joint drug task force; however, police departments have become more innovative with shared resources to develop other specialty teams. One example of a task force that blends multi-jurisdictional capacity with federal components is the High-Intensity Drug Trafficking Areas, or HIDTA (Holcomb et al. 2018).

Law enforcement also works within communities to offer public awareness and information programs. A common example is that of DARE, a drug education program focused in the school setting. Here, law enforcement officers speak directly to elementary school-age students in an attempt to familiarize them with both the legal and health dangers of drug use. This program originated in Los Angeles in the 1980s and quickly received national popularity. Studies on the program's effectiveness, however, are mixed. While the percentage of minors who engage in alcohol and cigarette use has declined over the past three decades, drug rates have remained relatively unchanged (Shoemaker 2018). Meanwhile, states have adopted dramatically different positions regarding drug treatment and recovery programs for offenders, with some states maintaining robust programs and others concentrating on incarcerating or otherwise punishing drug offenders.

Several iterations of DARE have also emerged that are geared more toward older students. Pertaining to marijuana use, much like the previously described law enforcement trainings, general focus is placed on drug prevention. While DARE is not a marijuana-specific program, the fact remains that marijuana use remains somewhat common among middle and high school students over the past two decades. Self-report studies like Monitoring the Future commonly identify marijuana as the most commonly used illicit substance for students (Shoemaker 2018). Research based on Monitoring the Future data suggests that between 1997 and 2017, nearly 1 in 4 high school seniors reported using marijuana at least once in the last 30 days. What is more, data from the American Academy of Pediatrics suggest that college-age students are increasingly using marijuana. This trend extends to marijuana usage in the last 30 days and over the past year. Regardless of the perceived failures or successes of the program, DARE remains a visible presence in many schools nationwide.

LOCAL, STATE, AND FEDERAL MARIJUANA LAWS

Statutory regulations can also impact law enforcement approaches to drug enforcement in a variety of ways. Following the passage of the Controlled Substance Act in 1970, possession, distribution, and manufacture of marijuana became federally prohibited. With this prohibition, marijuana was designated as a Schedule I controlled substance. Schedule I controlled substances are reserved for substances that have no accepted medical use and present a high likelihood of abuse, and illegal production, distribution, and use of Schedule 1 drugs are subject to severe legal penalties, including long prison sentences (Ward, Lucas, and Murphy 2019). Local or state law enforcement can only allocate so many resources to drug enforcement as they also must address other community problems outside of this issue. With federal statutes in place, however, federal law enforcement agencies such as the Drug Enforcement Agency have a mandate to dedicate toward combating large-scale drug trafficking operations.

Such operations commonly involve the importation of illicit substances from outside the United States. In 1970, the Racketeer Influenced and Corrupt Organizations (RICO) statute was instituted to fight against forms of organized crime. This gave federal prosecutors a new means of prosecuting offenses such as conspiracy and extortion that are indicative of organized crime including drug trafficking (Reid 2018). Asset forfeiture is a common result of those found in violation of RICO statutes. In response to federal RICO laws, individual states also implement similar statutes that could be used in nonfederal investigations. It is now common to see asset forfeiture, normally a civil process, used in conjunction with federal- and state-level investigations involving marijuana and other drugs (Holcomb et al. 2018).

Law enforcement can also use statutory authority to act on drug offenses with a wide array of discretions. One such example is the controversial Stay Out of Drug Areas (SODA) and Stay Out of Areas of Prostitution (SOAP) in Seattle,

Washington. Initially, such areas were designated due to increases in vagrancy, loitering, and vice. As a means of addressing the growing homeless population, local legislatures granted law enforcement officials the discretion to enforce civil processes such as trespassing notices and banishment. Whether intended by legislatures or not, enforcement of these measures by local police yielded increased arrests for, among other things, simple drug possession (England 2008; Beckett and Herbert 2009; Engel, Smith, and Cullen 2012).

Other statutes can implicitly affect marijuana policing—especially state-level marijuana legalization. In 2013, Colorado legalized both medicinal and recreational marijuana use (Ellison and Spohn 2017). While many other states have followed suit, the Controlled Substance Act still carries the threat of federal prosecution for marijuana offenses.

States that have legalized forms of marijuana use have also created unintended consequences for neighboring states. Law enforcement agencies in neighboring states where marijuana use has not been legalized now experience increased arrests of individuals leaving legalized areas. For instance, one 2017 study in Nebraska, where marijuana use is illegal, found that arrests and incarceration for marijuana offenses increased in counties along the Colorado border following Colorado's legalization of recreational and medicinal marijuana use (Ellison and Spohn 2017). Further, perceptions of marijuana use in law enforcement agencies outside of Colorado became more negative. Researchers examined several law enforcement agencies in Kansas, Nebraska, and Wyoming, where marijuana use of any kind was illegal. They found that law enforcement began to view legalization in neighboring states negatively. This negative attitude toward marijuana enforcement developed as focus and resources were dedicated solely to the handling of marijuana calls for service—leaving fewer departmental resources for other law enforcement activities (Ward et al. 2019). These approaches provide only a snapshot of the resources available to law enforcement in the enforcement of drug offenses. Several studies suggest the estimates for such enforcement resources have reached upward of $44.1 billion since the start of the War on Drugs (Ward et al. 2019). This is a massive undertaking that local, state, and federal law enforcement agencies must navigate. As legalization efforts progress, law enforcement agencies will continue to adapt to the changing landscape of the communities they police.

Jason T. Callahan

See also: Colorado; Confidential Informants; Drug Abuse Resistance Education (DARE); Drug Enforcement Administration (DEA); Law Enforcement Efforts, Marijuana Control; Weed and Seed Programs.

Further Reading

Beckett, Katherine, and Steve Herbert. *Banished: The New Social Control in Urban America.* New York: Oxford University Press, 2009.

Elliot, Luther, Andrew Golub, and Eloise Dunlap. "Off the Street and into 'the Cut': Deterrence and Displacement in NYC's Quality of Life Marijuana Policing." *International Journal of Drug Policy* 23 (2012): 210–219.

Ellison, Jared, and Ryan Spohn. "Borders Up in Smoke: Marijuana Enforcement in Nebraska after Colorado's Legalization of Medicinal Marijuana." *Criminal Justice Policy Review* 28, no. 9 (2017): 847–865.

Engel, Robin, Michael R. Smith, and Francis T. Cullen. "Race, Place, and Drug Enforcement: Reconsidering the Impact of Citizen Complaints and Crime Rates on Drug Arrests." *Criminology and Public Policy* 11(2012): 603–635.

England, Marcia. "Stay out of Drug Areas: Drugs, Othering and Regulation of Public Space in Seattle, Washington." *Space and Polity* 12, no. 2 (2008): 197–213.

Holcomb, Jefferson E., et al. "Civil Asset Forfeiture Laws and Equitable Sharing Activity by the Police." *Criminology & Public Policy* 17, no. 1 (2018): 101–127.

King, Ryan S., and Marc Mauer. "The War on Marijuana: The Transformation of the War on Drugs in the 1990s." *Harm Reduction Journal* 3, no. 1 (2006): 6.

Reid, Sue T. *Crime and Criminology.* 15th ed. New York: Wolters Kluwer, 2018.

Shoemaker, Donald. *Juvenile Delinquency.* 3rd ed. Lanham, MD: Rowman and Littlefield, 2018.

Ward, Kyle C., Paul A. Lucas, and Alexandra Murphy. "The Impact of Marijuana Legalization on Law Enforcement in States Surrounding Colorado." *Police Quarterly* 22, no. 2 (2019): 217–242.

M

Marihuana Tax Act (1937)

The Marihuana Tax Act of 1937 was the first federal legislation to regulate cannabis at the federal level, and it remained so until the passage of the Controlled Substances Act of 1970. One of the motivations behind the passage of the 1937 legislation was to perpetuate the position that cannabis did not have medical value. Furthermore, the legislation was designed to place a prohibitive tax on cannabis to discourage use.

When the Harrison Narcotic Act of 1914 was being developed, some members of Congress sought to include cannabis as well. However, cannabis was not included in that legislation, for at the time, few people knew what cannabis was or perceived it as a problem (Musto 1999). Indeed, both the National Association of Retail Druggists and the American Pharmaceutical Association opposed cannabis's inclusion within the Harrison Narcotic Act (Bonnie and Whitebread 1999). At that time, the primary uses for cannabis were corn plasters, veterinary medicine, and nonintoxicating medicaments (Musto 1999).

While cannabis would not be regulated at the federal level at that time, many states were enacting legislation that regulated cannabis. A year prior, in 1913, Maine prohibited the sale of cannabis without a prescription. In the next five years, Massachusetts (1914), Vermont (1915), and Rhode Island (1918) enacted similar legislation. By 1937, nearly every state either directly prohibited the recreational use of cannabis or had passed versions of the Uniform Narcotic Act. This act included cannabis as a prohibited substance (Bonnie and Whitebread, 1999).

The two most important individuals in convincing Americans that cannabis was a "demon drug" were Harry Anslinger (1892–1975) and William Randolph Hearst (1863–1951).

Anslinger was the first commissioner of the Federal Bureau of Narcotics, a position he held from 1930 to 1962, while Hearst was a newspaper magnate who ranked as one of the most powerful media figures of the day. Both men spread many wild tales of the effects of cannabis and argued that smoking the drug led to violence and insanity among users. Furthermore, both men tried to associate the plant with Mexican immigrants in order to take advantage of racist sentiments among white Americans. This included even abandoning the English spelling of *marihuana* for the Spanish spelling *marijuana*.

As pressure mounted to enact federal controls on cannabis, some people argued that the proper response was to simply amend the Harrison Narcotic Act and classify it alongside cocaine and opiates. However, such a tactic provided a dilemma. For one, the Harrison Narcotic Act had spawned countless lawsuits and the courts had to consider the constitutionality of the legislation on several occasions including several decisions by the U.S. Supreme Court. Furthermore, some people argued that by including cannabis in the Harrison Narcotic Act it might indicate to some people that the federal government was admitting that cannabis had medical utility—another situation the government hoped to avoid (Bonnie and Whitebread 1999).

In 1937, however, a Supreme Court decision on an unrelated issue—gun control—provided advocates of criminalizing marijuana with guidance for them to follow in crafting a bill. In *Sozinsky v. United States* (1937), the Supreme Court considered the constitutionality of the National Firearms Act. At issue was whether the annual tax on firearms dealers who sold machine guns, silencers, and rifles or shotguns with barrels less than 18 inches was constitutional. Many firearms dealers, angered about the cost of the tax, contended that it was essentially an unconstitutional penalty on their businesses. The Court disagreed, ruling that the legislation was a permissible extension of Congress's national taxing power.

Thus, to regulate cannabis, Congress settled on a $1 tax per ounce of cannabis for people who were registered with the federal government and a $100 tax per ounce for those who were not. In a move that would probably come with little surprise, the federal government allowed few people to register for the lower price. Thus, anyone who wished to purchase cannabis without such approval was forced to pay $100 tax per ounce—a considerable sum of money in that era (Bonnie and Whitebread 1999; Musto 1999). In *United States v. Sanchez et al.* (1950), the Supreme Court upheld the constitutionality of the Marihuana Tax Act (Griffin et al. 2013).

With the passage of the Marihuana Tax Act, federal drug regulators seemingly got what they wanted: it gave no acknowledgment of cannabis as a substance with medically advantageous properties, and it imposed a large tax that discouraged use. However, the legislation did have one problem. Since a person could legally obtain cannabis under the bill's provision, there was no presumption of illegality (at least at the federal level). Thus, if federal law enforcement officers caught a person in possession of cannabis, they could not presume that the people illegally possessed the plant. In *Leary v. United States* (1969) and *United States v. Covington* (1969), the Supreme Court ruled that it violated a person's Fifth Amendment guarantee from compelling self-incrimination if asked by federal law enforcement if the person in possession of cannabis had legally obtained it. The Court ruled differently in the case of a person who had sold cannabis to an undercover police officer. To comply with terms of the Act, any legal sale should have included the proper forms and stamps for a legal purchase (Griffin et al. 2013). The Marihuana Tax Act remained in effect until the passage of the Controlled Substances Act of 1970, which classified cannabis as a Schedule I drug—one deemed by the government to be dangerous and without any recognized medical value.

O. Hayden Griffin, III

See also: Anslinger, Harry (1892–1975); Comprehensive Drug Abuse Prevention and Control Act (1970).

Further Reading

Bonnie, Richard J., and Charles H. Whitebread. *The Marijuana Conviction: A History of Marijuana Prohibition in the United States.* 2nd ed. New York: Lindesmith Center, 1999.

Gahlinger, Paul. *Illegal Drugs: A Complete Guide to their History, Chemistry, Use and Abuse.* New York: Plume, 2004.

Griffin, O. Hayden, Alexis Lynn Fritsch, Vanessa H. Woodward, and Richard S. Mohn. "Sifting through the Hyperbole: One Hundred Years of Marijuana Coverage in the New York Times." *Deviant Behavior* 34 (2013): 767–781.

Musto, David F. *The American Disease: Origins of Narcotic Control.* New York: Oxford University Press, 1999.

Marijuana Opportunity Reinvestment and Expungement Act of 2019 (MORE Act of 2019)

The MORE Act (Marijuana Opportunity Reinvestment and Expungement Act of 2019) was introduced to the U.S. House of Representatives by New York's Democratic Representative Jerrold Nadler on July 23, 2019. The act's main goal is to officially decriminalize marijuana and end its prohibition at the federal level (Congress.GOV 2020). Its passage in the House in December 2020 marked the first time in U.S. history that either chamber of Congress had passed a bill to legalize marijuana at the federal level—though the measure did not become law because the Republican-controlled Senate did not bring the bill for a vote in that chamber.

Marijuana is classified as a Schedule 1 drug under the Comprehensive Drug Abuse Prevention and Control Act of 1970. All Schedule 1 drugs are considered as having high abuse potential and no recognized medical utility. This classification means that marijuana is illegal at the federal level. The MORE Act proposed removing marijuana from the list of scheduled substances, thus eliminating federal criminal penalties for manufacturing, distributing, or possessing marijuana. Currently, the designation of marijuana as a Schedule 1 controlled substance means that federal law conflicts with the laws of 47 states and the District of Columbia in which medical marijuana, recreational marijuana, or both are legal. The MORE Act would have resolved this conflict if it had become law.

In addition to ending the prohibition of marijuana at the federal level by removing marijuana's classification as a "controlled substance," the MORE Act also called to end the current practice of denying federal benefits to a person because of cannabis-related convictions. It also prohibited the denial of benefits and protections under immigration laws because of cannabis-related convictions or involvement in the cannabis industry, provided the industry was operating legally under state laws. The MORE Act also proposed to establish a process to expunge, or erase, convictions for federal marijuana offenses and conduct sentencing review hearings related to federal offenses. In addition, the MORE Act proposed to address several other issues that have hampered the development of the rapidly growing $19 billion cannabis industry (Wallace 2020). For example, cannabis-industry businesses are unable to secure loans or services that other small business often use. The MORE Act included provisions to open Small Business

Administration loans and services available to cannabis-related businesses, provided the business was operating lawfully in states that had legalized marijuana.

The MORE Act also proposed to address the social costs of the War on Drugs, which had disproportionately affected poor communities and communities of color. The MORE Act proposed a 5 percent tax on cannabis products that would be deposited into a trust fund to help pay for programs and services for individuals and businesses in communities impacted by the War on Drugs. Finally, the MORE Act proposed a symbolic change in federal law by requiring all references to *marijuana* or *marihuana* be replaced with *cannabis* and requiring federal agencies to publish demographic data on cannabis business owners and employees (Congress.Gov 2020).

The U.S. House of Representatives passed the bill on Friday, December 4, 2020, with a vote of 228 to 164. This was the first time that a chamber of Congress ever voted on a stand-alone cannabis bill. After passing the House, the bill was sent to the U.S. Senate on December 7, 2020, where it was referred to the Committee on Finance. Since the bill was not signed into law by the time the 116th Congress adjourned on January 3, 2021, the bill will need to be reintroduced. Experts believe it is unlikely the MORE Act will pass in the U.S. Senate (Broker 2020; Wallace 2020); even if the MORE Act does not ultimately pass, however, the passage of the Act in the U.S. House of Representatives is considered a significant and promising milestone by legalization advocates and the legal cannabis industry.

James Hawdon

See also: Comprehensive Drug Abuse Prevention and Control Act (1970); Marihuana Tax Act (1937); Medical Marijuana and the Law; Recreational Marijuana Laws.

Further Reading

Broker, Tyler. "An Historic Vote on the MORE Act." Above the Law, December 7, 2020. https://abovethelaw.com/2020/12/an-historic-vote-on-the-more-act/

Congress.Gov. 2020. "H.R.3884-More Act of 2020." https://www.congress.gov/bill/116th-congress/house-bill/3884

Wallace, Alicia. "Cannabis Got a Big Win in Congress, but Legal Weed Isn't around the Corner." CNN Business, December 4, 2020. https://www.cnn.com/2020/12/04/business/cannabis-more-act-house-vote/index.html

Marijuana Policy Project (MPP)

The Marijuana Policy Project (MPP) was founded in 1995 with the mission to change federal and state laws prohibiting marijuana in favor of state regulations that would be similar in many respects to current laws governing the production, sale, and use of alcohol. Like many other advocacy groups, the organization is formally split into two wings—the MPP itself is primarily responsible for lobbying, and the MPP Foundation is a tax-deductible nonprofit. As a national organization, the group has only provisional ties to specific states, forming ad hoc leadership structures for individual campaigns.

In 2019 alone, MPP had primary responsibility for voter initiatives authorizing medical and legal marijuana in Colorado, Alaska, Maine, Massachusetts, Nevada, and Michigan, as well as a role in California's, Vermont's, and Illinois's policy changes (MPP 2019). With the marijuana industry out in the open, MPP economists have estimated that marijuana could account for over $20 billion in economic activity by 2020 (MPP 2019).

By framing laws criminalizing the use of marijuana as a form of prohibition akin to the early twentieth-century prohibition of alcohol in the United States, MPP has supported widescale efforts to not only end criminal punishment for marijuana possession and use but also expunge all criminal records associated with past marijuana-related infractions. For instance, in Michigan, MPP has supported Governor Gretchen Whitmer's plan to expunge past marijuana convictions. A key aspect of MPP efforts has been to highlight studies, polls, and other resources indicating that marijuana is considered less dangerous than other similar substances such as alcohol and tobacco by medical experts, voters, and public opinion polls. MPP mobilizes around legislative change by tracking state laws, encouraging movement activity in receptive states, and modeling policy reform efforts for other contexts. For instance, MPP offers sample legislation for replacing criminal procedures with civil fines, taxes, and medical regulation (MPP 2019).

Due to its focus on both medical and legal marijuana use, MPP has also been involved in directing public sentiment around changing norms around the shifting status of marijuana. For instance, while earlier efforts focused almost exclusively on decriminalizing marijuana and allowing medical use, MPP has supported efforts to legalize marijuana use for adults, broadly (Fracassa 2017; Khazan 2018). The limited protections offered by medical institutions enabled the movement of the marijuana industry from illicit to a partially legal realm. However, MPP has continued to push for federal change and a widespread shift to a fully legalized but sensibly regulated recreational marijuana industry.

Given the support for these policies at a state level, under the Obama administration, U.S. agencies de-emphasized enforcing federal laws criminalizing marijuana prohibition. In 2018, Attorney General Sessions reversed this policy; however, the majority of enforcement actions by the Trump administration have been limited to immigration policy. Without legislative change at the federal level, both medical and recreational economies at the state level remain at risk. There is growing bipartisan support for legislation, such as the "Strengthening the Tenth Amendment through Entrusting States (STATES)" Act, which capitalizes on conservatives' support for states' rights with a widespread liberal approach to dismantling marijuana prohibition (Matthews and Staggs 2018).

Mario Alberto V. Espinoza-Kulick and Alex Espinoza-Kulick

See also: Alaska; California; Colorado; Medical Marijuana and the Law.

Further Reading

Dockray, Heather. "4/20 Isn't Just a 'Stoner' Holiday. It's an Opportunity for Activism." Mashable, April 20, 2019. https://mashable.com/article/legal-marijuana-activism/

Fracassa, Dominic. "Some Dispensaries to Require State IDs for Medical Pot Patients." *San Francisco Chronicle,* December 31, 2017. https://www.sfchronicle.com/bayarea/article/Some-dispensaries-to-require-state-sanctioned-IDs-12462675.php

Khazan, Olga. "Did the Trump Administration Just End Medical Marijuana, Too?" *The Atlantic,* January 5, 2018. https://www.theatlantic.com/health/archive/2018/01/sessions-medical-marijuana/549719/

Lowrey, Annie. "America's Invisible Pot Addicts." *The Atlantic,* August 20, 2018. https://www.theatlantic.com/health/archive https://www.theatlantic.com/ideas/archive/2018/08/americas-invisible-pot-addicts/567886/

Marijuana Policy Project (MPP). "Marijuana Policy Project: We Change Laws." 2019. www.mpp.org

Matthews, Mark, and Brooke Staggs. "California's Legalized Marijuana Would Be Federally Lawful under Bill Introduced by Cory Gardner, Elizabeth Warren." The Californian, June 7, 2018. https://www.thecannifornian.com/cannabis-news/nation-world/californias-legalized-marijuana-federally-lawful-bill-introduced-cory-gardner-elizabeth-warren/

Marley, Bob (1945–1981)

Robert Nesta Marley (1945–1981) was a Jamaican Rastafarian musician who famously promoted Rastafarian marijuana use globally through reggae music. Marley's career as a singer and songwriter began in the early 1960s and ended with his death from cancer in 1981. During these decades, he distinguished himself as an advocate for peace, social justice, oppressed groups, and a Jamaican religious movement called Rastafari. Rastafarians perceive marijuana as a sacrament used in spiritual rituals that assist in meditation, philosophy, and understanding the world. Marley's use of marijuana is rooted in his Rastafarian spiritual beliefs. As a Rastafarian, Marley used marijuana as a medium to create music and to encourage people to contemplate religion, politics, social justice, peace, and African anticolonialism—all themes that regularly appeared in his music. Moreover, Marley's impact has been felt long after his death. He left a legacy as a global ambassador for Jamaica, Rastafarianism, resistance movements, anti-imperialism, peace, and marijuana use, and as of 2015, more than 75 million Marley albums have been sold around the world. That same year, *Billboard* magazine asserted that he ranked as "arguably the planet's most-recognized musician" (Meschino 2015). At the same time, his advocacy for marijuana led him to become an enduring global icon for the drug.

Robert Marley was born on February 6, 1945, in Jamaica to a white Englishman and an African Jamaican woman. He spent his adolescent years in Trenchtown, a poor housing development in the urban area of the Jamaican capital of Kingston. He received little formal education, and his upbringing directly exposed him to the problems of poverty, inequality, police brutality, and harassment of Rastafari (primarily due to their use of marijuana). He soon discovered that music was a way that he could escape the suffering of everyday life. Together with his friends Bunny Livingston (Neville O'Riley Livingston) and Peter Tosh (Winston Hubert McIntosh), they formed a reggae group, *The Wailers*. The group signed with small Jamaican labels throughout the 1960s. Bob Marley met his wife, singer Rita Marley (Alfarita Constania Anderson), in Trenchtown in the 1960s; they were married in 1966. Their music began to reach a wider audience when they collaborated with African American musician Johnny Nash. After signing with Island Records in the early 1970s, Marley's music became popular with global audiences. Marley soon came to be renowned as a musical genius, prophet, peacemaker, unifier, troublemaker, advocate for an African homeland for the descendants of slavery, voice for those oppressed under colonialism and neocolonialism, and psalmist for the Rastafarian religion. He became known worldwide as a leading voice for reggae music, Jamaican culture, political and social activism in music, and marijuana use.

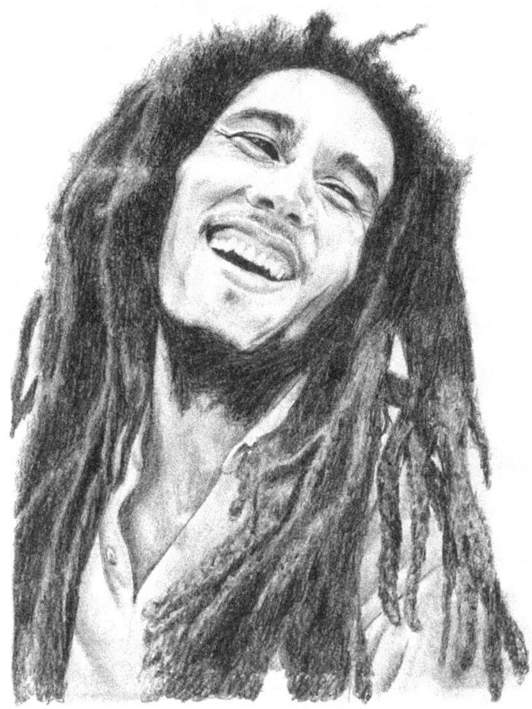

Bob Marley was a pioneer in reggae music, bringing it to an international level. Born in Nine Mile, British Jamaica, in 1945, Marley was the front man and founder of Bob Marley and the Wailers. Marley sang about overcoming oppression and violence as well as calling for the legalization of marijuana. He became a national hero in Jamaica during the late 1970s and after his death in 1981. (Abdul Rahman Rangkuti/Dreamstime.com)

As a practicing Rastafarian, Marley grew his hair in dreadlocks and smoked *ganja* (marijuana). Rastafarianism arose in Jamaica in the 1930s, blending South Asian and Central African beliefs in the Caribbean context. Rastafarians practice weed smoking for spiritual purposes, as a means for bringing themselves closer to the Judeo-Christian God, whom they call Jah. They regarded Emperor Haile Selassie of Ethiopia as God. Furthermore, they view Africa as their true spiritual home and believe that someday they will embark on a spiritual or physical exodus to return there (Farley 2006). They represented an anticolonial, anti-imperial mindset, and Rastafari gradually became the religion of the oppressed, the displaced, and the falsely accused. Rastafarians were social outcasts in Jamaica by the 1970s, often living in the margins of society. Rasta musicians were routinely harassed by the police, since vigorous enforcement of marijuana laws was one of the primary ways the Jamaican government tried to repress the Rastafarian movement. Livingston, Tosh, and Marley all eventually spent time in Jamaican prisons for marijuana offenses (Marley spent a month in jail in 1968 for marijuana possession). The group turned such incidents into material on which they based their songs.

Marley was introduced to Rastafarianism by his spiritual guide Mortimer Planno (Mortimo St George Planno), a Rastafarian elder who influenced his conversion from Catholicism. Planno took Marley to Rastafarian enclaves scattered across Kingston, including Jones Town, where he met members of the Twelve Tribes of Israel, or the twelve sons of the biblical patriarch, Jacob. The Rastafari members spent long hours in discussions of philosophical and theological ideas that were accompanied with praying, drumming, chanting, and smoking. Marley shortly became a member of the Twelve Tribes of Israel under the tribe Joseph. As a Rastafarian, Marley practiced weed smoking for spiritual purposes and for contemplation. Like many Rastas, he believed that marijuana was a "wisdom weed" and was key to achieving world peace and understanding:

> Now, herb is the healing of the nation. Going through all of this alien education that everybody's mind is being programmed, the only way some of us can get away from it is through meditation. The only way you can meditate in a place full of confusion is by using herb. So when you smoke the herb, you can meditate through a lot of traffic, a lot of noise, a lot of this. (quoted in Farley 2007, 152)

Marley further argued, "Herb is not a drug. Herb is a plant that grow. And God made it so that mankind can take it" (quoted in Farley 2007, 152). He used marijuana as an agent to create and write music that was rooted in Rastafarian philosophy and political ideas of his time.

Marley's viewpoints about politics, society, economics, and marijuana use can be seen throughout his music career. His 1972 album *Catch a Fire* helped bring the Wailers to the mainstream and change the way reggae was marketed. Marley and his band targeted American college students and European youths who embraced the genre as well as the radical political messages in his lyrics. Aesthetically, the album made a political statement about the use of marijuana, with an album cover featuring Marley "smoking a large cone-shaped spliff [marijuana cigarette]" (Moskowitz 2007a, 21). His album changed the perceptions of reggae music, the Rastafarian movement and marijuana use.

Marley's 1973 album with the Wailers, *Burnin'*, went even further to reflect interests in Rastafarianism and Jamaican politics. The album cover displayed a picture of Marley, Tosh, Livingston, and others at the front, and the back of the record had another large picture of Marley smoking a large spliff. Lyrically, the album was a call to action to Jamaica's oppressed classes to take charge of their own destinies, because the government was not going to do so. This message was reflected in songs such as "Rasta Man Chant" and "Get Up, Stand Up."

In 1978, Marley released another album that took his marijuana advocacy to a new level. He named his album *Kaya*—a Jamaican term for marijuana. Marley explained, "Kaya means herb. It's a password some of the brethren use in JA [Jamaica]. So 'Kaya' is really dealing with togetherness and humanity and peace, [because] the things of peace travel through the earth now" (quoted in Moskowitz 2007b, 87). The words of the first song on the album, "Easy skankin," begin with the words "cuse [excuse] me while I light my spliff" (Moskowitz 2007a, 48). His title track, "Kaya," was an ode to Rastafari and the use of marijuana by followers of the religion to seek wisdom. The song featured lyrics such as "got to have Kaya now" and alluded to the liberal use of marijuana as empowering (Moskowitz 2007a). His message to the audience is that they must relax, enjoy marijuana, and dance to reggae music.

Marley's use of weed as a ritual sacrament for clarity, truth-seeking, and understanding the world was reflected in his sociopolitical activism. Marley's role as a musician was didactic in other ways, which promoted social, political, or economic justice or Rastafarian teachings. In doing so, Marley helped shift the Rastafarian movement from a strong focus on mysticism and idealism toward real-world social and political activism (Campbell 1987).

Marley also used his music to send out messages about peace and unity. This is exemplified in the One Love Jamaican Peace Concert held in 1978 in Kingston, Jamaica, in which he brought leaders of the Jamaica Labor Party and the People's National Party on stage to help restore peace to the country in a polarizing political environment. It is also reflected in his calls for the liberation and unity of Africa in his music. In particular, his support of Zimbabwe's anticolonial guerilla movement was evident, both in his song "Zimbabwe" and his participation in the inaugural Independence Day celebration in Zimbabwe. At the latter event, Marley sang about Zimbabwe's liberation and also called for the liberation of South Africa from minority rule.

Marley continues to be both a reggae icon and ambassador for marijuana usage. His brand products, which often feature products with his image smoking marijuana, include products such as coffee, audio equipment, apparel, and lifestyle goods. Additionally, his family started also *Marley Natural*, a global marijuana brand in his honor. Products include the Jamaican cannabis strain that Marley himself enjoyed, smoking accessories, creams, lotions, and other marijuana-sourced items.

Sitinga Kachipande

See also: Beatles, The; "420"; Rastafarianism.

Further Reading

Campbell, Horace. *Rasta and Resistance: From Marcus Garvey to Walter Rodney*. Trenton, NJ: Africa New World Press, 1987.

Carrier, Neil, and Gernot Klantschnig. "Quasilegality: Khat, Cannabis and Africa's Drug Laws." *Third World Quarterly* 39 no. 2 (2018): 350–365.

Duvall, Chris. S. *Cannabis*. London, UK: Reaktion Books, 2014.

Farley, Christopher John. *Before the Legend: The Rise of Bob Marley*. New York: Amistad, 2006.

King, Stephen A., and P. Renee Foster. "'No problem, mon': Strategies Used to Promote Reggae Music as Jamaica's Cultural Heritage." *Journal of Nonprofit & Public Sector Marketing* 8 no. 4 (2001): 3–16.

Marley, Bob. *Listen to Bob Marley: The Man, the Music, the Revolution*. New York: Open Road Media, 2012.

Meschino, Patricia. "The Music and Marketing Genius of Bob Marley, 34 Years After His Passing." *Billboard,* May 11, 2015. https://www.billboard.com/articles/business/6561234/music-and-marketing-genius-of-bob-marley-34-years-after-his-passing

Moskowitz, David Vlado. *Bob Marley: A Biography*. Westport, CT: Greenwood Press, 2007a.

Moskowitz, David Vlado. *The Words and Music of Bob Marley*. Westport, CT: Greenwood Publishing Group, 2007b.

Steffens, Roger. *So Much Things to Say: The Oral History of Bob Marley*. New York: WW Norton & Company, 2017.

White, Timothy. *Catch a Fire: The Life of Bob Marley*. London, UK: Macmillan, 2006.

Martha and Snoop's Potluck Dinner Party

Martha and Snoop's Potluck Dinner Party started airing on VH1 in November of 2016. The series is a cooking/talk show combination that brings together some of the most unexpected personalities from across the entertainment industry. But the show is more than just recipes and frivolous banter; *Martha and Snoop* has opened a door through which people from all walks of life can come together, cook a meal, and share a laugh around the dinner table. The appeal of this show stems from the seemingly bizarre pairing of Martha Stewart and Snoop Dogg and their surprisingly genuine friendship.

For more than 30 years, Martha Stewart built an empire of cookbooks, lifestyle magazines, home and kitchen merchandise, and television shows about crafts, gardening, cooking, decorating, and entertaining. Despite a stain on her reputation—felony convictions related to a case of securities fraud and a five-month prison sentence—the Martha Stewart brand is defined by the tastes and spirit of a wealthy, sophisticated, straight-laced white woman from New England, hence, the fascination with her relationship with Snoop Dogg, one of the world's most successful musicians—a gangsta rapper, singer/songwriter, actor, and producer from Long Beach, California, who is also notorious for his longtime love of marijuana. Fans are captivated by the charming juxtaposition of their friendship.

The show's first episode, appropriately titled "Putting the Pot in Potluck" (Stewart et al. 2016), introduces the pair as "The King of Kush and the Queen of Cuisine." From the very beginning, the series promises to bring you "the *best* of high society and the best of *high* society." Throughout the series, marijuana feels like an omnipresent third host of the show. Stewart's unexpected tacit approval of Snoop's marijuana use and the freedom with which the hosts and their guests openly talk about smoking is what makes the show unique.

Each episode begins with a cocktail and demonstration on how to prepare it. Once the beverage is ready, Snoop invites Stewart and the rest of the audience to raise their glasses for a toast. The dinner party begins when the episode's guests arrive—typically well-known entertainers from the worlds of popular music, film, or television. After dinner, Stewart, Snoop, and their guests participate in an icebreaker-style game designed to break down stereotypes and expose surprising similarities. These conversations often revolve around issues of race, class, gender, and sexuality. Fans of the program assert that the inclusivity and intersectionality of the guest list makes it stand out as one of the most diverse on television.

Fans perceive that, among other things, it is Stewart's silent endorsement of marijuana use that leads Snoop and other men of color to often congratulate Martha on becoming a symbolic member of the Black community. Snoop himself often refers to Stewart as "gangsta" as a way to proclaim his respect for her and to honor all the ways she defies the stereotype of an upper-class, privileged, white, professional homemaker.

Martha and Snoop is an unusual type of cooking show as it openly celebrates marijuana consumption. Although she declines every blunt, bong, or brownie that Snoop offers her, Martha welcomes everyone who smokes and is willing to learn the slang, norms, and practices they share. For example, when Martha asked Snoop to help her with a wine decanter, he joked, "Oh, so I get to hit the bong on TV?!" (Stewart et al. 2017b). She explained, "It's sort of like a bong, but not exactly. You need to add this to your bong collection. Snoop gave me a bong last season, and I have it out—I've been using it for flowers. It's really kind of pretty for flowers." Snoop never misses an opportunity to draw parallels between Martha's mealtime instructions and his favorite pastime. "You got to put some greens on your plate, too. You got to have greens with everything you do. Martha taught me that, man. We always smoke 'em, but sometimes you got to eat 'em" (Stewart et al. 2017a). Some observers believe that this casual banter about pot use serves to normalize marijuana consumption, softening the image of marijuana users and giving the audience a window into a subculture that has traditionally been heavily criminalized.

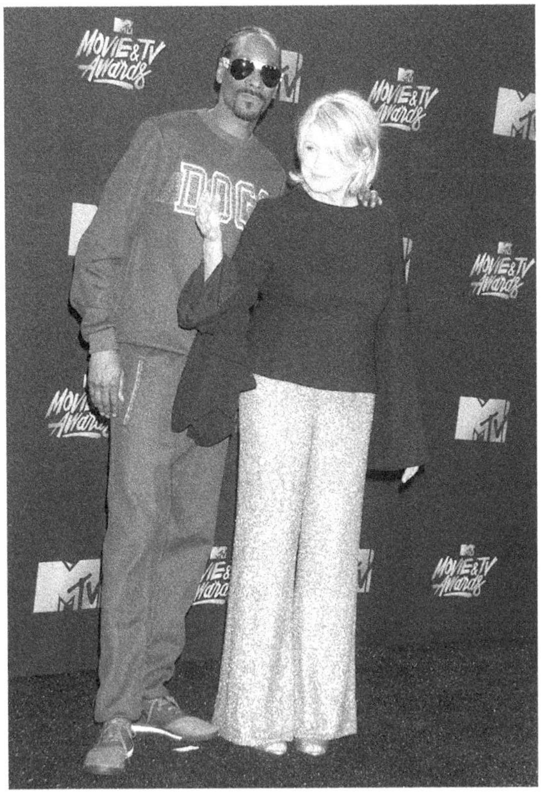

Martha Stewart and Snoop Dogg began hosting Martha and Snoop's Pot Luck Dinner Party in November of 2016. Airing on VH1, it was a combination of cooking and talk show. The series promised viewers the best of Martha Stewart's "high (i.e. rich) society" and Snoop's "high (i.e. stoned) society." (Featureflash/Dreamstime.com)

Martha and Snoop's Potluck Dinner Party had a three-year run (the last as *Martha and Snoop's Potluck Party Challenge*) before broadcasting its last episode in February 2020.

Kristin Richardson

See also: Edibles; Snoop Dogg (1971–).

Further Reading

Grossbart, Sarah. "Inside Snoop Dogg's Fascinating, Unlikely Relationship with Martha Stewart." E! Online, April 3, 2019. https://www.eonline.com/news/1028872/inside-snoop-dogg-s-fascinating-unlikely-relationship-with-martha-stewart

Jean-Philippe, McKenzie. "How Snoop Dogg and Martha Stewart Became the Ultimate Celebrity Best Friends." *O, The Oprah Magazine*, April 8, 2019. https://www.oprahmag.com/entertainment/tv-movies/a27055720/snoop-dogg-martha-stewart-friendship/

Judkis, Maura. "Martha Stewart and Snoop Dogg's Cooking Show Is the Cultural Exchange America Needs." *Chicago Tribune*, October 16, 2017. https://www.chicagotribune.com/lifestyles/home-and-garden/ct-martha-stewart-snoop-dogg-tv-20171016-story.html

Judkis, Maura. "The Buzz is True: Martha Stewart Partners with Canadian Cannabis Company." *Washington Post*, March 1, 2019. https://www.washingtonpost.com/news/voraciously/wp/2019/03/01/the-buzz-is-true-martha-stewart-partners-with-canadian-cannabis-company/

Shapiro, Katie. "Martha Stewart on How Snoop Dogg Got Her into the Cannabis Business, Her New CBD Line, and Aging Well." *Forbes*, June 24, 2019. October 16, 2020. https://www.forbes.com/sites/katieshapiro/2019/06/24/martha-stewart-on-how-snoop-dogg-got-her-into-the-cannabis-business-her-new-cbd-line-and-aging-well/#2097f81456d2

Stewart, Martha, et al. "Joy to the Wizorld!" In *Martha and Snoop's Potluck Dinner Party*. Studio City, CA: Sequential Brands, Merry Jane, and 495 Productions, 2017a.

Stewart, Martha, et al. "Pasta La Vista, Baby." In *Martha and Snoop's Potluck Dinner Party*. Studio City, CA: Sequential Brands, Merry Jane, and 495 Productions, 2017b.

Stewart, Martha, et al. "Putting the Pot in Potluck." In *Martha and Snoop's Potluck Dinner Party*. Studio City, CA: Sequential Brands, Merry Jane, and 495 Productions, 2016.

Maternal Reproductive Health

Maternal reproductive health is a major public health issue in the United States and abroad. Importantly, maternal health is not only linked to individual behavior but to policies and practices enacted at the local and national levels. Marijuana use is one behavior that can have significant impact on a woman's reproductive health.

While recreational use of most drugs has declined over the course of the 2010s, marijuana use has increased. Almost 4 percent of all pregnant women reported using marijuana over the past month in a 2017 national survey, which marks an almost 1.5 percent increase from 2002 (Brown et al. 2017). The reasons for this increase are most frequently attributed to more widespread societal acceptance of marijuana, decriminalization/legalization of pot, and documented health benefits of marijuana use.

Researchers warn, however, that marijuana use by expectant mothers may lead to several health risks. While research into the role of marijuana use in humans, both in the short and long terms, is limited, there is a growing knowledge base on how marijuana impacts fertility, pregnancy, birth, and development. These health risks are generally connected to how marijuana use interrupts appropriate endocrine functioning.

The endocrine system is a collection of glands that produce hormones. Hormones are molecules in the body that are transported via the blood stream to specific organs to regulate physiological functions. These hormones are critical for appropriate body functioning including growth, metabolism, tissue and sexual functioning, sleep, and behavior.

During pregnancy, mothers send blood, oxygen, and nutrients to their unborn child through the placenta. The placenta also regulates fetal development via growth hormones in the endocrine system, including insulin-like growth factor (IGF) and glucocorticoids. Hormones are secreted and delivered to the child through the placenta by the blood stream (Murphy et al. 2006). Given the importance of the endocrine system on human health and development, substances that are influential, either positively or negatively, on this system need to be explored.

Marijuana is considered a teratogen—a substance that can cause disruptions in the development of an embryo by "passing through" the placenta. The active ingredient in marijuana is tetrahydrocannabinol (THC), which affects the body through the endocannabinoid system (ECS). The ECS consists of cannabinoid receptors (named CB1R and CB2R) that increase in activity when THC is consumed and binds with the receptors (Brents 2016).

It is possible that marijuana might have a negative impact on the human endocrine system. THC has been found to disrupt multiple hormonal systems including the adrenal, growth, prolactin, and thyroid systems. THC has also been shown to reduce the level of prolactin production in pregnant females. However, studies do not find consistent evidence for alteration of other hormones (Cservenka, Lahanas, and Dotson-Bossert 2018; Mendelson and Mello 1984). Much of this research has been conducted on nonhuman animals, and extensions of these studies on humans have produced mixed results. Further, there have been differences in the effects of marijuana in humans based on the frequency of use (short- or long-term use) and tolerance. Keeping this in mind, some research does show some negative consequences of marijuana use on the human endocrine system.

To begin, marijuana has been found to disrupt normal ovulation and hormone secretion. This ovulation irregularity has been linked to increased infertility. Additionally, THC's impact on the ECS increases the chance of ectopic pregnancy and miscarriage. In one study, mothers who smoked marijuana during pregnancy were twice as likely to have a stillbirth. Interestingly, the impact of marijuana on infertility might actually decrease over time as tolerance develops (Brents 2016).

In pregnancies resulting in birth, marijuana has been shown to decrease gestational length. In one study, mothers who consumed marijuana gave birth up to 2.2 weeks earlier, on average, than non-marijuana consumers. Marijuana consumers were also more likely to have preterm labor, which is defined as birth after less than 37 weeks' gestation (Brents 2016). Over the life course, individuals who were exposed to THC in utero are also more likely to experience long-term negative consequences including inattention, impulsivity, antisocial behavior, cognitive impairment, and learning deficits (Huizink and Mulder 2006).

To date, research on the effects of marijuana on human growth and development is rare. Part of this is due to the difficulty of using humans in scientific experiments (randomly assigning people into groups of smokers and nonsmokers), but nonexperimental designs have shed light on potential negative consequences of marijuana use during pregnancy. However, this use has not been definitively linked to abnormal child development in humans. More research on marijuana and its influence on endocrine system functioning is needed.

Chad Posick

See also: Dependence; Gender; Medical Uses; Tetrahydrocannabinol (THC).

Further Reading

Brents, Lisa K. "Focus: Sex and Gender Health: Marijuana, the Endocannabinoid System and the Female Reproductive System." *The Yale Journal of Biology and Medicine* 89, no. 2 (2016): 175.

Brown, Qiana L., et al. "Trends in Marijuana Use among Pregnant and Nonpregnant Reproductive-aged Women, 2002–2014." *JAMA* 317, no. 2 (2017): 207–209.

Cservenka, Anita, Sarah Lahanas, and Julieanne Dotson-Bossert. "Marijuana Use and Hypothalamic-Pituitary-Adrenal Axis Functioning in Humans." *Frontiers in Psychiatry* 9 (2018): 472.

Huizink, Anja C., and Eduard J.H. Mulder. "Maternal Smoking, Drinking or Cannabis Use during Pregnancy and Neurobehavioral and Cognitive Functioning in Human Offspring." *Neuroscience & Biobehavioral Reviews* 30, no. 1 (2006): 24–41.

Mendelson, Jack H., and Nancy K. Mello. "Effects of Marijuana on Neuroendocrine Hormones in Human Males and Females." *NIDA Research Monograph Series* 44 (1984): 97–114.

Murphy, Vanessa E., Roger Smith, Warwick B. Giles, and Vicki L. Clifton. "Endocrine Regulation of Human Fetal Growth: The Role of the Mother, Placenta, and Fetus." *Endocrine Reviews* 27, no. 2 (2006): 141–169.

Medical Marijuana and the Law

Medical marijuana refers to using the marijuana plant, or its extracts, as medical treatment for various ailments. Medical marijuana has been shown to have a positive impact when used for treatment of certain diseases and illnesses. However, long-term use and misuse of some cannabinoids extracted from marijuana may have serious health-related consequences. The legality of medical marijuana use varies greatly by state, although many states have passed laws legalizing medical marijuana since 2010. Due to a lack of quality research and mixed findings, however, the U.S. Food and Drug Administration (FDA) has only approved a handful of cannabis-related medications.

Marijuana has been used as medicine by people from all parts of the world for centuries. The ancient Chinese used marijuana to treat problems related to loss of appetite and digestive issues (Marion 2018, 164). The Greeks, Egyptians, Africans, and Romans all also used marijuana to treat a myriad of both serious and minor health-related problems including gout, foot pain, hemorrhoids, malaria, and snake bites (Marion 2018, 165). In the United States, Christopher Columbus was said to have brought various strains of cannabis with him on the *Mayflower*, and marijuana was readily prescribed as a pain reliever by medical professionals until the end of the nineteenth century. In fact, marijuana was listed as a recognized medicine in the *United States Pharmacopeia* from 1850 to 1942. However, Marijuana was classified as a Schedule 1 drug under the Comprehensive Drug Abuse Prevention and Control Act (Controlled Substance Act) of 1970. As such, currently, the United States Drug Enforcement Agency (DEA) considers marijuana to be a substance that has a high potential for abuse and no accepted medial value.

The alleged medicinal benefits of marijuana have received increased attention, however, since that 1970 classification. With the passing of the Compassionate Use Act in 1996, California became the first state to permit the use of marijuana for medicinal purposes since 1970 (Pacula and Smart 2017, 402). As of November 2020, 35 states, the District of Columbia, Guam, Puerto Rico, and the U.S. Virgin Islands had all passed legislation that permits the medicinal use of marijuana

(National Conference of State Legislatures 2020). Typically, these laws set regulations on who can grow, cultivate, sell, and purchase marijuana-related medications. The approved drug products are available only to those who receive a "prescription" (e.g., recommendation) from a licensed health-care provider. Further, most statutes require that marijuana be purchased from a licensed dealer and prohibits, or restricts, individual growth of the plant. Medical marijuana is not paid for by health insurance providers because federal law still prohibits the possession and use of the drug.

The federal U.S. government has, generally speaking, conceded to state law and not pushed back against states legalizing medical marijuana. The FDA has also approved two medications containing cannabinoids—dronabinol and nabilone (National Institute on Drug Abuse 2020). Both of these medications are used to help increase appetites among patients suffering from weight loss caused by chemotherapy and AIDS.

The medicinal effects of marijuana come from cannabinoids, which are chemicals found in cannabis. Scientists have found more than 100 different cannabinoids in the marijuana plant. Cannabinoids bind to cannabinoid receptors located in the body, which then produce a variety of effects, many of which are still being studied. Cannabinoids can be extracted from the marijuana plant and used to create medications (National Institute on Drug Abuse 2020).

REGULATING CANNABINOIDS

The two main cannabinoids that are of medical interest are delta-9-tetrahydrocannabinol (THC) and cannabidiol (CBD). THC is the chemical in marijuana that produces the euphoric feeling that many users experience and associate with the "high." From a medical perspective, THC can increase appetite and reduce pain, inflammation, and nausea. CBD lacks the psychoactive properties that THC has, and CBD has a much broader medical use (Pacula and Smart 2017, 405). Further, in clinical trials CBD has been found to produce a therapeutic effect while also countering the psychoactive effects of THC. As such, many states have begun implementing CBD-only laws, which restrict the medical use of marijuana to medications in which CBD is the active cannabinoid (Pacula and Smart 2017, 405).

The affect particular strains of marijuana have on a user vary due to the ratio of THC to CBD found in each strain. The marijuana plant has been found to have over 400 constituent chemicals, each of which can produce different effects on the body (Atakan 2012, 241–254). These effects can further be altered by the method of consumption (e.g., inhalation via smoking, inhalation via vaporizing, oral ingestion). Consuming marijuana edibles allows for a slower and less potent intake of the cannabinoids. When inhaled, however, the chemicals are able to travel through the bloodstream and reach the brain much more quickly, leading to a more intense physiological reaction—especially in strains that are high in THC.

Medical marijuana is becoming a popular treatment for a variety of ailments including AIDS, alcohol withdrawal, Alzheimer's disease, cancer, depression, fibromyalgia, glaucoma, high blood pressure, insomnia, multiple sclerosis, nausea, neuropathic discomfort, vomiting, seizures, and general pain management.

The efficacy of marijuana as treatment varies greatly by condition. Marijuana acts on two neurotransmitters; the first is located in the central nervous system and the second is active during the inflammatory response. For patients using medical marijuana to treat glaucoma, it has been shown to reduce intraocular pressure. Further, by stimulating the production of prostaglandins (lipids produced in areas where there is infection or damage to tissue), marijuana is able to alter muscle contractions, reduce inflammation, modify blood pressure, and produce various other physiological effects. Due to these effects on the nervous system, medical marijuana usage is noted as an effective treatment for two types of epilepsy, Dravet syndrome and Lennox-Gastaut syndrome (Food and Drug Administration 2018).

Marijuana has been found to alleviate various forms of chronic pain, including pain experienced from fibromyalgia and rheumatoid arthritis. It has also been shown to be an effective treatment for multiple sclerosis. Additionally, research indicates that medical marijuana is a promising treatment for side effects associated with chemotherapy. These positive effects come from its ability to stimulate appetite, relieve nausea, and alleviate pain. For chronic illnesses such as HIV and AIDS, smoking marijuana can help increase weight and reduce nausea. Marijuana extracts have also been found to help shrink and kill certain types of cancer cells and to improve the behavior and appetite of Alzheimer's patients.

There are, however, several adverse side effects associated with the use of medical marijuana. Short-term side effects include impaired coordination, memory, and judgment; paranoia; and psychosis. Consequently, driving while under the influence of marijuana is not recommended due to these side effects. Some strains of marijuana have also been found to exacerbate mental health conditions, especially when taken by adolescents. Other short-term side effects may include anxiety, nausea, hallucinations, and dry mouth.

Long-term side effects include insomnia, increased anxiety and irritability, altered brain development, cognitive impairments, poor educational outcomes, psychosis, chronic bronchitis, and diminished perceptions of quality of life. Further, there is some research suggesting that marijuana may be addictive—at least psychologically (National Institute on Drug Abuse 2020). Withdrawal symptoms from long-term marijuana use are reported to be similar to those experienced from discontinuing tobacco use and include insomnia, anxiety, intense cravings, and irritability. It is estimated that approximately four million people have symptoms of marijuana dependency (National Survey on Drug Use and Health 2020).

Jenae McGill and Nathan E. Kruis

See also: Anxiety; Casual Users, Health Effects; Medical Uses; Mental Illness; Neurological Effects.

Further Reading

Atakan, Zerrin. "Cannabis, a Complex Plant: Different Compounds and Different Effects on Individuals." *Therapeutic Advances in Psychopharmacology* 2, no. 6 (September 2012): 241–254.

Food and Drug Administration (FDA). "FDA Approves First Drug Comprised of an Active Ingredient Derived from Marijuana to Treat Rare, Severe Forms of Epilepsy." 2018. https://www.fda.gov/news-events/press-announcements/fda-approves-first-drug-comprised-active-ingredient-derived-marijuana-treat-rare-severe-forms

Marion, Nancy E. *Drug Policy and the Criminal Justice System*. Durham, NC: Carolina Academic Press, 2018.

National Conference of State Legislatures (NCSL). "State Medical Marijuana Laws." 2020. https://www.ncsl.org/research/health/state-medical-marijuana-laws.aspx

National Institute on Drug Abuse (NIDA). "Is Marijuana Addictive?" 2020. https://www.drugabuse.gov/publications/research-reports/marijuana/marijuana-addictive.

National Survey on Drug Use and Health. *Results from the 2018 National Survey on Drug use and Health*. Substance Abuse and Mental Health Services Administration. Office of Applied Studies, 2020. https://www.samhsa.gov/data/sites/default/files/cbhsq-reports/NSDUHDetailedTabs2018R2/NSDUHDetailedTabs2018.pdf

Pacula, Rosalie Liccardo, and Rosanna Smart. "Medical Marijuana and Marijuana Legalization." *Annual Review of Clinical Psychology* 13, no. 1 (May 2017): 397–419.

Medical Uses

Historically, marijuana has been used to treat a wide array of illnesses across a multitude of cultures. However, around the early 1900s, marijuana was criminalized, later classified as a Schedule 1 drug at the onset of the War on Drugs (1971). This classification not only made any type of medical use or prescription illegal but also placed substantial limitations on the ability to conduct research on potential uses of marijuana for medical conditions. In the twenty-first century, however, public opinion has slowly but steadily shifted toward a more favorable view of marijuana, and as of 2020, it has been legalized for medicinal and/or recreational use in several states. In fact, marijuana is being used to treat glaucoma, wasting syndrome, nausea, pain, migraines, Parkinson's disease, ALS, epilepsy, and dementia. However, studies of its effectiveness are largely inconclusive, and more research is needed to determine what level of utility actually exists.

The use of cannabis for healing ailments is speculated to predate history, with some of the first accounts of its use found in Chinese medicine, ancient Egyptian society, and Indian Ayurvedic, an ancient form of healing science. Cannabis pollen was said to have been found on the mummy of the Egyptian pharaoh Ramesses II, and there are some arguments that the anointing oil used by Jesus was cannabis based. In all of these cultures, as well as Persian, French, Roman, Greek, British, and American societies, marijuana has been utilized for the treatment of glaucoma, gout, rheumatism, vomiting/nausea, parasitic infections, muscle spasms, menstrual cramps, diabetes, dysentery, diarrhea, hay fever, leprosy, incontinence, convulsive disorders, insanity, excessive menstrual bleeding/uterine bleeding, tetanus, typhus, arthritis, inflammation, malaria, edema, earaches, cramped joints, and chronic ulcers. It has also been used in various cultures as both an anesthetic and an analgesic. Cannabis has reportedly been used to help both suppress sexual longing and treat impotence, to stimulate the appetite, and to suppress it. Marijuana has also been used for a variety of mental ailments such as relief from anxiety, help in concentration, as a counter to alcohol and opiate addictions, and to fight insomnia and absentmindedness. By the time marijuana made its way into the American colonies, Pharmacopeia, a text listing medicinal drugs, their effects, and directions for use, patented tinctures were sold to treat ailments

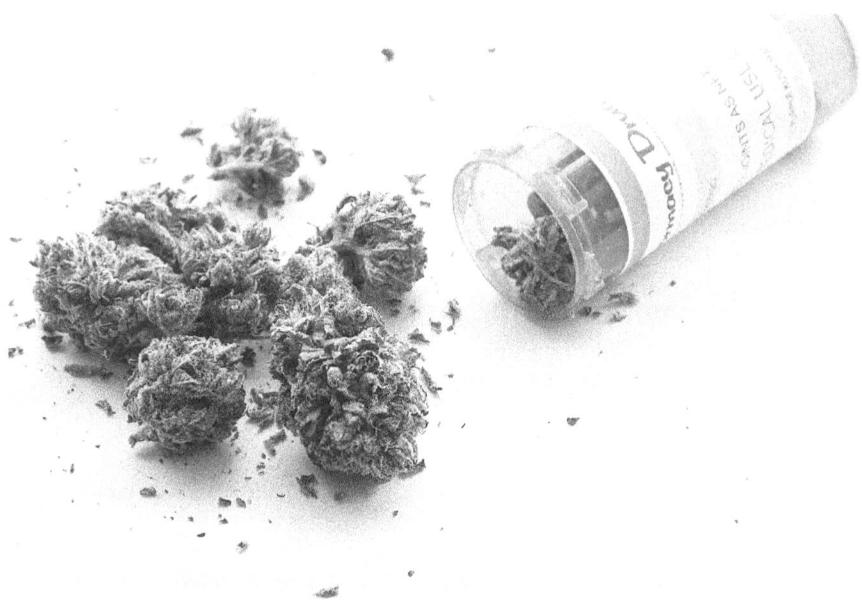

Prescription-grade medical marijuana. States began legalizing medical marijuana in 1996 and 36 states legalized it by 2020. Marijuana is commonly used to treat glaucoma, nausea, pain, anxiety, and a host of other aliments. (Atomazul/Dreamstime.com)

including rabies, and one manufacturer was marketing marijuana cigarettes as a remedy for asthma.

However, the moral panic that led to the passage of the Federal Marijuana Tax Act in 1937 began a shift away from the dispensing of cannabis for medical purposes by physicians and pharmacists. Though this law did not legally prohibit medical distribution, it made physician reporting requirements so cumbersome that it discouraged them from doing so and led to a decline in prescriptions. In 1942, marijuana was removed from the U.S. Pharmacopeia.

With the passage of the Federal Controlled Substance Act of 1970, cannabis was defined as a Schedule 1 substance. This classified it with drugs such as heroin and LSD as a controlled substance with no acceptable medical use, no safe level of use, and a high risk of abuse and addiction. The law also made both recreational and medical use of marijuana illegal and created barriers to researching potential medical benefits of marijuana. For example, any cannabis that is to be used for research in the United States must be obtained from the NIDA (National Institute on Drug Abuse) Drug Supply Program. While this may not be problematic in and of itself, NIDA's mission is focused on understanding the causes and consequences of drug use and addiction rather than possible therapeutic uses of drugs. Moreover, the institute also funds the majority of NIH (National Institute of Health) sponsored cannabis research. As a result, funding for research on the medical utility of marijuana is difficult to obtain. In addition to obtaining the cannabis to study, researchers also need approval from a variety of local, state, and federal agencies, institutions, or organizations. The difficulty in successfully navigating these hurdles can discourage many researchers from applying for grant funding or pursuing research efforts over the years.

All of the cannabis provided by NIDA to investigators is sourced from the University of Mississippi, which has been the sole source for such research since 1968. This is problematic because the cannabis available from the University of Mississippi may not include the types and variety of cannabis currently used in the general population, may not have comparable potency, and may be old and have been stored for years (which could also reduce potency) due to restrictions on production and the ebb and flow of supply and demand. Therefore, research done using this product may not relate to other contexts.

In the last decade, changes in policy at the state level and the more widespread acceptance of cannabis use have increased interest in its potential as a medical treatment for an array of conditions. However, cannabis remains illegal at the federal level, and the feral government continues to enforce strict regulations that limit research that could illuminate both therapeutic and adverse effects of marijuana use. Without this research, there is a lack of evidence-based information available to patients, health-care providers, and policy-makers that would allow them to make the best decisions possible regarding the use of marijuana for medical treatment. Despite these obstacles, however, some research has been completed, and medical marijuana is once again being used to treat a variety of illnesses, some of which have evidence to support claims of success in treatment and some of which do not.

Medical marijuana can be administered through smoking, vaporization, eating, tinctures, or salves. Medical marijuana is currently prescribed to some patients as an analgesic (for migraines and general pain relief), to ease nausea and vomiting after chemotherapy, and to stimulate patients' appetites in wasting illnesses (HIV/AIDS patients, dementia/Alzheimer's patients, and anorexics)—although this latter use is contentious. Advocates also assert that marijuana can relieve symptoms of neurological disorders, including muscle spasticity in patients with multiple sclerosis or spinal cord injuries, tremors and other movement disorders in patients suffering from Parkinson's disease, Huntington's disease or Tourette's syndrome, and epilepsy.

It also has been utilized in the treatment of glaucoma and mental illnesses such as anxiety, depression, and post-traumatic stress disorder (PTSD). Because cannabinoids are believed to serve as an anti-inflammatory and boost the immune system, there is an interest in using them to decrease and potentially alter the course of neurodegenerative conditions, such as dementia. Similarly, amyotrophic lateral sclerosis (ALS), which has no existing curative treatment, appears to be affected by neuroinflamation and immune dysregulation, making cannabis of interest as a potential treatment. Research with mice has shown slower progression of the disease with synthetic marijuana, but these findings have yet to be translated to treatment in humans.

The FDA has only approved two cannabinoids for the treatment of nausea and appetite stimulation as of 2020, and high-quality evidence exists only for the use of marijuana to treat chronic pain, neuropathic, pain, and spasticity associated with multiple sclerosis. Other indications have inconclusive research or have revealed potential health risks such as worsening of psychiatric illnesses, alongside the potential benefits.

Christine McCown

See also: Anxiety; Chronic Pain; Medical Marijuana and the Law; Mental Health; Mental Illness; Moral Panics.

Further Reading

Briscoe, Joshua, and David Casarett. "Medical Marijuana Use in Older Adults." *Journal of the American Geriatrics Society 66*, no. 5 (2018): 859–863.

Carliner, Hannah, Qiana L. Brown, Aaron L. Sarvet, and Deborah S. Hasin. "Cannabis Use, Attitudes, and Legal Status in the U.S.: A Review." *Preventive Medicine* 104 (2017): 13–23.

Compton, Michael T. *Marijuana and Mental Health*. Arlington, VA: American Psychiatric Association Publishing, 2016.

Eversman, Michael H. "Feeding on Fear: Edible Marijuana and Disproportionality in US Media." *Drugs: Education, Prevention & Policy* 23 no. 6 (2016): 462–470.

Hill, Kevin P. "Medical Marijuana for Treatment of Chronic Pain and Other Medical and Psychiatric Problems: A Clinical Review." *JAMA: Journal of the American Medical Association* 313 no. 24 (2015): 2474.

National Academies of Sciences, Engineering, and Medicine. *The Health Effects of Cannabis and Cannabinoids: The Current State of Evidence and Recommendations for Research*. Washington, DC: National Academies Press, 2017.

"Reports on Marijuana Usage Findings from Columbia University Provide New Insights (Use of Marijuana Exclusively for Medical Purposes)." *Mental Health Weekly Digest*, March 18, 2019: 434. https://www.worldcat.org/title/mental-health-weekly-digest/oclc/240898026

Vigil, Daniel I., Mike Van Dyke, Katelyn E. Hall, Alexandra Elyse Contreras, Tista S. Ghosh, and Larry Wolk. "Marijuana Use and Related Health Care Encounters in Colorado before and After Retail Legalization." *International Journal of Mental Health and Addiction*, no. 4: (2018): 806.

Warf, Barney. "High Points: An Historical Geography of Cannabis." *The Geographical Review*, no. 4 (2012): 414.

Mental Health

The impact of marijuana use on mental health remains largely unknown. Evidence suggests that marijuana slows down cognitive function, impacts short-term memory, and reduces inhibition (Compton 2016; Hill 2015). While some evidence ties marijuana use to a reduction of anxiety and improvement in mood (Iversen 2019), other researchers have found evidence that marijuana can cause anxiety and trigger panic attacks (Eversman 2016; Hill 2015). Still other findings suggest that marijuana may actually cause/contribute to suicide and psychosis (Eversman 2016; Hill 2015; Briscoe and Casarett 2018). The reasons for these varied findings lie just as much with the variation in methods of sampling and measurement as they do with the variations in individuals who use it—cannabis has varied effects on different people (Zablocki et al. 1991). In order to reach more definitive conclusions, additional research needs to be conducted.

Existing evidence suggests that marijuana use may impact mental health both positively and negatively. Initially, marijuana intoxication is associated with euphoria and heightened perception, while higher doses may lead to decreased motor activity, relaxation, and a sense of calm (Iversen 2019). In fact, relaxation and relief of anxiety are the most commonly reported motivations for using marijuana, and some evidence indicates that cannabidiol (CBD) found in marijuana even has antipsychotic properties (Iversen 2019; Walsh et al. 2017). Other studies have found increases in positive self-concept associated with marijuana use, suggesting a similarity to positive psychological benefits that occur with moderate use of alcohol (Zablocki et al. 1991). Some research recommends the use of marijuana to improve mood and sense of well-being among those with medical conditions.

Research studies, however, have also found that marijuana intoxication can negatively impact cognitive assessment in such areas as short-term memory and attention, ability to retain information, motor coordination, and judgment. Some methods of administration and high doses of tetrahydrocannabinol (THC), the main psychoactive compound that causes the "high" sensation so closely associated with marijuana consumption, may also cause anxiety, confusion, hallucination, paranoid ideation, unpleasant perception distortions, and psychotic symptoms. Early adolescent use among these younger individuals (whose brains are still developing) may negatively impact IQ and increase the risk of anxiety and depression in adulthood (Compton 2016; Hill 2015).

Regular marijuana use is associated with an increased risk of depression, anxiety, and psychotic illness—though the direction of this association is unclear, marijuana use can worsen these conditions, so use of medical marijuana (or recreational) must be monitored closely (Walsh et al. 2017). Similarly, marijuana dependence is associated with psychosis and the onset of schizophrenia, but causality remains unclear. Withdrawal symptoms from cessation of regular marijuana use may also be detrimental to mental health and can include anxiety, irritability, insomnia, dysphoria, and craving (Compton 2016; Hill 2015).

According to some research, there is a greater risk of suicide associated with chronic marijuana use. However, the direction of causality is again unknown, and like most previously mentioned indications for mental health, the findings are conflicting (Briscoe and Casarett 2018). Some studies tentatively show a decreased rate of suicide among males who are registered users of medical marijuana (Walsh et al. 2017), and others indicate that suicide typically occurs among younger individuals who have a history of chronic abuse (Briscoe and Casarett 2018). This finding has not been duplicated among individuals utilizing medicinal marijuana in a responsible fashion, and cannabis use has not been shown to increase the risk of self-harm or harm to others (Briscoe and Casarett 2018).

Existing research has focused primarily on negative consequences associated with illicit nonmedical use of cannabis, which is difficult to generalize to those using marijuana for therapeutic purposes. Regardless of whether use is medical or recreational, it has been suggested that marijuana use is not associated in the same way for all users. It fulfills a variety of functions such as coping with environmentally induced stress, masking the discomfort of preexisting psychological difficulties, the desire to enhance sensory pleasure, or simply use in a recreational capacity (Compton 2016; Hill 2015; Zablocki et al. 1991). As such, these individuals may experience the drug differently and may, as a result of these varying purposes and experiences, feel very different positive and/or negative emotions than one another (Zablocki et al. 1991).

Research has shown that the association between mental health and marijuana use differs between subgroups of users based upon not only the desired function of the drug but also the different characteristics of the users. For example, individuals with highly introspective personalities have been shown to experience psychological distress when using marijuana, as opposed to those with low introspectiveness who experience more perceptual distortions and sensorimotor sensations (Zablocki et al. 1991). Like other medications, older adults may be more sensitive to adverse effects of marijuana—this subgroup has not been examined (Briscoe and Casarett 2018).

Mental health, itself, has social determinants, and those factors (the circumstances surrounding a person's socialization and environment) have impacts on marijuana and other substance use (Compton 2016). While many studies show marijuana use being associated with higher rates of distress, marijuana use is also associated with instability in adult role performance and the use of other illicit drugs. This makes it difficult to separate the effects of cannabis from other drugs and to determine whether or not the psychological distress is a symptom of the marijuana use (or other drugs) or the role instability. Because early-onset long-term marijuana use can impact IQ and has been linked to poor school performance, marijuana use can, in turn, impact social determinants of mental health. If educational outcomes are affected, there might be an impact on employment status or income, which may in turn have an effect on an individual's sense of well-being or life satisfaction (Compton 2016).

Therefore, while marijuana use can have an impact on mental health, it is challenging to separate those impacts from other social, biological, and psychological factors. Marijuana has been associated with mental health problems, but does not by itself cause or cure them. Rather, it is a component cause—not necessary for the illness to develop and insufficient to cause it by itself. So, while marijuana use doubles the risk of schizophrenia in adolescent users, that may be more problematic for high-risk youth (adolescents with a family history of psychosis or environmental contributors such as a history of child abuse), and individuals who fall into that category might consider abstaining from use (Walsh et al. 2017; Compton 2016).

Alternative explanations for the association between marijuana and mental health problems include the self-medication hypothesis (people with symptoms of mental illness seek out marijuana to relieve them or decrease the unpleasant side effects of their medications), the hastening hypothesis (marijuana use hastens/speeds up the onset of psychosis in individuals who were genetically prone to developing the disorder at some point), and the shared diathesis model (genetic or other factors predispose the same individuals to mental illness and to marijuana or other drug abuse).

Mood disorders (major depressive disorder and bipolar disorder) and anxiety disorders (including social anxiety disorder, panic disorder, and generalized anxiety disorder) are the most prevalent psychiatric disorders across age groups. Marijuana is the most commonly used illicit drug. Therefore, comorbidity is highly likely and of interest, not only as a potential cause but also as a potential treatment.

Christine McCown

See also: Anxiety; Medical Uses; Mental Illness.

Further Reading

Briscoe, Joshua, and David Casarett. "Medical Marijuana Use in Older Adults." *Journal of the American Geriatrics Society66*, no. 5 (2018): 859–863.

Compton, Michael T. *Marijuana and Mental Health.* 1st ed. Arlington, VA: American Psychiatric Association Publishing, 2016.

Eversman, Michael H. 2016. "Feeding on Fear: Edible Marijuana and Disproportionality in US Media." *Drugs: Education, Prevention & Policy* 23 no. 6 (2016): 462–470.

Eversman, Michael H., and Jason D. P. Bird. "Moral Panic and Social Justice: A Guide for Analyzing Social Problems." *Social Work* 62 no. 1 (2017): 29.

Hill, Kevin P. "Medical Marijuana for Treatment of Chronic Pain and Other Medical and Psychiatric Problems: A Clinical Review." *JAMA: Journal of the American Medical Association 313* no. 24 (2015): 2474.

Iversen, Leslie. *The Science of Marijuana.* New York: Oxford University Press, 2019.

Walsh, Zach, et al. "Medical Cannabis and Mental Health: A Guided Systematic Review." *Clinical Psychology Review 51* (2017):15–29.

Zablocki, B., A. Aidala, S. Hansell, and H. White. "Marijuana Use, Introspectiveness, and Mental Health." *Journal of Health and Social Behavior 32* no. 1 (1991): 65–79.

Mental Illness

Medical marijuana has been used to treat mental illnesses including depression, anxiety, post-traumatic stress disorder (PTSD), bipolar disorder, psychosis/schizophrenia, and anorexia. However, due to confounding effects of not knowing whether self-treating the symptoms of mental illness with marijuana or the use of marijuana came first, caution should be used in treating individuals with mental illnesses and more research should be conducted—specifically to include individuals who have only used marijuana in the medical sense as opposed to also using it recreationally. Additionally, caution should be exercised as the effects of the drug differ by person, based on various factors (Compton 2016).

Marijuana has proven to be beneficial in treating various physical ailments, so its utility in treating mental illnesses is worth exploring. However, concerns have been raised, especially by individuals and organizations opposed to the legalization of marijuana, that the drug may worsen these conditions and, in some cases, even have a causal association with them. As it stands, mental health conditions are one of the most prominent reasons for medical cannabis and self-prescribed recreational cannabis use.

People who have anxiety disorders may experience a wide array of symptoms—and because it affects individuals so differently it can be difficult to determine the best course of treatment. Some studies suggest that marijuana can reduce symptoms of anxiety and help with sleep. Others suggest that, depending on the individual, marijuana can enhance symptoms and potentially cause greater anxiety. Research on treatment of PTSD with cannabis has been the most promising with potential for improving sleep and reducing flashbacks for treatment-resistant patients. However, there is concern that the effects of cannabis on PTSD may be similar to those of anxiety (with potential for worsening symptoms rather than relieving them) and that treating a marijuana addiction among PTSD patients would prove to be very challenging.

Some studies have found that those who use medical marijuana once a week or less had less depression, more positive effects, and fewer complaints about body aches and pains than nonusers. Other studies have shown little evidence of medicinal marijuana doing anything to help with depressive symptoms. Still other studies have shown that heavy habitual marijuana use increased the risk of subsequent depressive episodes, including suicidal ideation and attempts. Bipolar disorder has had some success in being treated with marijuana, and medical marijuana has been used as a supplement to lithium to allow for reduced consumption or for relief of the side effects produced by lithium. Marijuana also offers a more natural alternative in treatment for patients who might want to avoid the side effects of lithium and other drugs altogether. However, other studies indicate that marijuana may exacerbate mood disorder symptoms. Bipolar disorder and marijuana use are both associated with cognitive impairment, and it is unclear whether combining marijuana with bipolar disorder would enhance that impairment. Some findings indicate that it alleviates symptoms, while others find it to be confounding.

Marijuana that is available via dispensaries is generally high in THC, which makes it risky for those with psychotic disorders to use. Higher concentrations of THC have been linked to intensified symptoms of psychosis, so those who have a disorder or are at risk of the disorder should consider avoiding it.

Anorexia nervosa is a psychiatric disorder in which individuals experience body dysmorphia and starve themselves. Individuals who suffer from anorexia have been treated with marijuana in the hopes of increasing hunger in order to avoid excessive weight loss and more severe impacts on physical health. Unfortunately, THC has not proven effective in this endeavor. In fact, some studies have shown that increasing the appetite actually intensifies the conflict between food refusal and hunger and causes more dysmorphia and emotional anguish. These patients may also have underlying psychiatric disorders that could potentially make the use of cannabis even more ill advised.

Conflicting evidence exists concerning whether mental health is positively or negatively associated with marijuana use. Additionally, different people have different reasons for using marijuana. These motivations may impact their experience of the drug in either a positive or negative way, just as much as the extent and characteristics of their mental illness (if present) and the social factors surrounding it. Existing research has focused primarily on negative consequences associated with illicit nonmedical use of cannabis, making it of limited usefulness in studying the effects of marijuana that is used for therapeutic purposes (see Compton 2016). There are also interactions between some pharmaceuticals and marijuana. Marijuana can cause hypomania when combined with some antidepressants and have an additive affect when mixed with alcohol and other depressants.

All of these factors considered, it is worth noting that the side effects of many prescription medications issued for mental illnesses can cause some of the same issues as marijuana and can be equally challenging to cease using. Like any other medication, the potential side effects of medical marijuana in the treatment of mental illness should be discussed and weighed against the benefits. In order to be able to provide the most accurate information about both positive and negative outcomes, more conclusive research needs to be conducted.

Christine McCown

See also: Anxiety; Medical Uses; Mental Health.

Further Reading

Briscoe, Joshua, and David Casarett. "Medical Marijuana Use in Older Adults." *Journal of the American Geriatrics Society* 66, no. 5 (2018): 859–863.

Compton, Michael T. *Marijuana and Mental Health.* Arlington, VA: American Psychiatric Association Publishing. 2016.

Hill, Kevin P. "Medical Marijuana for Treatment of Chronic Pain and Other Medical and Psychiatric Problems: A Clinical Review." *JAMA: Journal of the American Medical Association* 313 no 24. (2015): 2474–2483.

Joy, Janet E., Stanley J. Watson, John A. Benson, and Institute of Medicine (U.S.). *Marijuana and Medicine: Assessing the Science Base.* Washington, DC: National Academies Press, 1999.

Walsh, Zach, et al. 2017. "Medical Cannabis and Mental Health: A Guided Systematic Review." *Clinical Psychology Review* 51 (February): 15–29.

Middle East

The Middle East has a long tradition of using cannabis, with evidence of use in Persia dating back to circa 700–600 BC (Hawdon 2005). Cannabis's popularity as an intoxicating drug spread throughout the Middle East and permeated broader Islamic culture within a few centuries. The popularity of marijuana and other drugs such as opium in the Middle East has been attributed to the Islamic prohibition against alcohol. The Middle East has among the highest rate of cannabis consumption in Asia (UNODC 2018).

In Lebanon, a 2018 drug report from the United Nations found that approximately 6.4 percent of the adult population uses marijuana. Similarly, the United Arab Emirates reports that 5.3 percent of its adult population are annual cannabis users, approximately 4.3 percent of Afghanistan's adult population use cannabis, and Pakistan and Kuwait report that between 3.0 percent and 4.0 percent of their adults use cannabis. Other Middle Eastern nations report very low rates of use. Jordan and Oman report below-average rates of cannabis use. Iran, Saudi Arabia, Qatar, and Bahrain report some of the lowest rates of use documented in United Nations' data, with reported rates ranging from 0.3 percent to 0.6 percent (UNODC 2018). Throughout most of the Middle East, penalties associated with the possession and use of cannabis remain harsh, and the death penalty is allowed for drug offenses in a majority of Middle Eastern nations (Blackman and Samti 2018).

An exception to the general pattern of use in the Middle East is found in Israel, the only non-Arabic state in the region. Israel reports the highest rate of use in the region, and a 2018 UN study reported that Israel has the highest rate of cannabis use in the world. In 2017, 27 percent of Israeli adults reported using marijuana within the last year, a rather dramatic increase from the slightly less than 9 percent of the adult population reporting annual cannabis use in 2008 (UNODC 2018). Much of this increase is attributed to legalization of medical marijuana and a thriving medical marijuana research industry (Schwartz 2017). Recreational marijuana use, which was decriminalized in Israel in 2019, has long been associated with the young and youthful tourists from Europe and the United States. The use of marijuana by tourists in Israel has been reported since immediately following the 1967 Six-Day War. After the Six-Day War, a pattern emerged wherein older Israelis and Arabs living in Israel who used marijuana were likely to follow the tradition of smoking hashish resin in a hookah or water pipe while young Israelis were more likely to smoke marijuana cigarettes or joints (Palgi 1975; Hawdon 2005).

James Hawdon

See also: Africa; Central Asia; China and Southeast Asia; Europe; India and South Asia; Latin America.

Further Reading

Blackman, Alexandra, and Farah Samti. "Is Marijuana Decriminalization Possible in the Middle East?" *Washington Post,* April 20. 2018. https://www.washingtonpost.com/news/monkey-cage/wp/2018/04/20/is-marijuana-decriminalization-possible-in-the-middle-east/

Hawdon, James. *Drug and Alcohol Consumption as Functions of Social Structures: A Cross-Cultural Sociology*. No. 47. Lewistown, NY: Edwin Mellen Press, 2005.

Palgi, Phyllis. 1975. "The Traditional Role and Symbolism of Hashish among Moroccan Jews in Israel and the Effect of Acculturation." In *Cannabis and Culture*, edited by Vera Rubin. Chicago: Aldine, 1975, 207–216.

Schwartz, Yardena. "The Holy Land of Madical Marijuana." *U.S. News & World Reports,* April 11, 2017. https://www.usnews.com/news/best-countries/articles/2017-04-11/israel-is-a-global-leader-in-marijuana-research

United Nations Office on Drugs and Crime (UNODC). *World Drug Report 2018.* Oxford, UK: Oxford University Press, 2018.

Military Use

The pivotal role drugs played during war is an often overlooked reality in history. Militaries around the world tolerated drug use to enhance military performance and provided soldiers with alcohol to enhance their fighting courage. Prior to the mid-twentieth century, it was common for soldiers to fight while intoxicated. During the American Civil War, morphine was used as a painkiller and to treat gastrointestinal issues. During World War I, soldiers were provided cigarettes, and this caused a spike in tobacco use in America. Cocaine was also used by soldiers to increase energy and support war-related mental health problems. Amphetamines were used by United States, Japan, Britain, and Germany during World War II to make soldiers march for a longer time and to alleviate pain. In Vietnam, dextroamphetamine (aka speed), codeine, steroids, sedatives, and neuroleptics were administered for medical purposes. Heroin, opium, and cannabis were also widely used as coping mechanisms.

For most of U.S. military history, American civilians who volunteered to enlist and admitted to cannabis use in the previous five years would not be allowed to serve. Since the legalization of cannabis in several U.S. states, the military was faced with the question of how to treat enlistees from states where cannabis is legal. The U.S. Armed Forces eventually decided to address such situations by approving a waiver of admission of pre-enlistment cannabis use. A noticeable increase is evident in the number of waivers being submitted and approved since this new policy went into effect.

However, even though the U.S. military loosened its stance on past cannabis use, the zero-tolerance policy while active in the military remains strong. Military personnel are randomly drug tested. Harsh penalties are dealt to soldiers caught using cannabis. It does not matter if usage was recreational or medical. Military spouses are allowed to consume cannabis in states where it is legal, but they are not allowed to bring marijuana home if they live on base.

Similarly, U.S. military veterans face a different environment from active duty military personnel when it comes to marijuana use. Since 2010, veterans are not penalized for cannabis use. Previously, if a veteran was identified as using drugs, including cannabis, they could lose their government-funded health care. Loss of health care for cannabis use is not something veterans have to worry about today.

Despite this regulatory change, the Veterans Administration (VA) government health-care provider is not allowed to recommend or write prescriptions for medical cannabis. The VA will also not fill or pay for medical cannabis prescriptions. Veterans working for the VA are drug tested, and cannabis is not allowed at VA health facilities, even in states where cannabis is legal. This stance stems from the fact that the VA is bound by federal law and not state law, and cannabis remains illegal under federal law.

The American Legion, a veteran-focused group with almost two million members, has urged the American government to allow the VA to accept cannabis use for medicinal purposes. Veterans tend to have higher levels of pain, traumatic brain injuries (TBI), post-traumatic stress syndrome (PTSD), and opioid addictions as compared to the general population. Cannabis is known to be useful in alleviating these and other health issues that members of the veteran community face.

The American Legion also wants more research on the use of cannabis in treating PTSD. As of 2020, cannabis is still listed under the federal law as a Schedule I drug that is dangerous and has no health benefits (alongside heroin and LSD). Given this classification, the VA maintains that it is not yet ready to allow medical professionals to recommend or prescribe cannabis to patients. In states where cannabis is not legal, veterans who use cannabis—even to treat PTSD or other ailments—are committing a crime. Veterans are working diligently to influence the law.

The military in The Netherlands takes an approach similar to Americans and maintains a zero-tolerance policy. In Canada, the opposite is true. Military personnel are allowed to use cannabis, although some limitations are in place. Cannabis use is not allowed for personnel using weapons or vehicles or if the serviceman or servicewomen is on duty. It is also not allowed when working abroad or before completing certain sensitive and complex duties, such as aircraft or parachute work. Each of these limitations has various time periods attached to the cannabis use restriction. In Italy, only the military is allowed to grow cannabis, and the military does all of the work necessary to get cannabis to the pharmacies that fill prescriptions for cannabis.

To date, a significant number of military men and women have been kicked out of the military or received less than honorable discharges because of cannabis use while serving. This is an unfortunate, yet continuous pattern in countries with strict cannabis use policies for military personnel.

Margot Gage Witvliet

See also: Anxiety; Incarceration, Use during; Mental Illness.

Further Reading

American Legion. "Medical Marijuana Research." n.d. Accessed August 23, 2021. https://www.legion.org/mmjresearch

Government of Canada. "Cannabis Use in the Military." n.d. Accessed August 23, 2021. https://www.canada.ca/en/department-national-defence/services/benefits-military/health-support/staying-healthy-active/addiction/cannabis.html

Kamienski, Lukasz. "Combat High: How Armies Throughout History Used Drugs to Make Soldiers Fight." *Military History Now,* May 8, 2018. https://militaryhistorynow.com/2018/05/08/combat-high-a-sobering-history-of-drug-use-in-wartime/

Kamienski, Lukasz. *Shooting Up: A Short History of Drugs and War.* New York: Oxford University Press, 2016.

Martin, William. "Martin: Support Veterans by Backing Medical Marijuana." *Houston Chronicle,* November 7, 2014. https://www.chron.com/opinion/outlook/article/Martin-Support-veterans-by-backing-medical-5878990.php

Martin, William. "War without End." *Texas Monthly,* June 2014. https://www.texasmonthly.com/politics/war-without-end/

Martin, William, and Katharine Neill Harris. "Marijuana as Medicine." *Baker Institute Report* 4 (2019): 1–11.

Momigliano, Anna. "In Italy, The Army Provides Medical Marijuana. And That's a Problem." *Washington Post,* November 29, 2017. https://www.washingtonpost.com/world/europe/in-italy-the-army-provides-medical-marijuana-and-thats-a-problem/2017/11/29/339e027e-d454-11e7-9ad9-ca0619edfa05_story.html

Monkees, The

The Monkees was a popular American TV show that ran from 1966 to 1968 about a fictional rock/pop band, also known as The Monkees. However, despite it being about a fictional rock band, the show spawned the creation of an actual rock/pop group of the same name that actually outsold the Beatles and the Rolling Stones combined in 1966 and 1967, when the band released several hit songs including "Last Train to Clarksville" and "Daydream Believer." The Monkees comprised Davy Jones, Mike Nesmith, Micky Dolenz, and Peter Tork. The show followed the (mis)adventures of the band members and was well known for its wacky plots and goofy central characters. In 1967, the TV show won an Emmy for outstanding comedy series. There was also a movie, *Head*, starring the band members, which was released in 1968. Their popularity waned after the cancellation of the TV show in 1968 and when the band disbanded, but the band nonetheless had successful tours in the 1980s and 2011 when the members reunited.

Although *The Monkees* did not, at the time, explicitly state they used marijuana, there were insinuations that they did use the drug. During one press conference, members deflected questions about whether they smoked marijuana by responding, "No, we barbeque it slowly for two hours." Some viewers have suggested that one of the episodes of their TV show, "Mijacogeo" (aka "The Frodis Caper"), used "Frodis" as a code for marijuana. There were also rumors that they smoked marijuana occasionally in a lounge, nicknamed the "Frodis Room" built off the soundstage where the series was filmed.

Micky Dolenz did publicly recount a time he smoked marijuana with Paul McCartney of the Beatles. Mike Nesmith also acknowledged his experiences with marijuana, both smoking and using edibles, in his memoir. Additionally, Peter Tork was arrested and sentenced to three months in an Oklahoma jail for hashish possession in 1972.

Of the four members of *The Monkees*, only Micky Dolenz and Mike Nesmith were alive as of 2020. Peter Tork died on February 21, 2019, at age 77 from cancer. At age 66, Davy Jones died on February 29, 2012 from a heart attack. His autopsy did find cannabinoids (which include marijuana) in his system, but these were not found to have played a role in his death.

Veronyka James

See also: Beatles, The.

Further Reading

Dolenz, Micky, and Mark Bego. *I'm a Believer: My Life of Monkees, Music, and Madness.* New York: Cooper Square Press, 2004.

Jones, Davy. *They Made a Monkee Out of Me.* Fort Collins, CO: A Book's Mind, 2014.

Nesmith, Michael. *Infinite Tuesday: An Autobiographical Riff.* New York: Crown Archetype, 2017.

Moral Panics

Humans have used marijuana for millennia for a variety of reasons. Many have celebrated its use as a beneficial medicine, a spiritual tool, or a source of recreation. However, others have questioned its benefits and challenged the claim that marijuana is harmless. At times, those opposing its use have grounded their claims in evidence, but there have been many other times when the dangers of marijuana have been exaggerated (Bostwick 2012). From its association with Mexican immigrants after the Mexican revolution and Federal Bureau of Narcotic's Commission Ansliger's "gore file" to its central role in the "War on Drugs," marijuana has frequently been part of sociopolitical debates (Berkey 2011). At times, these debates seem to lead to a disproportionate amount of concern given the harms or potential harms marijuana poses to society. The moral panic framework (Cohen 1972) can help explain why some issues are disproportionately focused on and stigmatized while other equally or even more harmful behaviors are widely tolerated or even ignored. While moral panics aim to right some perceived harm in society, the panic may be more damaging than the actual issue itself.

Cohen described moral panic as a "condition, episode, person or group of people who emerge to become defined as a threat to societal values and interest; its nature is presented in a stylized and stereotypical fashion by the mass media" (Cohen 1972, 1). During a moral panic, the threat the alleged problem poses to society is exaggerated. This is most often a result of sensationalized media. Once the problem is constructed, there is a heightening of stigmatization surrounding it and those who are associated with it lose political power. Simultaneously, other problems—often of a more serious nature—are ignored.

To be considered a moral panic, the problem should adhere to the following three criterion: there is an identifiable enemy, an alleged victim, and a widespread consensus to act. The problem becomes associated with the identifiable enemy, or what Cohen called the "folk devil," and the folk devil is depicted as a grave threat to the alleged victims. Often, the alleged victims are children, average citizens (i.e., the middle classes), or the society at large. The panic created by tying the problem to both victim and enemy incites a feeling that action (generally in the form of legislation) is necessary to safeguard against the perceived large-scale societal danger.

Though there are several elements of a moral panic, disproportionality is key: politicians, media outlets with specific political and commercial interests, or other moral entrepreneurs (those who seek to influence a group to keep or adopt a norm) provide distorted claims and statistics to illustrate the extent of the problem and the risks it poses to the people they are trying to rouse. Disproportionate attention too is also paid to some problems instead of others. As this disproportionality focuses attention on the moral panic, it distracts from potentially more serious problems. Media coverage plays a particularly critical role in defining social problems as attention worthy and deviant. This heightened media attention can create a consensus that the threat is serious enough and requires something be done to curb the problem. The consensus often coalesces around the identified folk devil, thereby creating hostility toward them. Elite-engineered moral panics excel at creating hostility toward folk devils and diverting criticism aimed at them for failing to address other problems such as political or economic crises (Goode and Ben-Yehuda 2009).

Constructing moral panics around marijuana use has served the interests of several such groups, historically. The Mexican Revolution of 1910–1911 brought immigrants into the Southwestern United States who were fleeing violence. They brought cannabis with them, and as prejudice and hostility against these arrivals rose, their marijuana smoking became a focus of racist claims issued by sensationalist newspapers, lawmakers, government officials, and others. Mexican immigrants were indiscriminately blamed for property crimes, kidnapping children, and engaging in murder sprees. In response, the first laws against cannabis in the United States were passed in border towns with Mexico. As a result of this moral panic, El Paso passed a local ordinance banning the sale and possession of marijuana.

Newspaper tycoon William Randolph Hearst (1863–1951) was a particularly important individual in driving moral panic about marijuana and those who used it. An owner of dozens of leading newspapers and magazines, Hearst launched a propaganda campaign against marijuana and published some of the most outlandish stories linking violent acts to cannabis consumption. It has been speculated that Hearst was motivated by his considerable financial interests in the lumber and paper industries since hemp, the fiber of the cannabis plant, can also be used to make paper, textiles, rope, and other products that compete with paper. Regardless of his motives, his campaign against marijuana worked, and public support for criminalizing marijuana increased. Since the law never effectively differentiated between hemp and marijuana, the war on hemp probably contributed to the overt war on marijuana (Warf 2014). In addition to those in the lumber and synthetic rope industries, cotton growers were also concerned about the competition from hemp and were major proponents of criminalizing cannabis.

Harry Anslinger (1892–1975), the commissioner of the Federal Bureau of Narcotics, was another major player in the creation of a moral panic over marijuana. Anslinger asserted that marijuana caused insanity and pushed people toward horrific criminal acts. He rejected clinical analyses that the drug neither incited violent behavior nor led to the use of more addictive drugs. Through the sensationalist media of the time (including Hearst newspapers and periodicals), Anslinger linked marijuana to jazz, which he despised largely because of its association with African American musicians. As one historian noted, "The discourses surrounding the war against marijuana reveal how particular gender and ethnic categories are selectively deployed in deliberately inaccurate ways, often invoking racist imagery" (Warf 2014, 430).

During the 1930s, the popular film *Reefer Madness* portrayed marijuana destroying the lives of young adults by sending them down paths to murder, rape, and criminal insanity. Through the fanning of these fears, along with ones asserting that marijuana caused racial minorities to commit crimes and white women to seek sexual relations with racial minorities, local and state governments cracked down on marijuana, and Congress passed the Marihuana Tax Act of 1937. This federal law put cannabis under the regulation of the Drug Enforcement Agency and criminalized possession throughout the United States.

During the 1960s, however, there was a shift in marijuana usage from low-income minority populations to middle-class, college-educated, white youth, popularized by the liberal political climate of the civil rights, women's rights, environmental, and anti-Vietnam war movements. As this generation grew older, some of them worked to reduce penalties for marijuana and other drug use in the 1970s. Nonetheless, the Federal Controlled Substance Act of 1970 defined cannabis as a "Schedule 1" substance, which made medical and recreational cannabis use illegal.

In 1972, President Nixon appointed the National Commission on Marijuana and Drug Abuse, which concluded that the drug should be decriminalized; however, he rejected their findings and continued to frame marijuana as a danger to American youth in particular and society in general. In 1975, the United States began spraying herbicide over Mexican marijuana fields, which had the unintended consequence of boosting domestic production of pot with much higher THC content. In 1982, President Reagan launched a federal "War on Drugs" that included the enforcement of stringent marijuana laws and numerous claims about the dangers posed by marijuana, both on its own and as a "gateway" to even more destructive drugs (Hawdon 2001).

As of 2021, there has never been a documented instance in which marijuana abuse has resulted in loss of life; the federal government continues to classify marijuana as a Schedule I controlled substance. Americans arrested for marijuana-related offenses continue to be disproportionately from poor/working class communities and communities of color.

Nonetheless, however, public opinion and policy toward legalizing marijuana have become more favorable, with several states legalizing medical use of marijuana and several states legalizing recreational use of marijuana. In many quarters, the moral panic that once surrounded marijuana seems both quaint and ridiculous. Yet, even states that have legalized recreational marijuana have strict antidrug policies, with regular mandatory drug testing for the work place, for example. Additionally, moral panic about marijuana use and abuse can still be found, such as in media coverage that exaggerate the danger and toxicity of edibles (Eversman 2016). These accounts distorted the danger posed by edible marijuana and increased the stigma and stereotypes surrounding its use. This same phenomenon has been extended to synthetic cannabinoids, "bath salts," and other drugs (see Miller et al. 2015). Some critics contend that concerns raised about such marijuana use qualify as moral panics because they end up being more harmful than the drugs themselves—by further stigmatizing and labeling marginalized groups, by causing people to doubt all claims of danger and potential risks when people do not see these claims actualized, and by making it more difficult for America to reform its criminal laws regarding marijuana.

Christine McCown

See also: Anslinger, Harry (1892–1975); Anti-Marijuana Campaigns in Popular Press; Comprehensive Drug Abuse Prevention and Control Act (1970); Medical Uses; *Reefer Madness.*

Further Reading

Berkey, Michael. "Mary Jane's New Dance: The Medical Marijuana Legal Tango." *Cardozo Public Law, Policy & Ethics Journal* 9, no. 2 (2011): 417.

Bostwick, J. Michael. "Blurred Boundaries: The Therapeutics and Politics of Medical Marijuana." *Mayo Clinic Proceedings 87,* no. 2 (2012): 172–186.

Carliner, Hannah, Qiana L. Brown, Aaron L. Sarvet, and Deborah S. Hasin. "Cannabis Use, Attitudes, and Legal Status in the U.S.: A Review." *Preventive Medicine 104* (2017): 13–23.

Cohen, Stanley. *Folk Devils and Moral Panics: The Creation of the Mods and Rockers.* Sociology and the Modern World. London, UK: MacGibbon and Kee, 1972.

Eversman, Michael H. "Feeding on Fear: Edible Marijuana and Disproportionality in US Media." *Drugs: Education, Prevention & Policy 23,* no. 6 (2016): 462–470.

Eversman, Michael H., and Jason D. P. Bird. "Moral Panic and Social Justice: A Guide for Analyzing Social Problems." *Social Work 62,* no. 1 (2017): 29.

Goode, Erich, and Nachman Ben-Yehuda. *Moral Panics: The Social Construction of Deviance.* 2nd ed. Chichester, UK: Wiley-Blackwell, 2009.

Hawdon, James E. "The Role of Presidential Rhetoric in the Creation of a Moral Panic: Reagan, Bush, and the War on Drugs." *Deviant Behavior 22*, no. 5 (2001): 419–445.

Miller, Bryan, John Stogner, Laura Agnich, Amber Sanders, Joseph Bacot, and Shanna Felix. "Marketing a Panic: Media Coverage of Novel Psychoactive Drugs (NPDs) and Its Relationship with Legal Changes." *American Journal of Criminal Justice 40*, no. 3 (2015): 523–541.

Warf, Barney. "High Points: An Historical Geography of Cannabis." *The Geographical Review* 104, no. 4 (2014): 414.

N

National Institute on Drug Abuse (NIDA)

The National Institute on Drug Abuse (NIDA) is a federal research institute formed in 1972 by the Drug Abuse Office and Treatment Act. The institute was established within the National Institute on Mental Health and, once operational, became one of the three institutes in the Alcohol, Drug Abuse, and Mental Health Administration. The stated goal of NIDA is to "advance science on the causes and consequences of drug use and addiction and to apply that knowledge to improve individual and public health." To do so, NIDA supports and conducts clinical research on drug use and its consequences and disseminates scientific research findings on substance abuse treatment. The research conducted by NIDA has been publicized in a bimonthly newsletter since 1985, as well as in numerous peer-reviewed journals and other academic outlets. NIDA also produces educational material for teenagers and parents on the dangers of drug use. Today, NIDA is the world's largest research institute dedicated to funding research on drug abuse, drug use prevention, and the treatment of substance abuse.

In the midst of the AIDS epidemic in the mid-1980s, NIDA began receiving substantial funding. The 1988 passage of the Anti-Drug Abuse Act similarly led to large funding increases for NIDA. The growing revenue stream allowed NIDA to start its Medications Development Program, with the goal of developing pharmaceutical drugs to treat symptoms of drug abuse. Work in the Medications Development Program additionally focused on developing drugs to block the effects of abused drugs, reduce drug cravings, mitigate drug withdrawal, reverse the deleterious effects of drugs, and prevent drug relapses (McCann, Acri, and Vocci 2008). For example, NIDA supported research that helped develop nicotine replacement mechanisms such as patches and gum that eventually led to the development of these products and widespread use by smokers seeking to quit the habit. NIDA has also funded research that developed synthetic cannabis for medical purposes, including the treatment of multiple sclerosis and HIV/AIDS (Onaivi et al. 2002).

An organizational shake-up hit NIDA in the 1990s. First, in 1990, NIDA was restructured to create the Medications Development Division, which was subsequently renamed the Division of Pharmacotherapies and Medical Consequences of Drug Abuse. Two years later, NIDA was transferred to the National Institute of Health. The reorganization strengthened the bond between NIDA and the Food and Drug Administration (FDA), as well as the pharmaceutical industry. After this transfer, NIDA placed additional emphasis on developing new medications for drug abuse treatment (McCann et al. 2008).

Although a well-funded government agency, NIDA's operations have attracted controversy as well. Notably, NIDA has a government-granted monopoly in the United States on the production of medical marijuana for research purposes. The organization has a contract with the University of Mississippi to grow the United States' only legal cannabis crop for medical and research purposes. This arrangement has sparked strong criticism from others who assert that NIDA should not have the right to determine who can study the medicinal effects of marijuana. Claims that NIDA has used its monopoly power to obstruct research that is not connected to the organization's research persist. In addition to concerns over the regulatory monopoly of NIDA, other researchers have charged the organization with using low-grade marijuana in its medical research. In fact, a report in *Mother Jones* (2005) described the cannabis used by NIDA in their research as brown, filled with seeds and stems, and of low potency. Medical marijuana researchers, however, tend to prefer high-potency cannabis with greater levels of the drug's psychoactive ingredient THC (Greenberg 2005). The effectiveness of the NIDA's anti-marijuana campaign has also been called into question. Westat, a research company hired by NIDA, found that the government's five-year ad campaign seeking to dissuade teenagers from using marijuana, costing more than $1 billion, was ineffective and maybe even counterproductive. Finally, two of the synthetic cannabinoid compounds developed by the researchers funded by NIDA to produce these substances for medical use eventually worked their way into the illegal drug scene and are found in the popular synthetic marijuana drugs K2 and Spice (Tatusov et al. 2015).

Despite these controversies, NIDA's $1.2 billion annual budget and status as the primary source of federal funding on drug research make it an important and powerful actor in the study of drugs.

Matthew Costello

See also: Chronic Pain; Medical Marijuana and the Law; Medical Uses; Mental Illness.

Further Reading

Greenberg, Gary. "Respectable Reefer." *Mother Jones*, November 1, 2005. https://www.motherjones.com/politics/2005/11/respectable-reefer/

Grim, Ryan. "A White House Drug Deal Gone Bad: Sitting on the Negative Results of a Study of Anti-Marijuana Ads." *Slate*, September 7, 2006. https://slate.com/technology/2006/09/a-white-house-drug-deal-gone-bad.html

McCann, David J., Jane B. Acri, and Frank J. Vocci. "Drug Discovery and Development for Reward Disorders: Views from Government." In *Animal and Translational Models for CNS Drug Discovery*, edited by Robert A. McArthur and Franco Borsini. Bethesda, MD: Academic Press, 2008, 23–40.

National Institute of Drug Abuse. *National Institute of Health.* n.d. Accessed August 23, 2021. https://www.drugabuse.gov/

Onaivi, Emmanuel S., et al. "Endocannabinoids and Cannabinoid Receptor Genetics." *Progress in Neurobiology* 66, no. 5 (2002): 307–344.

Tatusov, Michael, Maryann Mazer-Amirshahi, Lewis Nelson, and Jesse Pines. "6 Things Every EP Needs to Know about K2/Spice & the Synthetic Cannabinoid Epidemic." *Emergency Physicians Monthly*, October 23, 2015. https://epmonthly.com/article/6-things-every-ep-needs-to-know-about-k2spice-the-synthetic-cannabinoid-epidemic/

National Organization for the Reform of Marijuana Laws (NORML)

The National Organization for the Reform of Marijuana Laws (NORML) is a nonprofit marijuana-focused advocacy group. Founded in 1970 by lawyer Keith Stroup, NORML is a Washington, D.C.-based organization with chapters in North America, Europe, Asia, Africa, and Australia. In the 1970s, NORML was a leader of the marijuana decriminalization movement, helping to decriminalize marijuana in 11 states. NORML advised legislators on how to go about their decriminalization efforts and at times provided financial support to bring in expert witnesses.

NORML's influence on public policy became evident in its first years of existence. Stroup was close with some officials in President Jimmy Carter's administration, including presidential advisor Peter Bourne. Stroup's relationship with Bourne and the administration ended, however, after NORML sued the federal government over its endorsement of the use of a harmful herbicide in Mexican drug fields that was potentially harming marijuana users. In the 1980s, NORML found itself on the defensive due to the ramping up of the War on Drugs by President Ronald Reagan's administration. By the 1990s, however, NORML returned to the spotlight, revived by a rising debate over whether to legalize marijuana for some medical treatments.

Currently, NORML continues to advocate for decriminalization and legalization through many different parts of the organization. The Marijuana Research Library is filled with reports from NORML that summarize marijuana research related to many topics. The Marijuana Research Library also points those interested in the direction of research reports, public opinion surveys, health reports, NORML testimonies, crime statistics, and more.

NORML also operates nonprofits and organizations. The NORML Legal Committee (NLC) serves as NORML's legal arm. NLC is a team of defense attorneys that helps NORML stay on top of trends in marijuana law and provides advice on how NORML should address certain cases and policies. NLC's over 350 members have aided in the defense of those charged with marijuana-related citations and litigated cases that have set legal precedents for marijuana growers, sellers, and consumers.

Outside the courtroom, NORML works to get policy-makers to support the removal of marijuana prohibition laws. Through NORML PAC, NORML's nonpartisan political action committee, the organization provides financial support to legislators and candidates for public office who support NORML's goals. NORML believes that in order to become a serious actor in politics it needs to demonstrate power through strength in fundraising and donations.

The policies NORML advocates for center on marijuana decriminalization and legalization. On decriminalization, NORML supports removing all penalties for the private possession and responsible use of marijuana while maintaining penalties for those who sell and/or traffic large quantities. On legalization, NORML supports the move to allow adults to possess and cultivate marijuana on a small scale. This includes advocating for a regulated marijuana market that would allow purchasing from safe legal sources and the power for states to experiment with different models of legalization without federal interference.

While NORML advocates for decriminalization and legalization, it is clear about only advocating for responsible use of the substance. In 1996, NORML adopted five principles of responsible use to demonstrate how they view marijuana consumption. The five principles concern advocating for only adult use; discouraging the use of the substance while operating machinery/driving; the importance of being mindful of one's mental, physical, and social circumstances; resisting abusive use; and respecting the rights of others.

Aubrey D. Johnson

See also: Alaska; California; Colorado; Decriminalization; Taxation; Vermont; Washington D.C.; Washington State.

Further Reading

Anderson, Patrick. *High in America: The True Story Behind NORML and the Politics of Marijuana.* New York: The Viking Press, 1981.

Clark, Claire D., and Emily Dutton. "Peter Bourne's Drug Policy and the Perils of a Public Health Ethic, 1976–1978." *American Journal of Public Health* 105, no. 2 (2015): 283–292.

Goode, Erich. "Mr. Marijuana Retires: A Profile of Keith Stroup." *Contemporary Justice Review* 10, no. 4 (2007): 383–391.

National Organization for the Reform of Marijuana Laws—NORML. Accessed August 23, 2021. https://norml.org/

Nelson, Willie (1933–)

Willie Nelson (1933–) is an accomplished singer, songwriter, musician, actor, philanthropist, activist, and businessman. He is a central figure in country music and was partially responsible for bringing elements of the 1960s and 1970s counterculture to country music in the form of the musical genre known as "outlaw" country. Nelson is also a longtime marijuana user and advocate, and there is no country music artist whose name is more widely associated with marijuana.

Willie Hugh Nelson was born in Abbott, Texas, on April 29, 1933, to Myrle and Ira Nelson. His parents were musicians, but they divorced soon after his birth and both he and his sister, Bobbie, were raised by their paternal grandparents. Nelson's grandparents, Alfred and Nancy Nelson, were church musicians who established, cultivated, and supported the musical talents of both grandchildren (Nelson 2012). As a youngster, Nelson was also influenced by the myriad of musical styles found in Abbott and the surrounding areas, including church music; Black field-workers' songs; Mexican guitar-and-marimba music; and even Czech polka. Finally, Nelson was influenced by the country, Western swing, big band, and jazz music that poured forth from local radio stations and high-powered stations in America and across the border in Mexico.

Nelson began playing in dancehalls in his early teens; however, neither the church of which he was a member nor his grandmother looked favorably upon the dancehall lifestyle. Nelson's grandmother always supported his music, though, and times were tough after her husband died. Nelson's grandmother eventually acquiesced to his dancehall performances because he could make more money

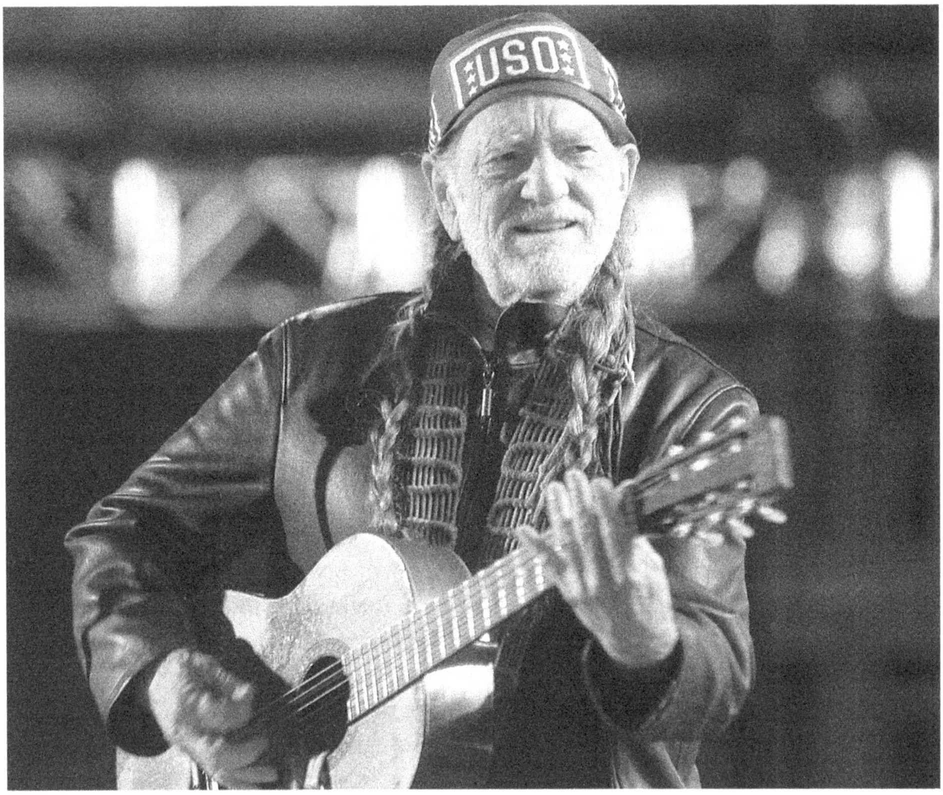

Willie Nelson, a country singer, musician, and songwriter whose prolific career spans more than 50 years, entertains service members and their families at Ramstein Air Base in Germany in May 2005. Nelson was born on April 29, 1933. In addition to his musical prowess, he is well known as an avid user of marijuana and a leading activist for its legalization. (PRNewsFoto/USO)

performing in dancehalls than working in the fields. However, she asked Nelson to honor his spiritual and religious roots.

Throughout his life, Nelson has never accepted the idea that his spirituality and his rowdy, "honky-tonk" lifestyle were incompatible. He has recorded many religious songs, and the first truly successful song he wrote, "Family Bible," was inspired by his grandmother (Nelson and Ritz 2015).

Throughout his teen years, Nelson played in dancehalls, worked in radio, and even organized a show featuring Bob Wills and His Texas Playboys. After high school, he preempted the draft by joining the air force but was soon discharged because of back problems. During the 1950s, Nelson held several odd jobs, worked as a DJ, and wrote and recorded songs, but he remained an obscure dancehall and honky-tonk performer.

However, in 1954, Nelson was introduced to something that would play an important part of his life—marijuana. Nelson was at a bar with his friend, Fred Lockwood, when Fred suggested they smoke. Nelson declined because he had seen the anti-marijuana film *Reefer Madness* and was concerned it would make him crazier than he was. Eventually, however, his friend convinced him to try it, and over the next several years, Nelson gradually became a regular pot smoker (Nelson and Ritz 2015).

In the 1960s, Nelson's songs finally began to achieve popular success. Although Nelson wrote "Family Bible" in the late 1950s, Claude Gray's rendition of the song did not become popular until 1960, which was the same year Nelson moved to Nashville. During the early 1960s, several other songs Nelson wrote became hits for other country artists, including Faron Young's "Hello Walls," Billy Walker's "Funny How Time Slips Away," Ray Price's "Night Life," Patsy Cline's "Crazy," and Roy Orbison's "Pretty Paper" (Nelson and Ritz 2015). In the early 1960s, Nelson recorded his first album, signed with RCA Victor, and joined the Grand Old Opry.

By the end of the decade, Nelson was increasingly drawn to peace-loving, pot-smoking, free-living ways of the 1960s counterculture. However, as Kinky Friedman, another iconoclastic country music artist, noted, Nelson's lifestyle changes and artistic shifts clashed with the "good ol' boy" network that ran Nashville, the center of the American country music scene, and saw marijuana as the "devil" (Nelson 2012). Moreover, Nelson's RCA records were not selling well; his second wife found out that he had impregnated his soon-to-be third wife; and his house in Nashville burned down in 1970. Nelson subsequently abandoned Nashville for Austin, Texas, a hotbed of countercultural activity and music in the Southwest (Nelson and Ritz 2015).

In the 1970s, Nelson became a central figure in "outlaw" country, a subgenre of country music that focused on themes of individualism, freedom, and the joys and challenges associated with living outside the law. Nelson recorded albums such as *Shotgun Willie*, *Phases and Stages*, and *Red Headed Stranger*. In 1975, *Red Headed Stranger* became Nelson's first album to reach number one on the *Top Country Albums* chart. This album included "Blue Eyes Crying in the Rain," which was his first song to reach the top of the *Hot Country Songs* chart. In 1976, Nelson contributed to a compilation called *Wanted! The Outlaws* with Waylon Jennings, Jessi Coulter, and Tompall Glaser. *Wanted!* also reached number one on the *Top Country Albums Chart*. The same year, Nelson released another number one album, *The Troublemaker*, which was highlighted by his cover versions of several Gospel classics (Billboard 2019).

In the 1970s, Nelson also became friends with Georgia Governor (and eventual U.S. President) Jimmy Carter and his family. Nelson campaigned for Carter during his 1975–1976 presidential campaign and later performed at the White House where he famously smoked marijuana with Jimmy Carter's son, Chip (James Earl Carter III), on the roof of the White House. Just prior to this, Nelson had been arrested and jailed by U.S. Customs during a trip to the Bahamas for having marijuana in his luggage (Doyle 2019). Over time, word of Nelson's arrests and exploits spread, which contributed to his association with marijuana.

From the 1970s through the 1990s, Nelson recorded many more successful songs and albums, and he remained a prominent figure in country music. In 1978, he released *Stardust*, which included cover versions of several popular songs, including "Georgia on My Mind" and "Blue Skies." In the 1980s, he released soundtrack albums from movies in which he acted, including *The Electric Horseman* and *Honeysuckle Rose*, and during the 1980s and 1990s, he starred as a preacher-turned-outlaw in the film *The Redheaded Stranger*, an outlaw in *Barbarosa*, and took minor roles in several other films (Nelson and Ritz 2015). Finally, he released several chart-topping albums, including *Always on My Mind*, *City of New Orleans*, *Me and Paul*, and *The Promiseland* (Billboard 2019).

Beginning in 1985, Nelson recorded and toured with a country "supergroup" called The Highwaymen. This group consisted of Nelson, Waylon Jennings, Kris Kristofferson, and Johnny Cash. They recorded the album *Highwayman*, which quickly rose to number one on the Top Country Albums chart. 1985 was also the year Nelson cofounded Farm Aid, an annual concert festival that supports family farms and farmers. In 1990, Nelson had much of his property and assets seized and auctioned by the Internal Revenue Service (IRS), which claimed that he owed $32 million in back taxes. Many of his friends helped Nelson by buying his property and returning it to him, but he also recorded and sold an album, *The IRS Tapes: Who'll Buy my Memories*, to pay back his debts (Nelson and Ritz 2015).

Although marijuana has been a part of Willie's life and persona for decades, it was rarely a prominent or explicit part of Nelson's work until his later years. Only in the twenty-first century did Nelson record songs such as "It's all going to Pot" with Merle Haggard or "Roll me Up and Smoke Me when I Die" with Kris Kristofferson, Jamey Johnson, and Snoop Dogg. Willie's house fire in 1970 is one of the events that made his marijuana use legendary. As everything he owned burned to the ground, Willie ran into the house to retrieve two guitar cases—one contained his beloved guitar, *Trigger*, and the other contained two pounds of marijuana. But, even then, marijuana was only a "supplement" for alcohol and cigarettes. It was not until the early 1970s that Nelson said he "fell in love" with marijuana. As he notes, alcohol agitated him while pot calmed him down, and, unlike cigarettes, smoking marijuana was a communal experience that brought people together. Finally, Nelson found that when it came to his two greatest pleasures—"making music and making love"—liquor made him "sloppy" while marijuana made those experiences "rapturous" (Nelson and Ritz 2015, Chapter 18).

Nelson continued to record albums and tour throughout the 1990s and into the twenty-first century, but his records did not achieve the same levels of success as his earlier work (Billboard 2019). He continued to act in films that emphasized his marijuana use, however, including roles as the "historian smoker" in *Half Baked* (1998), the pot-smoking Jesse Duke in *Dukes of Hazzard* (2005), and the pot-trading Farmer Bob in *Surfer, Dude* (2008). Furthermore, Nelson has made numerous television appearances on late-night talk shows, where his marijuana use is often highlighted.

Nelson also entered the legitimate marijuana trade when he launched his brand of marijuana called *Willie's Reserve* in 2015 (Doyle 2019). Nelson has been an activist for the reform of marijuana laws for much of his career, and he serves on the advisory board of the National Organization for the Reform of Marijuana Laws (NORML 2019). He has also performed for numerous benefits that support wildlife and environmental protection (Nelson and Ritz 2015). Nevertheless, his greatest achievement is his music, which has earned him many awards and the admiration of millions of fans.

C. Cory Lowe

See also: National Organization for the Reform of Marijuana Laws (NORML); *Reefer Madness*; Snoop Dogg (1971–).

Further Reading

Billboard. "Willie Nelson Chart History." 2019. https://www.billboard.com/music/willie-nelson

Doyle, P. "Willie Nelson: The High Life." *Rolling Stone,* April 29, 2019. https://www.rollingstone.com/music/music-features/willie-nelson-weed-issue-826290/

Nelson, Willie. *It's a Long Story: My life.* New York: Little, Brown and Company, 2015.

Nelson, Willie. *Roll Me Up and Smoke Me when I Die: Musings from the Road.* New York: HarperCollins, 2012.

NORML. "NORML Advisory Board." 2019. https://norml.org/advisory-board

Patoski, Joe Nick. *Willie Nelson: An Epic Life.* Hachette UK: Black Bay Books, 2008.

Neurological Effects

Several chemical compounds in marijuana exert effects throughout the body. Of these, the cannabinoid tetrahydrocannabinol (THC) is the most well-known compound in marijuana and is thought to be responsible for the majority of marijuana's psychoactive effects. THC exerts its psychoactive effects via the cannabinoid receptors in the brain. These effects may include euphoria, anxiety relief, sensory alterations, and mood changes. There are other cannabinoids in marijuana as well, such as cannabidiol (CBD), cannabigerol (CBG), and cannabichromene (CBC). These other cannabinoids may activate or inhibit cannabinoid receptors, but without many psychoactive effects. For example, they may activate or inhibit cannabinoid receptors in other parts of the body besides the brain. Research has implicated these cannabinoids in pain relief, seizure prevention, neurological plasticity, and reductions in inflammation (Silver 2019; Maroon and Bost 2018). Although less is known about these non-THC cannabinoids, research in this area is rapidly growing.

LOCATION OF CANNABINOID RECEPTORS IN THE BODY

Cannabinoid receptors are widely distributed throughout the brain, including in the cortex, hippocampus, connections of the basal ganglia, cerebellum, substantia nigra, and the caudate putamen (Silver 2019). There are few cannabinoid receptors in the brain stem, or medulla oblongata. Because this brain area controls basic and vital bodily functions such as respiration and heart function, fatal overdose on THC is essentially impossible (Silver 2019). Cannabinoid receptors are also located in the peripheral nervous system, heart, blood vessels, liver, lungs, digestive system, fat, and sperm cells (Silver 2019).

Endocannabinoids (Cannabinoids Native to Our Bodies)

Endocannabinoids are cannabinoids that are native to our bodies. The endocannabinoids that act upon cannabinoid receptors include anandamide (N-arachidonoylethanolamine, or AEA) and 2-AG (2-arachidonoylglycerol). Endocannabinoids regulate the release of other neurotransmitters such as γ-amino butyric acid (GABA), glutamate, and monoamines. These neurotransmitters are responsible for regulating many day-to-day psychological feelings such as anxiety/relaxation, happiness/sadness, and motivation. THC takes 20–30 hours to be reduced by only half of the amount that was consumed. In contrast to THC, endocannabinoids are very short-acting because they are metabolized by enzymes in the body quite quickly (Silver 2019). This short action makes the natural effects of these cannabinoids difficult to notice. This is the reason people do not typically feel the same "high" they get when they consume cannabis or THC.

CANNABINOID RECEPTORS

The two subtypes of cannabinoid receptors are generally considered to be CB_1 and CB_2. THC activates both of these receptor subtypes. Other cannabinoid receptors have been researched more sparsely. When THC binds to the CB_1 receptor, it inhibits the firing of certain neurons. For example, THC or other cannabinoid agonists can suppress the activation of neurons (Pertwee 2001; 2008). This inhibition is thought to be the mechanism by which marijuana (in particular, cannabidiol) may prevent seizures (Maroon and Bost 2018), which occur when too many neurons fire at once and at the same time.

Additionally, certain direct or downstream (secondary to the cannabinoid agonist's action on the receptor) effects are thought to be protective for neurons. The inhibition of glutamate transmission by cannabinoids is one such example. CB_1 receptors also mediate appetite by inhibiting neurons in the hypothalamus within the brain. This is because there are neurons that control satiety, or feeling full after a meal, located in the hypothalamus (Silver 2019). The CB_1 receptor is also expressed in many areas of the periphery, which are areas of the body containing nerves that are not part of the brain or spinal cord. In the periphery, the CB_1 receptors have been found in the heart, blood vessels, lungs, bladder, and gastrointestinal tract (Howlett 2002).

The CB_2 receptor is also a GPCR. Less is known about the CB_2 receptors and their distribution, but CB_2 receptors are generally only found in the periphery. CB_2 receptors are expressed primarily throughout the immune system, spleen, and tonsils (Pertwee 2001; Maroon and Bost 2018). Although these receptors are generally not distributed throughout the brain, they may play a role in neurological conditions such as Huntington's disease and Alzheimer's disease (Maroon and Bost 2018). Some of this involvement is mediated by CBD, rather than THC.

EFFECTS OF MARIJUANA OR THC

The psychological effects of THC include euphoria, stimulation of appetite and reduction of nausea, anxiolytic (anxiety reducing) effects, and pain relief. CBD may reduce the euphoric effect of THC when both are administered simultaneously (Dalton et al. 1976). THC mediates serotonin transmission via the 5-HT3 receptor (Maroon and Bost 2018). This mediation of serotonin is responsible for THC's ability to reduce nausea and partially responsible for THC's tendency to increase appetite.

The Addiction Research Center Inventory (ARCI) is a standardized test that is given to people when they consume a drug to determine what drugs have similarities and differences in the subjective feelings they result in. Drugs fall into different groups according to their psychological effects. For example, participants reporting "intellectual efficiency and energy" tend to score high on the benzedrine group (named after the stimulant drug benzedrine). Participants who are administered marijuana score lower on the benzedrine group relative to when they are administered placebo, indicating that they may feel less able to perform cognitive tasks like math when they consume marijuana (McDonald et al. 2003). In contrast, participants administered marijuana rate their subjective experience as higher along all other groups of items on this measure, which include euphoria (morphine-benzedrine group), stimulant-like effects (amphetamine group), dysphoria (a feeling of uneasiness) and somatic (bodily sensations) effects (LSD group), and sedation (pentobarbital-chlorpromazine-alcohol group). Other research has also directly shown impairment of some cognitive skills and working memory while under the effects of THC. There are also some negative effects on these skills with daily long-term use. However, effects of long term, but occasional use, are less clear.

A large body of evidence suggests that THC (and other cannabinoids such as CBD) provide pain relief, or analgesia. Analgesia from THC appears to stem from a wide range of neurological mechanisms, such as THC's (and other cannabinoids') effects on the opioid system. For example, when THC is administered to mice lacking the CB_1 receptor prior to administering the opioid drug morphine, the effects of morphine are blunted. This shows that the cannabinoid system may play a large role in controlling the opioid system—which has historically been a large focus of pain research. Many addictive pain drugs work directly on the opioid system. If THC is able to act upon the opioid system indirectly, it could provide an alternative to opioid drugs for pain relief. However, it is important to research whether THC or marijuana is also addictive.

MARIJUANA AND ADDICTION

The addictive properties of marijuana have been researched in nonhuman animals using drugs that block the effects of THC and the endogenous cannabinoids. In these procedures, THC is first repeatedly administered to animals for several days. Then, THC and the antagonist (the THC blocker) are administered together. If an animal displays a withdrawal syndrome, this indicates evidence of physical dependence. Withdrawal syndromes can include a lack of physical activity, change in appetite, and a change in grooming behavior, among other observable behaviors. Research on THC has shown that nonhuman animals do show a withdrawal reaction in these procedures, demonstrating that repeated administration of THC results in some level of physical dependence (Onaivi 2002). However, the withdrawal syndrome in humans after they stop regularly using marijuana is generally reported to be mild. There are no known reported overdose deaths from the physical effects of THC or from its withdrawal (Ashton 2001).

Chronic use (marijuana use that is repeated over several days) has been associated with lack of motivation, apathy, problems in completing tasks, and problems in pursuing long-term goals. Some studies have shown deficits in chronic and/or long-term (over the course of several years) users in terms of attention, memory, reaction time, and other cognitive measures compared to nonusers. There are very few studies demonstrating these effects in occasional users, unless they have consumed marijuana acutely prior to completing the cognitive tasks. That is, acute marijuana use impairs cognitive functions such as working memory, attention, and reaction time, and these effects are dose dependent. However, decrements in performance in occasional users return to normal after marijuana's effects have subsided. Additionally, the decreases in performance on cognitive tasks following marijuana use tend to be different from that of alcohol or other drugs. For some tasks, decreases in performance are less pronounced than those brought about by other drugs.

THC has downstream effects on neurotransmitters associated with the brain's reward system (e.g., dopamine), enhancing the firing of dopamine neurons in regions associated with reward (e.g., prefrontal cortex). Additionally, THC increases dopamine synthesis (creation of dopamine), release (from the neuron into the synapse, where it exerts its action), and turnover (amount of dopamine metabolized or converted by enzymes). It also inhibits the reuptake of dopamine, such that a greater amount of dopamine remains in the synapse of the neuron. This inhibition of dopamine reuptake is associated with reinforcing (similar to rewarding) effects.

The reinforcing effects of THC have also been studied in both human and nonhuman animal behavioral studies. Typically, increasing reinforcing effects are associated with greater chance of abusing a drug or becoming dependent upon it. In nonhuman animals, two common procedures used to demonstrate reinforcing effects of a drug include conditioned place preference (CPP) and self-administration. CPP involves administering the drug (i.e., THC), a placebo (control), or the drug's antagonist in distinct environments and then measuring the time spent in the environment associated with each drug. The drug is considered reinforcing if the time spent in the environment associated with the drug is greater than the time spent in the environment associated with the placebo and the antagonist. Self-administration procedures allow the animal to press a lever to produce intravenous infusions of the drug. In nonhuman animals, reinforcing effects of THC are difficult to demonstrate, with a wide variation between studies. Some studies have shown aversion to THC and its associated environments. That is, the animal sometimes spends more time in the environment associated with the antagonist or placebo and, in self-administration paradigms, may not self-administer THC (Onaivi 2002, 93–94). However, in contrast to nonhuman animals, many humans do find THC to be very reinforcing. Additionally, other nonhuman animal studies have shown that THC enhances the reinforcing effect of electrical brain stimulation and that the effects of THC on the brain's reward processes may depend upon genetic differences (Onaivi 2002, 82–83). Reinforcing effects also appear to be dependent upon timing of administration and dose of THC in both humans and nonhuman animals, with relatively lower doses of THC more likely to show reinforcing effects than higher doses, which often show aversive effects.

Marissa Turturici

See also: Anxiety; Dependence; Mental Health; Mental Illness.

Further Reading

Ashton, C. Heather. "Pharmacology and Effects of Cannabis: A Brief Review." *British Journal of Psychiatry* 178, no. 2 (2001): 101–106.

Dalton, William S., Robert Martz, Louis Lemberger, Bruce E. Rodda, and Robert B. Forney. "Influence of Cannabidiol on Delta-9-Tetrahydrocannabinol Effects." *Clinical Pharmacology & Therapeutics* 19, no. 3 (1976): 300–309.

Friedman, Daniel, Jacqueline A French, and Mauro Maccarrone. "Safety, Efficacy, and Mechanisms of Action of Cannabinoids in Neurological Disorders." *The Lancet Neurology* 18, no. 5 (2019): 504–512.

Howlett, Allyn C. "The Cannabinoid Receptors." *Prostaglandins and Other Lipid Mediators* 68–69 (2002): 619–631.

Maroon, Joseph, and Jeff Bost. "Review of the Neurological Benefits of Phytocannabinoids." *Surgical Neurology International* 9, no. 1 (2018): 91.

McDonald, Jennifer, Laura Schleifer, Jerry B Richards, and Harriet de Wit. "Effects of THC on Behavioral Measures of Impulsivity in Humans." *Neuropsychopharmacology* 28, no. 7 (2003): 1356–1365.

Onaivi, Emmanuel S., ed. *The Biology of Marijuana: From Gene to Behavior*. Boca Raton, FL: CRC Press, 2002.

Pertwee, Roger G. "Cannabinoid Receptors and Pain." *Progress in Neurobiology* 63, no. 5 (2001): 569–611.

Pertwee, Roger G. "Ligands That Target Cannabinoid Receptors in the Brain: From THC to Anandamide and beyond: Ligands That Target Cannabinoid Receptors in the Brain." *Addiction Biology* 13, no. 2 (2008): 147–159.

Silver, Robert J. "The Endocannabinoid System of Animals." *Animals* 9, no. 9 (September 16, 2019): 686.

Nixon Administration "War on Drugs"

Psychoactive substances have a very long history of human use. Up until the twentieth century, such drugs as opium, cannabis, and cocaine could be used in the United States without any restrictions. Laws regulating the production and use of psychoactive drugs started appearing in the early twentieth century. Over time, as illicit recreational drug use grew in its popularity, the restrictions evolved and intensified. They reached a new peak during the presidency of Richard Nixon (1969–1974) as Nixon declared drug abuse "public enemy number one" and launched a campaign of policies and programs to reduce illicit drug use across the country.

In 1909, the Smoking Opioid Exclusion Act became the first federal statute prohibiting the possession and use of opioids for smoking. In 1914, the federal government prohibited the production, use, and distribution of coca leaves and its derivatives, as well as opium, for any nonmedical purposes. At approximately the same time, several states, including Massachusetts, California, Maine, Wyoming, and Indiana, also enacted laws regulating marijuana usage. By 1933, 29 states had criminalized cannabis, and in 1937, the United States passed the Marijuana Tax Act, which federally prohibited the use of cannabis (Labate and Cavnar 2014).

Despite these laws, drug use and abuse remained prevalent in American society, although this was not perceived as a major threat until the second half of the twentieth century. From the beginning of the 1960s, many younger people started experimenting with drugs. Much of this increase stemmed from the rise of a counterculture movement that consisted of two main streams: the politically engaged "new left" and "hippies" who were less concerned with political activism and more focused on personal expression and living life by their own rules, norms, and philosophical values. Many of those views held by the hippies were contradictory to the ones of the ruling establishment. Psychedelic drugs were an important component of the counterculture movement; they were especially prevalent among the hippies who used them for recreation, self-exploration, and for achieving transcendental experiences. Various drugs such as cocaine, heroin, LSD, and marijuana became very popular among the youth. As illicit drug use was becoming more prevalent within the United States, it also became more prevalent among troops serving in Vietnam and other parts of the globe. In 1971, over 50 percent of all military personnel in Vietnam used marijuana on a regular basis (Savage and Gabriel 1976).

These trends alarmed the Nixon administration, which also saw political advantage in taking a hard line against illicit drug use. Nixon became the president of the United States at the peak of the counterculture movement. He strongly emphasized the problem of drug abuse and its disastrous impact on society. In 1970, President Nixon signed the Controlled Substances Act (CSA), which aimed to regulate lawful production, possession, and distribution of controlled substances at the federal level. This law classified substances under five schedules depending on how dangerous they were, how big was their potential for abuse and addiction, and whether they had medical value. Marijuana was classified as Schedule 1, or the most dangerous, drug along with MDMA (ecstasy), LSD, and heroin.

The CSA also established the National Commission on Marihuana and Drug Abuse, which aimed to evaluate the effects of actual and potential marijuana use on the American society. This was done mainly because Nixon's administration needed evidence in order to justify the classification of marijuana as a Schedule 1 drug. However, the Commission instead published a report in which it recommended decriminalization of marijuana. The Commission declared that marijuana poses "little proven danger of physical or psychological harm from the experimental or intermittent use of the natural preparations of cannabis, including the resinous mixtures commonly used in this country" (Kaplan 1972, 80). The Commission recommended that the use of marijuana be discouraged by means of prevention and treatment rather than criminalization and penalization of marijuana possession. Nixon ignored the recommendations of the Commission. Instead, in a special message to Congress in 1971, Nixon declared drug abuse "public enemy number one" and announced a campaign to combat illegal drug use—including marijuana—in the United States. Illustrative of that goal were significant changes in the funding allocated for the federal drug law enforcement; that funding increased from $36 million in 1969 to $257 million in 1974. This increased emphasis on combating drug use in the United States focused to a significant degree on marijuana, the most commonly used illicit drug. Marijuana arrests subsequently rose from 31 percent of all drug-related arrests in 1965 to 69 percent in 1975 (Gettman 2005).

Along with increasing funding for law enforcement agencies that were dealing with illicit drugs and introducing new laws and regulations, Richard Nixon also implemented institutional reforms that aimed to help the country in its "war on drugs." In 1973, he established the Drug Enforcement Administration (DEA), which merged all federal antidrug agencies under a single unified command under the direction of the U.S. Department of Justice, with its main task to enforce the CSA. At its inception, the DEA was assigned approximately 1,500 special agents and a budget close to $75 million (Chepesiuk 1999). This reorganization aimed to put an end to the interagency rivalries; to give the FBI a significant role in drug enforcement; to provide for better coordination of antidrug initiatives with state, local, and foreign authorities; to place a single administrator in charge of federal drug law enforcement; and to coordinate all federal efforts related to drug enforcement outside the Justice Department.

Four decades later, the war on drugs is still being fought, although with less intensity than in Nixon's years. In 2011, the Global Commission on Drug Policy published a report acknowledging the failure of government efforts to use criminalization of marijuana use and possession to stamp out demand for the product (The Global Commission on Drug Policy 2011). Most researchers and policy-makers also agree that the war on drugs has disproportionately affected minorities. Some researchers also believe that it has contributed to an overall increase in drug overdoses and strengthened drug cartels (Coyne and Hall 2017). At the moment, the legalization of marijuana is spreading across the United States. At the time of writing (November of 2020), 36 states have legalized medical marijuana, while 15 states have legalized marijuana for recreational use. It is expected that more states will legalize marijuana for medical or recreational use in the near future. Nevertheless, Nixon's War on Drugs has had significant impacts on American society, culture, and policy.

Stan Korotchenko

See also: American Presidents; "Drug Abuse Message to Congress" (President Carter, 1977).

Further Reading

Chepesiuk, Ron. *The War on Drugs: An International Encyclopedia*. Santa Barbara, CA: ABC-Clio, 1999.

Coyne, Christopher J., and Abigail Hall. "Four Decades and Counting: The Continued Failure of the War on Drugs." *Cato Institute Policy Analysis* 811 (2017).

Gettman, Jon B. *Crimes of Indiscretion: Marijuana Arrests in the United States*. Washington, DC: National Organization for the Reform of Marijuana Laws, 2005.

The Global Commission on Drug Policy. "War on Drugs: Report of the Global Commission on Drug Policy." 2011. https://www.globalcommissionondrugs.org/reports/the-war-on-drugs

Kaplan, John. *Marihuana: A Signal of Misunderstanding; First Report of the National Commission on Marihuana and Drug Abuse*. Washington, DC: US Government Printing Office, 1972.

Labate, Beatriz Caiuby, and Clancy Cavnar. *Prohibition, Religious Freedom, and Human Rights: Regulating Traditional Drug Use*. New York: Springer, 2014.

Nahas, Gabriel G, and Albert Greenwood. "The First Report of the National Commission on Marihuana (1972): Signal of Misunderstanding or Exercise in Ambiguity." *Bulletin of the New York Academy of Medicine* 50, no. 1 (1974): 55.

Nixon, Richard. "Remarks about an Intensified Program for Drug Abuse Prevention and Control." *The American Presidency Project*, June 17, 1971. https://www.presidency.ucsb.edu/documents/remarks-about-intensified-program-for-drug-abuse-prevention-and-control#axzz1PCJydjl5

Savage, Paul L., and Richard A. Gabriel. "Cohesion and Disintegration in the American Army: An Alternative Perspective." *Armed Forces & Society* 2, no. 3 (1976): 340–376.

Wesson, Donald R. "Psychedelic Drugs, Hippie Counterculture, Speed and Phenobarbital Treatment of Sedative-Hypnotic Dependence: A Journey to the Haight Ashbury in the Sixties." *Journal of Psychoactive Drugs* 43, no. 2 (2011): 153–164.

Wood, Evan, et al. "The War on Drugs—a Devastating Public Policy Disaster." *Lancet* 373, no. 9668 (2009): 989–990.

O

Obama, Barack (1961–)

Barack Obama (1961–) was the forty-fourth president of the United States, holding office from January 2009 to January 2017. In many ways, Obama's drug policies continued those of his predecessors. For example, the Obama administration did not pursue reclassifying marijuana under the Comprehensive Drug Abuse Prevention and Control Act, which is the primary federal law governing the control of drugs. Under this law's Title II or Controlled Substances Act, marijuana is defined as a Schedule I controlled substance that has a high potential for abuse, no currently accepted medical use in the United States, and lack of accepted safety standards for use under medical supervision. As a Schedule I drug, marijuana is illegal at the federal level, and the Obama administration did not change this classification or even try to change it. Yet, during Obama's time in office, many state laws regulating marijuana changed dramatically. Although a dozen states had legalized medical marijuana by the time Obama was sworn in as president, 16 others and the District of Columbia legalized medical marijuana during his tenure. In addition, beginning with Colorado and Washington in 2012, states began legalizing recreational marijuana use, and six additional states and the District of Columbia would legalize recreational marijuana use before President Obama left office. Although the federal laws regulating marijuana did not change under Obama, his administration's position on legalized medical and recreational marijuana at the state level changed several times over his time in office.

While campaigning for president, then-Senator Obama promised to end President George W. Bush's policy of raiding medical marijuana distribution centers in states that had legalized medical marijuana (Scherer 2012). Once elected, the Obama administration formally announced guidelines that adopted that position. In October 2009, Attorney General Eric Holder advised federal law enforcement officials to not pursue prosecution of medical-marijuana patients and their caregivers who were complying with state laws. However, the attorney general was also quick to note that "we will not tolerate drug traffickers who hide behind claims of compliance with state law to mask activities that are clearly illegal" (U.S. Department of Justice 2009). This position resulted in several states licensing medical marijuana dispensaries that would be regulated through state health departments (Dickinson 2012).

This initial position of the Obama administration changed somewhat abruptly in 2011. First, a number of federal prosecutors began issuing warnings that they would enforce the federal prohibition of marijuana even in states where medical marijuana was permitted and even prosecute state employees responsible for implementing state regulations for medical marijuana dispensaries (Dickinson 2012; Sullum 2015). Then the Justice Department formally reversed its earlier position when Deputy Attorney General James Cole updated the Guidance Regarding Marijuana Enforcement (U.S. Department of Justice 2013). The effect of this policy position paper was to more narrowly define areas where federal law enforcement would not aggressively enforce the Controlled Substance Act. Now, only those jurisdictions with "strong and effective regulatory and enforcement systems to control the cultivation, distribution, sale, and possession of marijuana" were to escape federal prosecution (U.S. Department of Justice 2013). The guidelines also defined "caregivers" as only those who provided care for individuals with cancer or other serious illnesses. This definition of caregiver clearly excluded medical-marijuana dispensaries, which were now open for federal prosecution. In addition to these changes at the Justice Department, the Drug Enforcement Administration (DEA) issued a statement saying that medical marijuana should not really be considered medicine, the Department of Housing and Urban Development prohibited medical marijuana patients from renting properties, and the Internal Revenue Service reiterated its stance that medical marijuana business could not deduct expenses related to the distribution of an illegal drug (Scherer 2012). These changes resulted in numerous federal raids on marijuana dispensaries, discouraged banks from working with marijuana dispensaries for fear of being prosecuted for money laundering or other federal drug crimes, and denied dispensaries tax deductions frequently used by other businesses. In fact, the federal government conducted more raids on medical marijuana dispensaries during Obama's first term as president (2009–2013) than had been conducted during the entire Bush administration two terms from 2001 to 2009 (Lindsey 2016). Obama claimed his administration had been consistent and defended his administration's actions by saying,

> What I specifically said was that we were not going to prioritize prosecutions of persons who are using medical marijuana. I never made a commitment that somehow we were going to give carte blanche to large-scale producers and operators of marijuana—and the reason is because it's against federal law. (quoted in Dickinson 2012)

The Obama administration's approach to marijuana then changed during his second term. First, in 2013, the Obama administration's Justice Department announced it would allow the sale of marijuana for recreational use in Washington and Colorado after those states legalized recreational use. This position paved the way for six additional states and the District of Columbia to legalize recreational marijuana before President Obama left office. The Obama administration also reversed their earlier approach toward medical marijuana dispensaries in 2014. Late that year, President Obama signed a new set of spending laws that disallowed raids on medical marijuana dispensaries in states where it was legal, and the law was upheld in 2015 by a federal court in California that ruled it was unlawful for the DEA to use federal funds to raid dispensaries operating legally under local and state laws (Lindsey 2016). Yet, despite these efforts, his administration did not pressure the DEA to change marijuana's classification as a Schedule I drug.

While the Obama administration's record on marijuana was disappointing to those who had hoped he would push for federal legalization, he was credited with liberalizing the federal approach toward illegal drugs more broadly. He refused to use the phrase "War on Drugs." He also tried to address one of the ways the War on Drugs had led to mass incarceration by urging U.S. attorney generals to not charge mandatory minimum sentences for drug offenses and backed the Fair Sentencing Act that reduced the sentencing disparity between crack cocaine and powder cocaine. He also granted clemency to over 1,300 people convicted of relatively minor, nonviolent drug offenses, thereby allowing them to leave prison early. Obama granted clemency to more people convicted of drug offenses than the previous 11 presidential administrations combined (Newman 2017).

James Hawdon

See also: Comprehensive Drug Abuse Prevention and Control Act (1970); Incarceration for Marijuana Offenses; Incarceration Rates; Medical Marijuana and the Law; Nixon Administration "War on Drugs"; Reagan Administration "War on Drugs"; Recreational Marijuana Laws; Trump, Donald (1946–).

Further Reading

Dickinson, Tim. "Obama's War on Pot." *Rolling Stone,* February 16, 2012. https://www.rollingstone.com/politics/politics-news/obamas-war-on-pot-231820/

Johnson, Kevin, and Raju Chebium. "Justice Department Won't Challenge State Marijuana Laws." *USA Today*, August 29, 2013. https://www.usatoday.com/story/news/nation/2013/08/29/justice-medical-marijuana-laws/2727605/

Lindsey, Nick. "Dispensary Raids Rise under Obama Regime." *Green Rush Daily,* February 24, 2016. https://greenrushdaily.com/news/politics/dispensary-raids-rise-obama-regime/

Newman, Tony. "Looking Back: President Obama's Historic Efforts to Roll Back the Drug War and Tackle Mass Incarceration." *Drug Policy Alliance*, January 18, 2017. https://drugpolicy.org/blog/looking-back-president-obamas-historic-efforts-roll-back-drug-war-and-tackle-mass-incarceration

Scherer, Michael. "What Is President Obama's Problem with Medical Marijuana?" *Time,* May 3, 2012. https://swampland.time.com/2012/05/03/what-is-president-obamas-problem-with-medical-marijuana/

Sullum, Jacob. "Is Obama Finally Ready to Dial Back the War on Drugs." *Forbes,* January 1, 2015. https://www.forbes.com/sites/jacobsullum/2015/01/01/is-obama-finally-ready-to-dial-back-the-war-on-drugs/?sh=3211a0293217

U.S. Department of Justice. "Attorney General Announces Formal Medical Marijuana Guidelines." *Justice News,* October 19, 2009. https://www.justice.gov/opa/pr/attorney-general-announces-formal-medical-marijuana-guidelines

U.S. Department of Justice. "Memorandum for all United States Attorneys: Guidance Regarding Marijuana Enforcement." August 29, 2013. https://www.justice.gov/iso/opa/resources/3052013829132756857467.pdf

Office of National Drug Control Policy

The Office of National Drug Control Policy (ONDCP) was formed with the passing of the Anti-Drug Abuse Act of 1988. The Anti-Drug Abuse Act was supported by President Ronald Regan as a part of his administration's so-called War on Drugs. This initiative comprised two major components: implementing policies for drug control in the United States and forming the ONDCP. Presented by

Robert Michel and Tom Foley, the bill received bipartisan support, passing with margins of 364-11 in the House and 87-3 in the Senate. The ONDCP was officially founded on October 27, 1989. It is led by a director, colloquially referred to as the Drug Czar, who oversees the office and advises the president.

The overarching goal of the ONDCP is to reduce drug use in the United States and to advise the Executive Office of the President on drug control. However, since its inception, the ONDCP's reach has expanded to international drug control. Domestically, there are three notable campaigns and programs funded by the ONDCP: the National Youth Anti-Drug Media Campaign (NYADMC), High-Intensity Drug Trafficking Areas (HIDTA), and Drug-Free Communities (DFC).

The ONDCP is responsible for the National Drug Control Strategy. This annual report is presented by the acting director of the National Drug Control Policy. It comprises detailed goals from the administration to support the overarching mission of the ONDCP. The report also provides an overview of illicit drug-related violence, crime, and health consequences as well as the manufacturing and trafficking of illicit drugs. A second major component of the ONDCP is the national federal drug control budget. During its first year, the fiscal budget was $7.864 billion dollars. By 2010, the budget had risen to $15 billion. The 2020 fiscal year budget offers $34.6 billion dollars. This budget covers the wide-reaching efforts of the ONDCP to include law enforcement, education, grants, and other drug control programs.

The Director of ONDCP is prohibited by law from supporting any initiatives to legalize illicit substances. Further, if a substance is listed as a schedule I drug, it is the director's responsibility to prohibit any ONDCP funds to be used for legalization efforts, including for medical purposes. Second, if the drug is not a schedule I substance, it must first be approved for medical use by the Food and Drug Administration prior to ONDCP support. This has complicated the push for legalizing marijuana as it is a schedule I drug and unapproved by the Food and Drug Administration. As such, the ONDCP actively campaigns against all marijuana use.

One such campaign is the National Youth Anti-Drug Media Campaign (NYADMC). Launched in July of 1998, it is the "largest national antidrug media campaign in US history" (Palmgreen et al. 2007). The primary focus of this program has been to target marijuana use among young people, though other illicit substances have been occasionally included. The NYADMC has sparked controversy for its alleged inefficacy and heavy-handed propaganda (Palmgreen et al. 2007).

Two large grant programs are managed in the ONDCP. The High-Intensity Drug Trafficking Area program was established in 1990 with a mission to coordinate drug control between various agencies at the local, state, tribal, and federal level to reduce and eliminate drug trafficking in specific areas across the United States. This program currently covers nearly 70 percent of the U.S. population. The second grant program is the Drug-Free Communities program. This provides communities with grants to reduce drug use in young people. The DFC program supports over 700 community programs in the United States.

On March 29, 2017, President Donald Trump signed an Executive Order for the Commission on Combating Drug Addiction and the Opioid Crisis, which is supported financially by the ONDCP. However, in 2018, the Trump administration proposed moving the ONDCP to the jurisdiction of the Justice Department. Some worried that this would cause a shift in the way drug control is handled and argued moving the ONDCP to the Justice Department would emphasize legal punishment over community-based interventions and control (Watkins 2018). However, the proposal was not passed.

Lyla Byers

See also: Anti-Drug Abuse Acts of 1986 and 1988; Reagan Administration "War on Drugs."

Further Reading

Drug Enforcement Administration (DEA). "High Intensity Drug Trafficking Areas (HIDTAs)." n.d. Accessed August 23, 2021 https://www.dea.gov/hidta

Michel, Robert, and Thomas Foley. "H.R.5210 - 100th Congress (1987–1988): Anti-Drug Abuse Act of 1988." Congress.gov, November 18, 1988. https://www.congress.gov/bill/100th-congress/house-bill/05210

"Office of National Drug Control Policy." WhiteHouse.gov, n.d. Accessed August 23, 2021 https://www.whitehouse.gov/ondcp

Office of the Commissioner. "FDA and Cannabis: Research and Drug Approval Process." U.S. Food and Drug Administration, FDA, n.d. Accessed August 23, 2021. https://www.fda.gov/news-events/public-health-focus/fda-and-cannabis-research-and-drug-approval-process

Palmgreen, Philip, et al. "Effects of the Office of National Drug Control Policy's Marijuana Initiative Campaign on High-Sensation-Seeking Adolescents." *American Journal of Public Health 97*, no 9. (2007): 1644–1649.

Watkins, Ali. "Trump Plan to Move Drug Prevention Program to Justice Dept. Prompts Protests." *New York Times,* February 6, 2018. https://www.nytimes.com/2018/02/06/us/politics/ondcp-hidta-grants-justice-department.html

Online Marijuana Markets

Cannabis is one of the most commonly used drugs in America (Hawdon 2005; McCance-Katz 2017). While recent trends toward medical and recreational legalization have increased the licit supply of cannabis in many U.S. states, continued legal restrictions federally and in many U.S. states preserve a robust illicit market for cannabis. The Dark Web—a set of overlay technologies that leverage the protocols of the internet and a network of volunteer machines to allow for anonymous web browsing (Dingledine, Mathewson, and Syverson 2014)—provides a convenient, secure, and effective way to access cannabis within the United States.

Cannabis has been one of the most frequently bought and sold drug on Dark Web cryptomarkets (Christin 2013; Soska and Christin 2015). One such marketplace, Silk Road, was dominated by cannabis sales. Of all listed items, 17.3 percent were dedicated to "cannabis" (3.6 percent) or "weed" (13.7 percent) in the early 2010s (Christin 2013, 216). For comparison, the next largest category of listings was "drugs," at 9 percent. Across a wider subsection of 35 different cryptomarkets, cannabis routinely makes up around 25 percent of all recorded sales (Soska and Christin 2015).

Sensational media accounts paint the Dark Web as a tool of unfettered drug procurement. Yet, the Dark Web as a facilitating technology for cannabis consumption depends on the age, location, and the consumption behaviors of users. Research leveraging Google Trend data as a proxy for interest in the Dark Web within U.S. states indicates three ways in which the Dark Web's utility as a means of procuring drugs is highly variable (Jardine and Lindner 2020).

First, Dark Web cryptomarkets make for comparatively poor means of drug procurement for youth. Any sort of moral panic about the Dark Web as a tool by which youth can access cannabis needs to seriously contend with the offline constraints involved in the typical cryptomarket drug-procurement crime script (Jardine and Lindner 2019). The full crime script to purchase drugs on a cryptomarket includes two steps—funding a cryptocurrency wallet and providing a secure physical world address to which drugs can be shipped—that are comparatively challenging for youth to complete. Combined with easier access to cannabis from local social networks, these constraints plausibly limit the use of Dark Web drug markets among youth. The limiting effect of the cryptomarket crime script on youth cannabis consumption is evident empirically. From 2011 to 2015, for example, Google Trends interest in a Dark Web index term did not correlate with self-reported cannabis consumption among those age 12–17, but did correlate with those age 18–25 or 26 plus (Jardine and Lindner 2020).

Second, early evidence (2011–2015) of trends in medical and recreational legalization of cannabis within the United States provide an interesting glimpse into how legal context interacts with consumption of cannabis via Dark Web markets. Medical legalization does not appear to change the generally positive and significant relationship between interest in the Dark Web and cannabis consumption within U.S. states. Interestingly, the same pattern does not hold for recreational legalization. Here, recreationally legalization actually amplifies the positive association between the Dark Web and cannabis use (Jardine and Lindner 2020). This pattern could be due to a lack of dispensary infrastructure in newly legalized states or a conflation of state-level legalization and U.S.-wide legalization, which might encourage users in recreationally legalized states to order cannabis from a cryptomarket and have it delivered via the U.S. Postal Service without realizing that such activity is likely to violate federal law.

Finally, while there is some evidence that cryptomarkets might act as a wholesale source for drugs (Aldridge and Décary-Hétu 2016), available evidence also suggests that the Dark Web may be used by those who consume cannabis frequently (past month, but not past year) and not at all by more infrequent casual users (past year) (Jardine and Lindner 2020), but only for those age 26 or older. Like the main results, the Dark Web simply might not be a useful tool for youth drug procurement, even for more frequent users.

New technologies certainly matter for cannabis consumption in the United States. Dark Web cryptomarkets are a prime example of one such system, as they promise additional protection from law enforcement, a reduction in gang-related drug violence, home delivery, and, in some cases at least, comparatively high-quality products (Aldridge, Stevens, and Barratt 2018). Yet, how the Dark Web might matter for cannabis use in the United States varies based upon demographics, location, and consumption patterns. The Dark Web amplifies use in some context but is not a tool of cannabis consumption among youth.

Eric Jardine and Andrew M. Lindner

See also: Dispensaries; Moral Panics; Medical Marijuana and the Law.

Further Reading

Aldridge, J., and D. Décary-Hétu. "Hidden Wholesale: The Drug Diffusing Capacity of Online Drug Cryptomarkets." *International Journal of Drug Policy* 35, Supplement C (2016): 7–15. https://doi.org/10.1016/j.drugpo.2016.04.020

Aldridge, J., A. Stevens, and M. J. Barratt. "Will Growth in Cryptomarket Drug Buying Increase the Harms of Illicit Drugs?" *Addiction* 113, no. 5 (2018) : 789–796. https://doi.org/10.1111/add.13899

Christin, N. *Traveling the Silk Road: A Measurement Analysis of a Large Anonymous Online Marketplace*. Paper presented at the Proceedings of the 22nd International Conference on World Wide Web, Rio de Janeiro, Brazil, 2013.

Dingledine, R., N. Mathewson, and P. Syverson. *Tor: The Second-Generation Onion Router*. Paper presented at the Proceedings of the 13th Conference on USENIX Security Symposium – Vol. 13, San Diego, CA, 2014.

Hawdon, J. *Drug and Alcohol Consumption as Functions of Social Structures: A Cross-cultural Sociology*. Lewiston, NY: Edwin Mellen Press, 2005.

Jardine, E., and A. M. Lindner. "The Dark Web and Cannabis Use in the United States: Evidence from a Big Data Research Design." *International Journal of Drug Policy* 76 (2020): 102627. https://doi.org/10.1016/j.drugpo.2019.102627

Jardine, E., and A. M. Lindner. *Does What Happens on the Dark Web, Stay on the Dark Web? Cryptomarkets, Drug Use and Drug Arrests in America*. 2019.

McCance-Katz, E. F. *The National Survey on Drug Use and Health: 2017*. Washington DC, 2017. https://www.samhsa.gov/data/sites/default/files/nsduh-ppt-09-2018.pdf

Soska, K., and N. Christin. *Measuring the Longitudinal Evolution of the Online Anonymous Marketplace Ecosystem*. Paper presented at the 24th USENIX Security Symposium. Washington, DC, August 12–14, 2015.

Operation Intercept

Operation Intercept was a large-scale, highly publicized anti-marijuana operation that was undertaken by the Nixon administration from September 21 to October 11, 1969. Timed to coincide with the peak of the annual marijuana harvest in Mexico, the initiative was designed to reduce the illegal importation of marijuana into the United States from Mexico. During the short time it was in place, the operation nearly shut down the border between Mexico and the United States. Nearly 2,000 federal agents were employed in the operation, and every car crossing the border to or from Mexico was thoroughly searched. Prior to Operation Intercept, approximately 1 in 20 cars were thoroughly searched. In the first week of the operation alone, over two million people were stopped at the 31 official border crossings (Gooberman 1974). Additional enforcement efforts came in the form of the expanded use of radar, high-speed aircraft, and patrol boats—all meant to intercept shipments of drugs into the United States (Craig 1980).

The operation, though temporarily effective in its primary purpose, was extremely unpopular with the Mexican government as well as with American businesses and border communities. The operation was effectively ended on October 2, 1969, after only 11 days. It was soon replaced with a far less severe plan named "Operation Cooperation." This program, and the subsequent coordinated work with Mexican officials, focused on large-scale smugglers and on finding and destroying the fields in Mexico where marijuana and poppies were grown.

The stated intent of Operation Intercept was to focus on the economics of the marijuana market rather than rely on punitive drug laws that were being used at the time. These laws, while unforgiving on paper, were quite forgiving in practice. At the time, only about 1 percent of those arrested for marijuana-related charges were brought to trial and convicted (Gooberman 1974). The hope was that the operation would create a shortage of marijuana in the United States and spur a large increase in the price. For those familiar with the principles of supply and demand, the idea was to decrease supply (shift the supply curve back), thus increasing the equilibrium price. Deputy Attorney General Richard Kleindienst told reporters at a news conference, "We hope to drive the price so high it will be unavailable to students in colleges and high schools . . . who are using it so commonly today" (Gooberman 1974).

According to most reports, Operation Intercept was very effective in achieving its goal. During the operation itself, 3,202 pounds of marijuana were seized. More importantly, the operation had a prolonged "chilling" effect on the import and attempted import of marijuana into the United States. Over the following year, shortages and scarcity of marijuana were reported across the United States (Gooberman 1974). The effect on prices varied, with prices rising everywhere and some cities seeing increases of 100 percent or more. The price of a pound of marijuana in New York City reportedly rose from about $60 to over $300 (Gooberman 1974).

As with a great deal of U.S. drug policy, Operation Intercept produced unintended consequences. First, with the availability of marijuana down and price up, users often turned to more easily accessible drugs or alcohol. Operation Intercept also had economic effects outside the marijuana trade—for both Mexican and U.S. businesses. The concerns expressed by these business interests, and the political power behind those interests, ultimately led to the operation's short life.

According to basic economic theory, as the price of one product rises, or if a product is simply not available, consumers are likely to switch their consumption to a lower priced or more available similar product. Several economic studies have shown, for example, that drug use is higher in counties where alcohol sales are prohibited. This theory played out in the aftereffects of Operation Intercept. A study that took place immediately after the operation found that 50 percent of those who reported difficulty in getting marijuana increased their consumption of alcohol as a direct result (McGlothlin, Jamison, and Rosenblatt 1970). Later studies, while mixed, generally support the idea that alcohol and marijuana are substitute products (DiNardo and Lemieux 2001). In the most comprehensive book written on the effects of Operation Intercept, Gooberman (1974) also asserted that the reduction in the availability of marijuana following Operation Intercept led some to increase their use of other "harder" drugs such as LSD, heroin, hashish, and amphetamine. Such lateral moves to other drugs clearly undermined the primary, public health-related intent of Operation Intercept.

Operation Intercept also had spillover effects. In economics, the concept of spillovers (or externalities) is rooted in the idea that economic actions or policies often have effects outside the primary sphere of the action or policy. In the case of Operation Intercept, this meant that the policy had profound effects on industries and communities outside the markets for drugs and those who engaged in those markets. Most notably, the operation harmed the economies of many border cities in both Mexico and the United States by effectively shutting down trade and tourism during the operation.

The effect on Mexico, where tourism is a key industry, was immediate and crushing. "As word of Intercept's long delays turned American tourists away by the thousands," noted one account, "business sales and hotel occupancies fell 40–70 percent" (Craig 1980). Needless to say, both businesses and politicians in Mexico quickly spoke out against the operation. America's political and economic relations with Mexico were also strained.

While generally supportive of the idea of Operation Intercept, businesses and communities on the U.S. side of the border soon faced their own, very significant unintended consequences of the operation. In a letter to the governor of Texas, the Mayor of Brownsville, Texas, where tourism from Mexico accounted for a substantial part of the economy, stated, "The cure will kill the patient because we are creating altogether too much ill-will and receiving very harsh criticism from the very people with whom we have been striving mighty hard to get along with." He added that the economic impact of the operation was "so severe that the City Commission . . . has instructed me to request of you that the Brownsville community be declared an economic disaster area" (Craig 1980). Another official claimed that "the architects of Operation Intercept failed to recall a small but very significant fact—there are two sides to this damn border" (Craig 1980). Similar sentiment became widespread, and U.S. businesses and communities quickly turned against the operation, arguing that the costs far outweighed the benefits. When national politicians, including some in Nixon's own cabinet, joined in the criticism, the end of Operation Intercept was inevitable.

Despite its success with regard to slowing the import of marijuana from Mexico, it became clear to U.S. officials that the costs, in terms of relations with Mexico and the economic impact on border communities in the United States, outweighed any potential benefits of the operation. Operation Intercept was effectively halted on October 2, 1969. It was officially replaced on October 11 by the gentler "Operation Cooperation."

Steve Trost

See also: Law Enforcement Efforts, Marijuana Control; Nixon Administration "War on Drugs"; Pricing.

Further Reading

Craig, Richard B. "Operation Intercept: The International Politics of Pressure." *Review of Politics* 42, no. 4 (1980): 556–580.

DiNardo, J., and T. Lemieux. "Alcohol, Marijuana, and American Youth: The Unintended Consequences of Government Regulation." *Journal of Health Economics* 20, no. 6 (2001): 991–1010.

Gooberman, Lawrence A. 1974. *Operation Intercept: The Multiple Consequences of Public Policy.* Elmsford, NY: Pergamon.

McGlothlin, W., K. Jamison, and S. Rosenblatt. "Marijuana and the Use of Other Drugs." *Nature* 228 (1970): 1227–1229. https://doi.org/10.1038/2281227a0

P

Petty, Tom (1950–2017)

Thomas Earl "Tom" Petty (October 20, 1950–October 2, 2017) was a multiplatinum-selling American singer-songwriter from Gainesville, Florida, who was the lead singer and frontman for the popular rock band Tom Petty and the Heartbreakers. In addition to intermittent solo endeavors, he was also a member of the short-lived late 1980s supergroup the Traveling Wilburys, which included Bob Dylan, George Harrison, Jeff Lynne, and Roy Orbison. Petty's musical style was perhaps best characterized as rock with a southern influence, but he and his band often incorporated elements from other genres, including folk, blues, and country music.

Growing up with an abusive father, Petty dropped out of high school at the age of 17 and moved to Los Angeles, California, to further pursue a musical career at the age of 23. He originally played bass guitar before forming the Heartbreakers in 1976 and switching primarily to guitar. He also frequently played the harmonica and ukulele on his albums and during live shows. In interviews, Petty gave credit to Elvis Presley and the Beatles for inspiring him to be a musician and the Rolling Stones for making his aspirations appear obtainable.

Over the course of his career, Petty recorded 13 studio albums with the Heartbreakers between 1976 and 2014, as well as three solo albums. He is estimated to have sold more than 80 million records and produced more than 50 singles of which more than a dozen appeared in the top ten on the US Billboard Charts, including "American Girl," "I Won't Back Down," "Learning to Fly," "Free Fallin'," and "Runnin' Down a Dream." Petty was nominated for 18 Grammy Awards and won 3. In 2002, Tom Petty and the Heartbreakers were inducted into the Rock & Roll Hall of Fame.

Petty was candid about his marijuana usage throughout his life and career. Both allusions and overt references to marijuana, in addition to other drugs, can be heard throughout many of his songs. The most notable is perhaps the iconic 1993 hit "Mary Jane's Last Dance" (sometimes mistakenly referred by its chorus as "Last Dance with Mary Jane") the lyrics of which appear to refer to the drug. However, Petty had never confirmed the true meaning of the song, and plausible alternative interpretations exist.

Following his divorce from his first wife in 1996, Petty became addicted to heroin. After struggling to quit, Petty was able to overcome his addiction through rehabilitation before marrying his second wife in 2001. In 2017, Petty died at the age of 66 from cardiac arrest after accidental overdose from mixed drug toxicity. Following his death, the Los Angeles County medical examiner reported finding fentanyl and fentanyl analogs, oxycodone, alprazolam, and citalopram in his system. In a statement released after his death, it was stated that Petty had been prescribed medications, including fentanyl, to address pain associated with several issues, including a severe hip fracture. His death came a week after he had finished a 53-show tour to celebrate the fortieth anniversary of the formation of The Heartbreakers. It was stated that Petty was suffering from severe pain from his fractured hip the entire tour.

John M. Eassey

See also: Beatles, The; Garcia, Jerry (1942–1995); Monkees, The; Nelson, Willie (1933–); Snoop Dogg (1971–); Woodstock.

Further Reading

Sweeting, Adam. "Tom Petty Obituary." *The Guardian,* October 3, 2017. https://www.theguardian.com/music/2017/oct/03/tom-petty-obituary

Zanes, Warren. *Petty: The Biography.* New York: Henry Holt and Company, 2015.

Zollo, Paul. *Conversations with Tom Petty.* New York: Omnibus Press, 2005.

Pricing

Like any product, there are numerous factors that impact the price of a gram of marijuana. Unlike other products, however, marijuana's status as a banned substance in many locations means that data on its price are difficult to obtain and highly variable. Moreover, its banned status for recreational use in some states also affects price, stemming both from the additional costs to the seller (the risk involved in carrying, transporting, and selling an illegal substance) and the risk and social stigma on the buyer (potentially lowering demand). This makes price data on illicit drugs extremely valuable for researchers, as it allows them not only to study the relative strength and influence of various elements on an illicit drug's price but also how changes in price affect consumer and seller behavior.

The traditional source of price data for illicit drugs in the United States has been the federal government. The Drug Enforcement Administration's (DEA) System to Retrieve Information from Drug Evidence (STRIDE) database collects information on confiscated illicit drugs sent to DEA labs for testing, but this data is restricted to internal researchers. The Office of National Drug Control Policy previously published aggregated reports on historical trends of illicit drug prices, demonstrating that overall marijuana prices were decreasing; however, their last published report only covered 1981 through 2007. Ultimately, some have criticized the government for not providing the necessary resources to study national trends in drug use (Casteel 2017).

In the late 2010s, however, research consultancy groups have sought to fill this information gap by increasing data availability on marijuana use specifically. For instance, in 2016 the GfK Knowledge Group began hosting a nationwide online survey of marijuana use (Pacula, Jacobson, and Maksabedian 2016), which was later supplemented with questions by RAND Corporation to gather self-reported data on prices paid for marijuana (Hunt and Pacula 2017). In contrast to the challenges involved in accessing illicit drug data in the United States, the European

Monitoring Centre for Drugs and Drug Addiction posts annual data on the price, purity, and potency of many illicit drugs.

Despite issues of data availability and accuracy, researchers continue to make progress in studying what determines the price of illicit drugs such as marijuana. Researchers have identified several main determinants common to both legal and illegal marijuana sales, including regional pricing differences, seller productivity, quality and purity, and bulk discounts (Clements and Zhao 2009). In areas where the sale of marijuana is illegal, there would be additional factors exerting pressure on price. First, unregulated marijuana is a pure "experience good," meaning that buyers may not know the quality and purity of a drug even after purchasing and consuming it (Caulkins 2007). This uncertainty makes it difficult not only for prospective buyers trying to evaluate a fair price but also for drug agencies trying to estimate black-market prices. Second, sellers (assuming they do not enjoy risk) would need to be compensated for the probability of incurring a criminal penalty from the sale of a banned substance, raising the cost of doing business and putting upward pressure on price (National Research Council 2010).

While the legalization of marijuana for recreational use would remove these additional costs, legalization would also introduce many other considerations and market forces. From a market power perspective, the less sellers there are in an area, the more those marijuana sellers will be able to raise price. Legalization could potentially lower the market power of incumbent sellers as new ones enter the market, making local markets for marijuana more competitive and putting downward pressure on price. However, there is no guarantee that a competitive marketplace and lower prices would persist in the long run, and it could take several years before prices begin to reflect a fully transitioned, legalized market (Hunt and Pacula 2017). On the demand side, legalization of marijuana for recreational use might increase its popularity among segments of the public as people adopt a more favorable view of marijuana use. Evidence that many new buyers would enter the market following legalization remains mixed (Pacula and Lundberg 2013); however, an increase in buyers would increase demand and put upward pressure on price.

The above considerations, coupled with limited instances of legalization and the fact that many states that legalize marijuana for recreational use already have robust medical marijuana markets (Hansen, Miller, and Weber 2017), make determining legalization's overall effect on price difficult. Hence, the decrease in the price of marijuana observed by the Office of National Drug Control Policy may not continue after legalization. Nevertheless, many researchers believe that the price of legalized marijuana would be lower than its black-market price (see Caulkins and Reuter 1998 for the most oft-cited example of this argument).

An additional price consideration that is less under control of buyers and sellers is that both local and state governments are likely to levy a tax on the sale of marijuana to generate government revenue. This would impose an additional cost on sellers, who are likely to pass on some of this cost to consumers via increased prices. For example, the state of Colorado imposes a 15 percent excise tax on marijuana retailers (which is often reflected directly in the sales price) in additional to a 15 percent retail marijuana sales tax. Both of these taxes contribute to higher recreational marijuana prices for the consumer (see Colorado Department of Revenue,

Taxation Division for more information). The exact degree to which buyers or sellers would bear the burden of these taxes would depend on how sensitive their relative behavior is to price changes (which economists call price elasticity), with the more price insensitive group shouldering the greater burden of the tax.

Although there is much to consider concerning what affects the price of marijuana, the primary consequence of these prices changes (whether it be through legalization, taxes, or other factors) is how it alters the amount of marijuana being bought and sold. Assuming a standard downward sloping demand curve, the more dramatically potential buyers react to price changes, the more new marijuana users there would be as price decreases. One meta study of youth marijuana use found that "policies that reduce the price of marijuana by ten percent therefore, will lead to a three to five percent increase in the number of new marijuana users among youth, all else equal" (Pacula and Lundberg 2013, 5). A later study using crowd-sourced transaction data found that a 10 percent reduction in price would lead to a 6.7–7.9 percent increase in new marijuana users when pooling all age groups (Davis, Geisler, and Nichols 2016). Ultimately, while the exact amount is disputed, all evidence indicates that there will be more buyers in the market as the price of marijuana decreases.

As a final counterpoint to the above discussion on marijuana price changes, it should be noted that researchers have found that in some markets the price of illegal illicit drugs may remain fairly constant over time, while the quantity offered per standard price will change (Caulkins and Reuter 1998; Caulkins 2007). However, this phenomenon would be unlikely to persist following legalization.

Thomas J. PlaHovinsak, II

See also: Taxation.

Further Reading

Casteel, Kathryn. "Data on Drugs Use Is Disappearing Just When We Need It Most." Fivethirtyeight.com, June 29, 2017. https://fivethirtyeight.com/features/data-on-drug-use-is-disappearing-just-when-we-need-it-most/

Caulkins, Jonathan P. "Price and Purity Analysis for Illicit Drug: Data and Conceptual Issues." *Drug and Alcohol Dependence* 90 (2007): S61–S68.

Caulkins, Jonathan P., and Peter Reuter. "What Price Data Tell Us about Drug Markets." *Journal of Drug Issues* 28, no. 3 (1998): 593–612.

Clements, Kenneth W., and Xueyan Zhao. *Economics and Marijuana: Consumption, Pricing and Legalisation.* Cambridge, UK: Cambridge University Press, 2009.

Davis, Adam J., Karl R. Geisler, and Mark W. Nichols. "The Price Elasticity of Marijuana Demand: Evidence from Crowd-Sourced Transaction Data." *Empirical Economics* 50, no. 4 (2016): 1171–1192.

Hansen, Benjamin, Keaton Miller, and Caroline Weber. *The Taxation of Recreational Marijuana: Evidence from Washington State.* No. w23632. Cambridge, MA: National Bureau of Economic Research, 2017.

Hunt, Priscillia, and Rosalie Liccardo Pacula. "Early Impacts of Marijuana Legalization: An Evaluation of Prices in Colorado and Washington." *The Journal of Primary Prevention* 38, no. 3 (2017): 221–248.

"Marijuana Taxes | File." 2014, July 14. https://www.urban.org/policy-centers/cross-center-initiatives/state-and-local-finance-initiative/state-and-local-backgrounders/marijuana-taxes

National Research Council. *Understanding the Demand for Illegal Drugs*. Washington, DC: The National Academies Press, 2010. https://doi.org/10.17226/12976

Pacula, Rosalie Liccardo, Mireille Jacobson, and Ervant J. Maksabedian. "In the Weeds: A Baseline View of Cannabis Use among Legalizing States and Their Neighbours." *Addiction* 111, no. 6 (2016): 973–980.

Pacula, Rosalie Liccardo, and Russell Lundberg. "Why Changes in Price Matter When Thinking About Marijuana Policy: A Review of The Literature on The Elasticity of Demand." *Public Health Reviews* 35, no. 2 (2013): 2.

R

Race

In the United States, marijuana criminalization and punitive enforcement bear a legacy of prejudice and fear associated with racial/ethnic minorities and the foreign born. During the first half of the twentieth century, most states and the federal government enacted anti-marijuana laws that targeted Black communities and Mexican migrants, stoking racism and popularizing largely unsupported claims about the threat and danger of the drug. At the federal level, this included the passage of the Marihuana Tax Act of 1937, which in practice severely restricted and made illegal the possession and sale of the drug. In the years that followed, state and federal anti-marijuana laws intensified in terms of both targeting minorities and punishment severity, while also contributing to the growth of and participation in illicit, underground drug economies (Thompson 2017; Vitiello 2019). The modern "War on Drugs," a defining feature of American law enforcement in the last three decades of the twentieth century, marked an escalation of those efforts, producing striking racial disparities in arrests, prosecutions, sentencing, and incarceration. The effects spilled over into the labor market as well, given the reluctance of employers to hire persons with a criminal record. This dynamic excluded minorities in disproportionate numbers from numerous economic and professional opportunities, including those in the more recent legalized marijuana industry.

First heralded by President Richard Nixon (1969–1974) in 1971, the War on Drugs represented a heavily politicized tough-on-crime stance. Nixon's policy initiatives in this instance only incrementally increased drug arrests and incarceration, but his public rhetoric of law and order did much to strengthen disparaging stereotypes connecting racial/ethnic minorities to drugs (Alexander 2020). The Nixon administration also classified marijuana as a Schedule I substance—a designation signifying high potential for abuse and no medical value assigned to such drugs as LSD and heroin. Under President Ronald Reagan (1981–1989), the War on Drugs sharply accelerated and expanded. Indeed, the Reagan administration prompted increased policing and surveillance of Black, Latino, and poor neighborhoods; stricter enforcement of drug laws; harsher penalties for drug offenses; and mandatory minimum sentences at all levels of government (Vitiello 2019). At the federal level, in particular, this included such powerful legislation as the Comprehensive Crime Control Act of 1984 and Anti-Drug Abuse Act of 1986. These laws established and lengthened mandatory minimum sentences for drug offenses, while also eliminating federal parole. Arrest and incarceration rates, in turn, skyrocketed during the 1980s and 1990s, and the state and federal prison population swelled from just under 330,000 inmates in 1980 to nearly 1.4 million in 2000 (Bureau of Justice Statistics 1980–2000). Over half of this growth was attributable to drug offenses, including marijuana.

Since California first legalized marijuana in 1996 for adult medical use, 34 U.S. states and the District of Columbia have followed suit. Additionally, since 2012, 15 states and the District of Columbia have legalized marijuana for adult recreational use. At least in part, this reflects a general softening of public perception and attitudes toward the drug. Over the last two decades, there has been a gradual but steady shift in support for marijuana legalization. In fact, in recent years, nearly two-thirds of Americans have supported legalization (Gallup 2019). Yet this shift in public opinion, as well as state and local policy changes, contrasts with current policing practices and the continued effects of the War on Drugs on Black and Latino communities. From 2012 to 2018, for instance, total U.S. arrests declined, but the proportion of drug arrests actually increased. For this same period, despite a relative decline in marijuana arrests, they consistently outpaced all other drug-related offenses, accounting for over 40 percent of an estimated 11 million drug arrests, with roughly 90 percent for simple possession (FBI Uniform Crime Report). Furthermore, although whites, Blacks, and Latinos use and sell marijuana at comparable rates, available data suggest racial/ethnic minorities are at far greater risk of being arrested (ACLU 2013), prosecuted, convicted, and incarcerated (Vitiello 2019) for marijuana offenses than whites. Importantly, disparate contact and experiences with the criminal justice system can impact and severely penalize minorities outside of it. Particularly salient here is the link to employment.

An extensive body of research demonstrates that U.S. Blacks and Latinos face frequent prejudice in the labor market, resulting in significant disadvantages (in earnings, job placement, promotions, etc.) compared to whites. Scholars suggest such inequality is at least in part a product of stereotypes of criminality projected by white employers on minorities (Pager, Bonikowski, and Western 2009). This is amplified by the numerous institutional barriers to employment created by a criminal record—barriers that disproportionately affect Black and Latino economic and professional opportunities given the unequal application and enforcement of the law. State and federal restrictions, for example, directly exclude persons with a felony conviction from licensing and employment in several hundred U.S. industries (Alexander 2020; Thompson 2017). In addition, thousands of state laws for occupational and business licensing contain provisions that take any criminal history and record into account (Slivinski 2016). Many of these laws include "good moral character" clauses that automatically bar individuals from licensing due to arrests (with or without formal charges) and misdemeanor charges (with or without conviction). Thus, even an incident without a conviction or prison time still carries lasting penalties and consequences.

Noticeably, the legal marijuana industry (medical and recreational) in most U.S. states contains laws with "good moral character" clauses that guide licensing procedures and outcomes. Many of these clauses focus specifically on drug-related offenses and criminal history. New York, for instance, legalized medical marijuana in 2014, but according to state law, any felony conviction for drug possession bars individuals from employment in the industry (Drug Policy Alliance 2017). Likewise, in Washington D.C., which legalized recreational marijuana in 2014, persons with drug-related misdemeanors are barred from licensing, whereas persons with other types of misdemeanor offenses (violent crime, theft, etc.) may still receive consideration (Thompson 2017). Such restrictions disproportionately impact Blacks and Latinos, limiting potential business ownership and employment access in the legal market.

Several states, including California, Colorado, and Oregon, have moved to reduce restrictions on licensing and participation in the industry in an effort to ease some of the enduring injustice and inequality that connects marijuana and the drug war to both the criminal justice system and mainstream economy (Thompson 2017). Even so, studies suggest whites are greatly overrepresented in the legal marijuana industry, and Blacks and Latinos represent only a small fraction of business owners and employees (Drug Policy Alliance 2017; Vitiello 2019). Given that U.S. minorities continue to be marginalized by the law and in the labor market, it is unsurprising that they face persistent institutional barriers and inequalities in the legal sale and production of marijuana.

Salvatore J. Restifo

See also: Conflict and Labeling Theories; Incarceration for Marijuana Offenses; Incarceration Rates; Racial Inequalities in Sentencing.

Further Reading

Alexander, Michelle. *The New Jim Crow: Mass Incarceration in the Age of Colorblindness.* 10th Anniversary ed. New York: The New Press, 2020.

American Civil Liberties Union (ACLU). *The War on Marijuana in Black and White.* New York: ACLU Foundation. 2013.

Bureau of Justice Statistics. *Prisoners Series.* Washington, DC: U.S. Department of Justice, 1980–2000. https://www.bjs.gov/

Drug Policy Alliance. *Marijuana Reform in New York: Diversity and Inclusion in the Marijuana Industry.* 2017. http://smart-ny.com/wp-content/uploads/2017/06/StartSMART_DPA_NY_Marijuana_Reform_Diversity_Inclusion_09.14.2017.pdf

Federal Bureau of Investigation, Uniform Crime Report. *Crime in the United States—Persons Arrested.* Washington, DC: U.S. Department of Justice, 2012–2018. https://ucr.fbi.gov/crime-in-the-u.s

Gallup. *Illegal Drugs.* 2019. https://news.gallup.com/poll/1657/illegal-drugs.aspx

Pager, Devah, Bart Bonikowski, and Bruce Western. "Discrimination in a Low-Wage Labor Market: A Field Experiment." *American Sociological Review* 74, no. 5 (2009): 777–799.

Slivinski, Stephen. *Turning Shackles into Bootstraps: Why Occupational Licensing Reform Is the Missing Piece of Criminal Justice Reform.* Policy Report: no. 2016-01. Tempe, AZ: Center for the Study of Economic Liberty at Arizona State University, 2016.

Thompson, Beverly Yuen. "'Good Moral Characters': How Drug Felons Are Impacted under State Marijuana Legalization Laws." *Contemporary Justice Review* 20, no. 2 (2017): 211–226.

Vitiello, Michael. "Marijuana Legalization, Racial Disparity, and the Hope for Reform." *Lewis & Clark Law Review* 23, no. 3 (2019): 789–821.

Racial Inequalities in Sentencing

Racial disparity in sentencing is an issue that has plagued the American criminal justice system for some time. This affects a multitude of stages within both the juvenile justice system and the adult correctional system. Disparities exist at all levels of the U.S. legal system, from the imposition of bail and assignments of public defenders through the formal sentencing of a convicted offenders. Implications based on race and the intersection of race and class remain prevalent in each of these judicial processes.

The Reagan-era "War on Drugs" emerged during the height of the crack cocaine epidemic. Designation of this issue as an epidemic was meant to elicit a fearful response from the public and a sense of doom if it was not confronted. Media attention focused on urban inner cities, as drug use and sale were largely cast in association with African Americans and other persons of color. The ensuing result of "get tough" policies catered to this public fear of crack cocaine spreading from the inner cities into suburban communities. The 100-to-1 sentencing guidelines emerged in response from such public fear. Guidelines facilitated through this legislation allowed for sanctioned differences in sentences based on the form and weight of cocaine an individual was found to be in possession of. Put another way, this legislation called for an individual convicted of possessing 500 grams of powder cocaine to receive the same sentence as an individual convicted of possessing 5 grams of crack cocaine. Such legislation focused more on the characteristics of a user rather than the pharmacological differences in the substances itself (Barak, Leighton, and Cotton 2015).

Such policies were implicitly derived on racial contexts, as crack cocaine use was largely associated with minority usage while powder cocaine was associated not only with white offenders but also with middle- to upper-class white offenders. Even with the crack cocaine epidemic subsiding well prior to the turn of the century, such federal laws remained in effect until 2010 when the Fair Sentencing Act of 2010 reduced the ratio disparity from 100:1 to 18:1 (Barak et al. 2015). While these laws and policies do not deal specifically with marijuana offenses, they show how legislative statutes can be implicitly shaped by the race and socioeconomic status of offenders.

Another controversial statue is that of the "3 strikes" laws that were passed in California and several other states in the 1990s. Following the trend of "get tough" criminal policy, the 3 strikes laws sought to curb recidivism rates among chronic offenders. This legislative effort was enacted to give harsher punishments for offenders who repeatedly committed offenses. The desired result would increase public safety for law-abiding citizens. Under these laws, however, lesser offenses such as minor property crimes and misdemeanor drug charges, such as marijuana possession, could lead to felonious punishments (Reid 2018).

As punishments for nonviolent offenses such as property crimes and possession of illicit substances grew, so too did the number of incarcerated offenders. California, which had implemented the 3 strikes laws in 1994, was impacted so drastically that in 2014, voters in the state passed Proposition 47, which reclassified certain offenses from felonies to misdemeanors. Offenses concerning some narcotics, controlled substances, cannabis, and property crimes were among those reclassified (Reid 2018). One 2018 study investigated the effects of Proposition 47 on racial disparities in arrest rates and found that white offenders had a significant proportion of felonious offenses reclassified as misdemeanors. For all offenders, felony drug arrests decreased, but due to the reclassification of offenses, white offenders saw the largest drop. This study also observed an overall decrease in racial disparities for drug use as a result of the implementation of Proposition 47 (Mooney et al. 2018).

Aside from the statutory language of the preceding examples, much of the racial inequalities in sentencing extends to a larger, systemic issue. Of paramount concern is the disproportionate minority contact found within the criminal justice system. Studies have found that racial disparities are exasperated when minority youth have contact with police at an early age (Crutchfield et al. 2009). Such contact yields higher rates of further contact and arrest later in life.

YOUTH POPULATIONS

Though commonly associated with the program initiated by Office of Juvenile Justice and Delinquency Program (OJJDP), disproportionate minority contact characterizes both the juvenile justice system and the adult criminal system (Shoemaker 2018). Efforts made by the OJJDP have focused on addressing the concerns of disproportionate minority contact through changes to the structural organization of the juvenile justice system. Several reforms such as interrupting the school-to-prison pipeline, conflict resolution over institutionalization, and incentivized alternatives to incarceration have been proposed and tried (Church II, Springer, and Roberts 2014).

Self-report surveys such as the Monitoring the Future study indicate that marijuana is the most common illicit substance used by high school age students. Marijuana-related offenses highlight the points already discussed concerning disproportionate minority contact and the racial disparities of law enforcement contact with juvenile offenders. In fact, marijuana offenses can further exacerbate these two systemic issues. For instance, one study found that in the early 2000s, approximately 60 percent of adjudicated juveniles participated in some type of substance abuse. Additionally, approximately 13 percent of all juvenile cases in 2013 were specifically related to drug offenses (Shoemaker 2018).

ADULT POPULATIONS

Upon arrest, one of the first judicial processes an arrestee faces is the bail determination hearing. In this step, a magistrate or court official weighs several factors to determine whether an arrestee is a flight risk or presents the potential to miss court. Several factors play into this decision, such as whether the defendant has any past criminal history or a record of failing to make court appearances. However, additional factors play a role such as financial assets, a stable job, and roots within the community. These latter economic characteristics merit further discussion as many argue that this portion of the bond hearing serves to criminalize characteristics of class rather than taking into account the alleged offense that brought the accused before the court (Donnelly and MacDonald 2019). A 2017 study, for example, suggested that pretrial confinement has a causal relationship with convictions (Menefee 2018). Further, minorities are disproportionately affected by pretrial detention, creating a disparity in representation (Williams 2017).

Once the accused progresses through the judicial process, he or she will appear in court for an arraignment. In this stage, a judge provides the defendant with an official reading of the formal charges brought by the state. If a defendant has not already obtained the services of an attorney, a judge can assign a public defender in the circumstances that the accused qualifies as indigent. This is a constitutional right guaranteed under the Sixth Amendment and subsequently adapted after the *Gideon v. Wainwright* (1963) Supreme Court ruling (Reid 2018). Similar to the preceding circumstances of a bail hearing, concerns of class and status emerge to influence the quality of defense one can secure. Public defenders are easily inundated with large caseloads and may not have the same time to dedicate to all clients the same way a private attorney may. Often with larger caseloads, public defenders may opt to accept a plea bargain from the prosecutor's office as an alternative to the time needed to prepare a case that goes to trial. As in the previous discussion of imposition of bail, the intersection of race and class becomes visible. The implications of both are further highlighted in the assignment of a public defender. Wooldredge, Goulette, and Travis III (2015) identify the impact of racial disparities at each of these stages of the judicial process from arrest to detention as a cumulative disadvantage that amplifies racial disparities as cases progress.

This discussion of plea bargains highlights the use of plea agreements as an alternative to bringing a case to trial. Often, this is a tool used to alleviate heavy court dockets and the increased number of cases assigned to both defense and prosecuting attorneys. Typically, such plea bargains may result in reduced punishments as an incentive to a defendant. The caveat with such plea deals is that the accused loses the right to appeal a conviction. It may seem as counterintuitive to think that an innocent person would accept a plea bargain. However, with the list of cumulative effects of pretrial imprisonment coupled with inadequate defense and the possibility of facing a full sentence if a plea agreement is not reached may be too daunting for some (Wooldredge et al. 2015). This has direct implications on the weight of pretrial detention, especially among minority offenders.

Jason T. Callahan

See also: Age; California; Incarceration for Marijuana Offenses; Incarceration Rates; Incarceration, Use during; Race.

Further Reading

Barak, Gregg, Paul S. Leighton, and Allison Cotton. *Class, Race, Gender, and Crime; Social Realities of Justice in America.* 4th ed. Lanham, MD: Rowman & Littlefield, 2015.

Church, Wesley T., II, David W. Springer, and Albert R. Roberts. *Juvenile Justice Sourcebook.* 2nd ed. New York: Oxford, 2014.

Crutchfield, Robert D., Martie L. Skinner, Kevin P. Haggerty, Ann McGlynn, and Richard F. Catalano. "Racial Disparities in Early Criminal Justice Involvement." *Race and Social Problems* 1, no. 4 (2009): 218–230.

Donnelly, Ellen, and John MacDonald. "The Downstream Effects of Bail and Pretrial Detention on Racial Disparities in Incarceration." *The Journal of Criminal Law and Criminology* 108, no. 4 (2019): 775–814.

Menefee, Michael R. "The Role of Bail and Pretrial Detention in the Reproduction of Racial Inequalities." *Sociology Compass* 12, no. 5 (2018): 1–9.

Mooney, Alyssa, et al. "Racial/ethnic Disparities in Arrests for Drug Possession after California Proposition 47, 2011–2016." *American Journal of Public Health* 108, no. 8 (2018): 987–993.

Reid, Sue T. *Crime and Criminology*. 15th ed. New York: Wolters Kluwer, 2018.

Shoemaker, Donald. *Juvenile Delinquency*. 3rd ed. Lanham, MD: Rowman and Littlefield, 2018.

Williams, Marian R. "The Effect of Attorney Type on Bail Decisions." *Criminal Justice Policy Review* 28, no. 1 (2017): 3–17.

Wooldredge, John, Natalie Goulette, and Lawrence Travis III. "Is the Impact of Cumulative Disadvantage on Sentencing Greater for Black Defendants?" *Criminology and Public Policy* 14, no. 2 (2015): 187–223.

Rastafarianism

Rastafarianism is a religious movement with roots in Jamaica. Founded by Leonard Percival Howell (1898–1981) and Kingston-area Black Jamaicans in the 1930s, Rastafarianism is heavily influenced by the radical ideas of Marcus Garvey (1887–1940), a Jamaican activist and intellectual who spread a message of Black pride and Africa as the Black homeland. The religion mixes Christian, Hindu, and traditional African religious practices. Africa and Ethiopia are at the center of the Rastafarian movement, with believers viewing Ethiopia as the faith's homeland.

The central figure of Rastafarianism is Haile Selassie I (1892–1975). Born Lij Tafari Makonnen and known as Ras Tafari Makonnen, Selassie was crowned emperor of Ethiopia on November 2, 1930. The coronation of Selassie lives on as the most important holiday in the Rastafarianism belief system. To the Rastafari, the coronation marks the return of Messiah, marking a new era that revealed the true leader of the African diaspora. It is believed that the Messiah will lead oppressed Black people out of Babylon (the current world of oppression) and into the homeland.

The Rastafarian movement has followers all over the world, although religious practices and interpretations vary across regions. One of the most well-known practices is the use of the Tree of Wisdom. The Tree of Wisdom is a term given to marijuana by Rastafarians. The roots of marijuana and Rastafarianism began in colonial Jamaica, and the relationship has evolved over time. Following the end of slavery in Jamaica, former masters found themselves without a work force. This led to the importation of Indian laborers. With these laborers came their practices, including Hinduism and marijuana use. Contact with these Indian laborers exposed Black Jamaicans to the potential of marijuana as a healing and spiritual plant.

The spiritual context in which Rastafarians use marijuana is best seen during "sessions." Sessions are occasions in which Rastafarians, traditionally men, gather in a

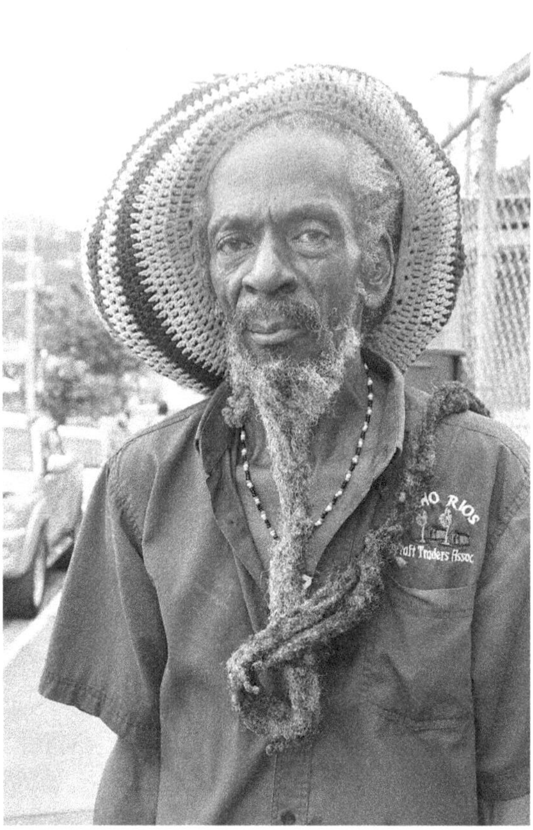

A follower of the Rastafarian religion in Jamaica. Rastafarianism is a religion that combines West African and Christian beliefs founded in Jamaica in the 1930s. It holds marijuana as a scared plant. Followers believe smoking marijuana brings them closer to God or Jah. (Pressfoto/Dreamstime.com)

circle to pass around a hand-rolled marijuana cigarette or a drink containing marijuana resin. During these sessions, participants discuss many aspects of the Black experience, and the plant is seen by participants as a tool for knowledge development and spiritual enlightenment.

The context of marijuana's status as the Tree of Wisdom in the Rastafari movement is tied to prohibition. With the rise of marijuana prohibition in Jamaica, aided by U.S. efforts, the Rastafari belief in marijuana as the Tree of Wisdom was strengthened. It was thought that whites and other upholders of Babylon wished to keep those in the Rastafari movement from this wisdom, thus hiding essential truths and blocking enlightenment. This dynamic led to marijuana becoming, in part, a symbol of Rastafarian's rejection of Babylon.

The worldwide spread of the Rastafari movement is attributed to the rise in popularity of reggae. Prominent reggae artists helped spread Rastafari symbolism and teachings to a worldwide audience with their mainstream success. Thus, reggae is responsible for turning the highly localized Rastafari movement into a global movement. Other ethnic and racial groups that faced colonial histories similar to Black Jamaicans found the empowering message of the religion to be particularly attractive and useful. The rise of Rastafarianism outside of Jamaica, however, led to issues concerning the relationship between marijuana prohibition and the religious freedoms of Rastafarians. These clashes between law and religious freedom continue today.

Like other religions containing an element of substance use, the Rastafari movement faces challenges, particularly in Western contexts. Rastafarians and advocates draw parallels between the Rastafarian movement and the Native American Church (NAC). Where the Rastafari use marijuana, the NAC uses peyote. Peyote is a cactus plant used by the NAC and other Native American groups in religious contexts that contains the psychedelic substance known as mescaline. Peyote has an overwhelmingly religious or sacred connotation, while marijuana is most known as a recreational drug. Thus, it is not a sacred substance that can be used without penalty. An example of this conflict comes in the form of the 1991 case of a Rastafari who was arrested for possession and importation of marijuana seeds at a Guam airport. The defense in the case argued that the use and importation was tied to his Rastafari beliefs and justified in the Rastafarian interpretation of the Bible. Thus, the case brought up arguments over religious freedoms. In September of 2000, the Superior Court of Guam ruled in the Rastafari's favor and his charges were dismissed. The ruling cited the Religious Freedom Restoration Act, which was established in 1993 to further ensure religious freedoms and has protected the rights of some religious minorities to incorporate substances in their religious practices. In 2001, the case was brought by the prosecution to the Ninth Superior Court, where it found that the Rastafari could still be tried on the importation charges. In response to this, the Rastafari appealed and claimed his religion requires him to travel with marijuana when necessary. These types of legal battles highlight the struggle of Rastafaris to have marijuana recognized as a sacred substance in the United States and its territories. The case did set a precedent, which allows for the religious smoking of marijuana on federally owned lands in the United States.

The United States is not alone in confronting this issue. Rastafarianism is a recognized religion in England and Wales; however, antidrug policies in the United Kingdom make it hard for Rastas to use marijuana without fear of legal penalties. Additionally, an Italian conviction was overturned in 2008 by the Italian Supreme Court in favor of a Rastafari who was charged with possession with intent to supply. When the case got to the Supreme Court, the judges upheld the precedent of religious rights and the protection of religious minorities. Thus, like the NAC, substance use associated with Rastafarianism brings up concerns about balancing religious freedoms with legal systems and antidrug policies.

Aubrey D. Johnson

See also: Race; Religion.

Further Reading

Benard, Akeia A. "The Material Roots of Rastafarian Marijuana Symbolism." *History and Anthropology* 18, no. 1 (2007): 89–99.

Gibson, Matthew. "Rastafari and Cannabis: Framing a Criminal Law Exemption." *Ecclesiastical Law Society* 12, no. 3 (2010): 324–344.

Urban, Hugh B. "Messianism, Music, and Ganja." In *New Age, Neopagan, and New Religious Movements: Alternative Spirituality in Contemporary America.* Oakland: University of California Press, 2015.

Reagan Administration "War on Drugs"

Ronald Reagan (1911–2004) was one of the most influential presidents regarding the criminalization and characterization of cannabis in the United States. Through his administration's policy and rhetoric, he advanced the country's view of marijuana as a dangerous drug that should be controlled at all costs. The Reagan administration's actions on this front influenced the American public's views on cannabis through the 1980s and 1990s, and its hostility toward marijuana still reverberates in public policy discussions concerning marijuana and other drugs today.

Reagan served as the nation's fortieth president from 1981 to 1989. Reagan summarized his views on cannabis in a preelection speech (1980) when he said, "Marijuana, pot, grass, whatever you want to call it, is probably the most dangerous drug in the United States" (Gerber 2004, 41–42). During his two terms in office, Reagan enacted several policies to enhance punishment for drug offenses and expand the "War on Drugs" that had been first launched in the early 1970s by the Nixon administration. One of Reagan's first significant actions as president was to expand the Domestic Cannabis Eradication/Suppression Program. This program was initiated in 1979 with the primary goal of eradicating all of cannabis in the United States. Before Reagan's presidency, it was only active in 7 states. By 1985, the program had spread to all 50 states (Massing 2000).

During this same time, Ronald Reagan's wife, Nancy Reagan (1921–2016), used her position as First Lady to further bolster the Reagan administration's war on drugs. The "Just Say No" national ad campaign, which Nancy Reagan championed, warned parents and children of the perils of using illicit drugs, particularly cannabis, for American youth. During her husband's two terms in office, Reagan traveled to 65 cities in 33 states to spread awareness of cannabis's alleged dangers. She also took her antidrug message to 9 foreign countries. Additionally, she appeared on several televised interviews and radio shows, held two international conferences, and gave numerous speeches on the issue.

Another Reagan administration antidrug initiative came in 1983, when it initiated the Campaign Against Marijuana Planting. This campaign became a massive eradication task force connecting numerous agencies from local police to the National Guard and utilizing federal resources such as U-2 spy planes (Balko 2013). The Reagan White House also made a change to the Posse Comitatus Act, which prohibits the use of the military in civilian law enforcement, by allowing the navy to engage in the domestic war on drugs by interdicting drug-smuggling vessels in international waters. Further, the budget for interdiction jumped dramatically during the 1980s, from $4 million at the start of Reagan's presidency in 1981 to over a $1 billion by the end of his final term in1989 (Chepesiuk 1999).

Reagan also applauded Congress's 1986 passage of the Anti-Drug Abuse Act of 1986. This act set in place mandatory minimum sentences for drug offenders and classified cannabis with other drugs such as heroin. It also gave life sentences to repeat offenders of various violent and nonviolent drug laws (Brown and Sefiha 2018). It was through acts like these that Reagan shaped the U.S. culture toward drug users. Reagan also began to push for more aggressive use of civil asset forfeiture, a tactic that would "not only [send] pot users to jail, but also '[forfeit] everything they own" (Gerber 2004, 41).

Though Reagan and his office viewed cannabis as a hard drug on par with heroin, administration officials struggled to find reputable studies supporting its position. Reagan's "Drug Czar," Carlton Turner, the director of the Drug Abuse Policy Office, believed that cannabis was causing crime and harm to people but struggled to find research to prove it. At one point, he resorted to connecting cannabis use with homosexuality (Gerber 2004). Turner's successor, Charles Schuster, reported fielding calls from a prominent GOP senator very soon after his appointment with questions asking why the millions spent by the agency had not yet found danger in cannabis—an attitude, Schuster reported, that soon changed to "[f]ind something wrong with marijuana" (Gerber 2004, 41). Schuster admitted that for several years after becoming Reagan's Drug Czar, the agency tried to find a connection between cannabis and brain damage, but was unsuccessful (Gerber 2004). From spending millions on efforts to connect marijuana with physical and criminal dangers to incarcerating millions for its consumption, Reagan's administration left a legacy of aggressive actions toward cannabis and its users.

Zachary Hutchinson and Ben Stickle

See also: American Presidents; "Drug Abuse Message to Congress" (President Carter, 1977); Nixon Administration "War on Drugs."

Further Reading

Balko, Radley. *Rise of the Warrior Cop: The Militarization of America's Police Forces.* New York: Public Affairs, 2013.

Brown, Stephen, and Ophir Sefiha. *Routledge Handbook on Deviance.* New York: Routledge, 2018.

Chepesiuk, Ron. *The War on Drugs: An International Encyclopedia.* Santa Barbara, CA: ABC-CLIO, 1999.

Gerber, Rudolph J. *Legalizing Marijuana: Drug Policy Reform and Prohibition Politics.* Westport, CT: Greenwood Publishing Group, 2004.

Massing, Michael. *The Fix.* Berkeley: University of California Press, 2000.

Recreational Marijuana Laws

In the early 2000s, marijuana was illegal in all 50 U.S. states. But while cannabis remains illegal at the federal level as of 2020, 15 states (Alaska, Arizona, California, Colorado, Illinois, Maine, Massachusetts, Michigan, Montana, Nevada, New Jersey, Oregon, South Dakota, Vermont, and Washington), as well as the District of Columbia and the U.S. territories of Guam and the Northern Mariana Islands, have legalized marijuana for recreational use by adults 21 and older. Sixteen states (excluding those listed above) have passed laws decriminalizing the possession of small amounts of cannabis, and 36 states (including those listed above) have legalized medical marijuana (Marijuana Policy Project n.d.-a). While state laws vary when it comes to how much cannabis an individual can possess or if residents are allowed to grow marijuana plants in their homes, it remains illegal to consume marijuana in a public place or on federal property. Experts predict that legalization will continue to spread throughout the United States as more Americans come to support legalization and states begin to recognize its potential to generate tax revenue.

Colorado and Washington were the first two states to end marijuana prohibition, with residents in both states approving ballot measures to regulate the production and distribution of cannabis during the November 2012 election. Both states allow adults to purchase up to an ounce of marijuana at a time from a state-licensed dispensary. Colorado residents are also allowed to grow up to six marijuana plants at home for personal use, but in Washington only medical marijuana patients are allowed to do so (Marijuana Policy Project n.d.-a).

Alaska and Oregon were the next two states to legalize marijuana, when voters in both passed ballot measures during the 2014 midterm election. Alaska's law, which went into effect on February 24, 2015, allows anyone 21 and over to possess up to an ounce of marijuana and grow up to six plants at home. Oregon's law, which went into effect on July 1, 2015, also allows adults to possess up to an ounce of marijuana in public, but it limits individuals to growing four plants at home (NORML n.d.). Washington, D.C., residents also voted to legalize marijuana in 2014, making it legal for adults to possess up to two ounces of marijuana and grow up to six plants at home. But unlike in other states, the District's law does not regulate marijuana sales, meaning it's still illegal to buy or sell marijuana anywhere in D.C. As a result, a sort of "gray" market has developed, where merchants sell regular items (such as hats and shirts) and "gift" a small amount of marijuana with it (D.C.'s law allows adults to transfer up to an ounce of marijuana to another person). D.C.'s local officials have tried to pass legislation allowing commercial sales, but they have not been able to get Congress to approve the move (since D.C. is a federal district and not a state, Congress must approve any legislation the District Council passes for it to become law) (Austermuhle 2019).

The next wave of marijuana legalization came in November 2016, when voters in California, Massachusetts, Nevada, and Maine approved ballot measures to end marijuana prohibition. Under California, Massachusetts, and Nevada's statutes, anyone 21 and older can possess up to an ounce of marijuana at a time; Maine's law allows residents to possess up to 2.5 ounces, more than twice the limit in most other states. While all four states allow residents to grow cannabis for their own personal use, Nevadans can only do so if there is no licensed dispensary within 25 miles of their home (Marijuana Policy Project n.d.-a).

Vermont and Michigan legalized recreational marijuana in 2018. Vermont's law, which went into effect on July 1, 2018, allows anyone 21 and older to possess up to an ounce of marijuana and grow up to two plants at home. Vermont was also the first state to end marijuana prohibition through the legislative process rather than at the ballot box; however, the Vermont law does not establish a legal market for the production and sale of cannabis like in other states. Legalization followed in Michigan a few months later, with voters approving a ballot initiative during the midterm election; dispensaries officially opened for business in the state in December 2019. Michigan's law is more permissive than that of other states, allowing adults to possess up to 2.5 ounces of cannabis and grow up to 12 plants at home (Marijuana Policy Project n.d.-a).

Illinois was the eleventh state to legalize marijuana. In May 2019, the state's General Assembly approved legislation ending prohibition, and the act went into effect on January 1, 2020. While Illinois is not the first state to legalize recreational marijuana through the legislative process, it is the first to legalize the commercial sale of it in this fashion (Marijuana Policy Project n.d.a). Illinois's law allows residents 21 and older to possess up to 30 grams of marijuana (there are lower limits for nonresidents), and like in Washington state, only medical marijuana patients are allowed to grow marijuana at home (NORML n.d.).

While marijuana legalization has spread across the United States over the past decade, many states have faced calls to repeal legalization and continue to struggle with black-market sales. For example, several Colorado towns and cities have passed laws restricting the sale and consumption of marijuana, and in 2018, a bill was introduced in the Washington state legislature to repeal the voter initiative that legalized marijuana. The bill, however, did not pass (National Conference of State Legislatures 2019). California's legal marijuana industry has also struggled. In a 2019 report, the state's Cannabis Advisory Committee estimated that nearly 80 percent of California's marijuana market remains illicit; licensed retailers cite high taxes as part of the issue, as well as the fact that about 75 percent of California's cities have banned retail marijuana shops (McGreevy 2019). While states have attempted to rectify these issues by adjusting tax rates and making it harder for towns to ban retail stores, only time will tell what effect, if any, these policy changes will have.

Looking ahead into the 2020s, experts predict that many more states will take up measures to legalize marijuana. During the 2020 election, voters in Arizona, New Jersey, Montana, and South Dakota passed legislation legalizing recreational marijuana for people 21 and over. South Dakota and Mississippi voters also passed initiatives to allow medical marijuana. These voter-approved initiatives are expected to go into effect in 2021 (Cannon 2020). New York governor Andrew Cuomo has also made legalization a top priority for his third term, although a reform bill has yet to pass in the state legislature; lawmakers did, however, pass a decriminalization bill, downgrading the possession of two ounces or less from a misdemeanor to a fine (McKinley and Wang 2019). Many 2020 Democratic presidential candidates also expressed support for legalization, and support has continued to build among the American public. According to a 2019 Pew Research Center study, the number of U.S. adults who opposed legalization dropped from 52 percent in 2010 to 32 percent in 2019 (Daniller 2019).

Katherine McCarthy

See also: Alaska; California; Coffeeshops; Colorado; Decriminalization; Edibles; Head Shops; Washington D.C.; Washington State.

Further Reading

Austermuhle, Martin. "D.C.'s Plans To Sell Recreational Weed Are Up in Smoke Thanks to New Spending Bill." *DCist*, December 17, 2019. https://dcist.com/story/19/12/17/d-c-s-plans-to-sell-recreational-weed-are-up-in-smoke-thanks-to-new-spending-bill/

Cannon, Jay. "These States Legalized Recreational Marijuana on Election Day." *USA Today*, November 4, 2020. https://www.usatoday.com/story/news/politics/elections/2020/11/04/recreational-weed-legal-arizona-new-jersey-south-dakota-montana/6160708002/

Daniller, Andrew. "Two-thirds of Americans Support Marijuana Legalization." *Pew Research Center*, November 14, 2019. https://www.pewresearch.org/fact-tank/2019/11/14/americans-support-marijuana-legalization/

Marijuana Policy Project. "State Policy." n.d.-a Accessed August 23, 2021. https://www.mpp.org/states/

Marijuana Policy Project. "2020 Statewide Ballot Initiatives." n.d.-b Accessed August 23, 2021. https://www.mpp.org/policy/ballot-initiatives/

McGreevy, Patrick. "California's Legal Pot Industry Is Stuck. Should Voters Step In?" *Los Angeles Times*, December 24, 2019. https://www.latimes.com/california/story/2019-12-24/two-years-california-legal-marijuana-industry-is-stuck

McKinley, Jesse, and Vivian Wang. "Marijuana Decriminalization Is Expanded in N.Y., but Full Legalization Fails." *New York Times*, June 20, 2019. https://www.nytimes.com/2019/06/20/nyregion/marijuana-laws-ny.html

Metropolitan Police Department (Washington, D.C.). "The Facts on DC Marijuana Laws." n.d. Accessed August 23, 2021. https://mpdc.dc.gov/marijuana

National Conference of State Legislatures. "Marijuana Overview." Last modified October 17, 2019. https://www.ncsl.org/research/civil-and-criminal-justice/marijuana-overview.aspx

NORML. "State Laws." n.d. Accessed August 23, 2021. https://norml.org/laws

Reefer Madness

Reefer Madness, originally titled *Tell Your Children*, is a propaganda film released in 1936 that relies on scare tactics to convince parents that marijuana is an addictive, soul-destroying drug that causes incurable insanity. The film was one facet of the anti-marijuana campaigns that rolled across the United States in the first half of the twentieth century, a movement that included passage of the Marijuana Tax Act of 1937. Contrary to its goal of demonizing marijuana, however, *Reefer Madness* was dismissed and ironically ascribed as an absurdity. It bombed at the box office and today lives on as a comedic cult classic (Kelley 2019).

The film begins with a lengthy prologue of the manic symptoms of using marijuana, such as uncontrollable emotions, lack of physical restraint, hallucinations, delusions, and violent behavior. The film then turns to the narrator, Principal Dr. Alfred Carrol (played by Josef Forte), telling a group of parents that marijuana, "not alcoholism, not opium, and not cocaine," is the "number one threat to today's youth." *Reefer Madness* then delves into the lives of several restless yet upstanding high schoolers. The bulk of the story focuses on two such high school siblings, Bill (Kenneth Craig) and Mary Lane (Dorothy Short).

While hanging out at the local diner, drug dealer Ralph Wiley (David O'Brien) invites Bill to a party at the home of Mae Coleman (Thelma White) and Jack Perry (Carleton Young). Mae and Jack's apartment is an epicenter for selling and using marijuana for the local adult and teen clientele. The smoke-filled apartment offers an enticing vibe, replete with laughter, dancing, piano playing, and kissing. Succumbing to the peer pressure, Bill is hooked on marijuana after one joint that is masked as a cigarette. Life spirals quickly out of control for Bill; he starts flunking out of school, dodging his family, and hooking up with girls. The movie reaches its climax when a concerned Mary goes looking for Bill at the reefer house. Welcomed by Ralph, Mary is tricked into smoking reefer. Mary's giggles and friendly encounter quickly turn precarious as Ralph sexually assaults her. Her brother is in the next room, fresh from a hazy sexual encounter, and hears Mary screaming. He runs to rescue her from Ralph's violent grip, but succumbs to hallucinations, moving in and out of consciousness. Jack also runs in to join the squabble, which takes an unexpected deadly turn. While knocking out Bill with the butt of his gun, Jack shoots and kills Mary and then attempts to frame Bill by making him think that he killed Mary. This prompts further madness, including murder and suicide. In the end, the truth is revealed, and drug-pushing antagonist Jack is charged as criminally insane and sent to a mental institution. The film cuts to a final warning by Principal Carrol, "The dread marijuana may be reaching forth next for your son. Or yours. Or yours! or YOURS!" (Ferranti 2018).

Courtney B. Ross

See also: Anti-Marijuana Campaigns in Popular Press; Gateway Drug Hypothesis; Moral Panics.

Further Reading

Ferranti, Seth. "When the Government Said Marijuana Made You Crazy." *OZY*, November 13, 2018. https://www.ozy.com/true-and-stories/when-the-government-said-marijuana-made-you-crazy/88232/

Kelley, Mary. "Reefer Madness: A Laughable Look at Past Attitudes." *The Scarlet*, September 21, 2019. https://thescarlet.org/16445/larts/reefer-madness-a-laughable-look-at-past-attitudes/

Religion

Many religions have used a wide variety of intoxicants in their ceremonies. In fact, religious use is likely one of the oldest, if not the oldest, reasons people used drugs. Anthropological evidence suggests Neanderthals used drugs in religious ceremonies more than 50,000 years ago, and there is similar evidence found in Neolithic sites more than 7,000 years old. In fact, almost all ancient peoples considered intoxicating and medicinal plants sacred, and these substances were often incorporated into their religious beliefs and practices. Cannabis was one of the many drugs used in ancient religions, and its use continues in some contemporary religions as well (Hawdon 2005).

Historical examples of cannabis being incorporated into religious settings and rituals are numerous. For example, according to Herodotus (fifth century BC), the Scythians who lived in present-day southern Siberia used hemp seeds during funeral rites to induce a trance among those attending the service. Cannabis was also allegedly used in early Taoism, the Chinese belief system originating in the fourth century BC. Early Taoist texts refer to the ritualistic burning of cannabis in incense burners to help eliminate selfish desire and achieve a mindful state of naturalness (Needham 1976).

Another common way drugs are used in religions is to induce religious visions and facilitate communication with spirits. Visions are culturally patterned and deeply engrained into the religious culture that experiences them so that similar visions are experienced by members of the religion. When a vision occurs, it is interpreted as communication from supernatural entities. While religious visions are not always drug induced, they often are. For example, Amerindians living near the Gulf of Mexico use marijuana, or la santa rosa, to induce visions such as the Hill of Gold or "the place where God always goes." Marijuana also assists them in religious contemplation and as a "stimulant to thought" (Williams-Garcia

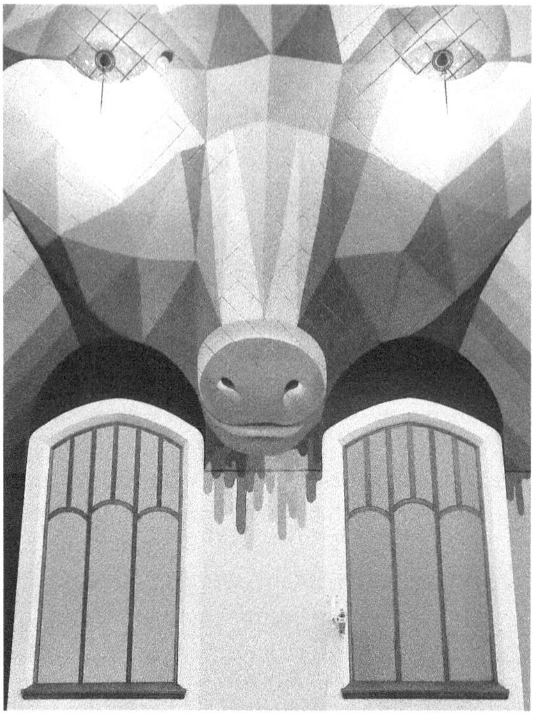

Stained glass dome of the International Church of Cannabis, home church for Elevationism, located in Denver, Colorado. Drugs, including cannabis, have been used in religious ceremonies since the dawn of human civilization. Many religions, including Hinduism, Rastafarianism, and the International Church of Cannabis, use marijuana in their rituals. (Faina Gurevich/ Dreamstime.com)

1975, 137). Similarly, Sufi mystics of Islam believe cannabis can reveal truth (Ferrara 2018).

Another way that marijuana is used in religious rituals is in the common practice of divination, or seeing the future by supernatural means. Several religions use marijuana in their divinatory practices, including Taoism. Numerous religions, including some found in North America as well as those of the Zulus and Pygmies of Africa, use marijuana as part of healing ceremonies. Zoroastrian shamans smoked cannabis to induce a state of ecstasy in an attempt to replicate the religious experiences of Zoroaster, and the religion's most important ancient text, *Avesta*, refers to hashish as a beneficial drug (Ferrara 2018; Hawdon 2006).

Researchers have also found evidence of cannabis being used by ancient Israelites in their religious ceremonies. Researchers investigating a well-preserved Judahite shrine in the ancient temple of Tel Arad found residues of teterahydrocannabinol (THC), cannabidiol (CBD), and cannabinol (CBN). While it is unclear exactly what function the cannabis played, the report's authors believe it was likely used as a deliberate psychoactive substance (Jean 2020).

Marijuana in its many forms, including hashish and bhang, is also deeply rooted in the Vedic tradition of ancient India. The *Rig Veda* and the *Atharva Veda* consider marijuana a "sacred grass" and "gods' food" and one of five hallowed plants. This tradition evolved in Hindu philosophy, and Brahmin priests use cannabis to help worshippers achieve a spiritual awakening or liberation. Cannabis holds a revered role in Hinduism, especially among those devoted to the god Shiva. Hindu traditions related to Shiva consider cannabis as being of divine origin. According to one story, Shiva and other gods churned the ocean making Amrita, the potion for eternal life. During this process, some Amrita dripped onto the earth, and cannabis sprouted where the drops fell. Shiva is often depicted smoking marijuana, which sustains him.

Some followers devoted to Shiva smoke marijuana as an offering during Shivratri, which is celebrated monthly, but particularly during the annual Maha

Shivaratri festival. The festival is a solemn remembrance of "overcoming darkness and ignorance" and involves prayers, fasting, and meditating. While not everyone involved smoke cannabis, thousands of people do to honor Shiva and aid in meditation (Fisher 1975; McLaren 2019). The Hindu festival of Holi, of the festival of spring, also involves the use of cannabis. During the festival, bhang drinks are consumed to enhance the spirit of the occasion.

Another religion in which marijuana assumes a prominent role is Rastafarianism, which is a Jamaican religious tradition based on interpretations of the Bible. Rastafarians believe cannabis is both a sacramental and beneficial plant, and smoking cannabis is one of the principal rituals of Rastafarianism. It is also consumed as a tea, as a spice, and as medicine. Rastafarians smoke marijuana to achieve an altered state of consciousness, especially during "groundings" or gatherings of like-minded people to discuss and consider current events through the prism of the religion's principles and tenets. Cannabis is believed to purify the heart and have healing powers, and it cultivates personal reflections and introspections that can help one discover his or her inner divinity.

According to Temple University religion professor Leonard E. Barrett, "The herb is the key to new understanding of the self, the universe, and God. It is the vehicle to cosmic consciousness" (Barrett 1988, 254–255).

Other religions have been founded in the past century that consider cannabis to be sacred, and some of these have cannabis at the center of their religious beliefs. For example, religions such as Temple 420, The First Church of Cannabis, and the THC Ministry consider cannabis to be a sacrament. For example, The First Church of Cannabis's twelfth "Deity Dozen" guideline put forth by the church states, "Cannabis, 'the Healing Plant' is our sacrament. It brings us closer to ourselves and others. It is our fountain of health, our love, curing us from illness and depression. We embrace it with our whole heart and spirit, individually and as a group" (Funaro 2015).

While cannabis is revered in many religions, there are numerous religions that either explicitly or implicitly forbid the use of cannabis. In other religions, whether marijuana is forbidden or acceptable is debated, and the interpretation of the sacred texts regarding intoxication varies by religious traditions within the religion. For example, some Buddhists interpret the Fifth Precept of Buddhism of "do not take strong drink" to refer to all things that cloud the mind, which would include cannabis; however, other Buddhist traditions believe the Fifth Precept applies only to alcohol (Yin-shun 1998).

James Hawdon

See also: Ancient Religions; Family Life; Military Use; Rastafarianism.

Further Reading

Barrett, Leonard E. *The Rastafarians: Sounds of Cultural Dissonance*. Vol. 795. Boston, MA: Beacon Press, 1988.

Ferrara, Mark S. *Sacred Bliss: A Spiritual History of Cannabis*. Lanham, MD: Rowman & Littlefield, 2018.

Fisher, James. "Cannabis in Nepal: An Overview." In *Cannabis and Culture*, edited by Vera Rubin. Chicago: Aldine, 1975, 247–256.

Funaro, Vincent. "Indiana Marijuana Church Releases Its Own Ten Commandments: The New Deity Dozen." *The Christian Post*, June 8, 2015. https://www.christianpost.com/news/indiana-marijuana-church-releases-its-own-ten-commandments-the-new-deity-dozen.html

Hawdon, James. *Drug and Alcohol Consumption as Functions of Social Structures: A Cross-cultural Sociology*. Lewistown, NY: Edwin Mellen Press, 2005.

Jean, Celia. "Cannabis Was Used in Ancient Israelite Ceremony, Researchers Find." *The Jerusalem Post*, May 31, 2020. https://www.jpost.com/judaism/first-known-evidence-of-cannabis-used-in-early-judaic-ceremony-found-629699

McLaren, Erik. How Hinduism's Cannabis God Fuels India's Weed-Loving Culture. *Herb* August 14, 2019. https://herb.co/news/culture/shiva-india-ganja-culture/

Needham, Joseph. *Science and Civilisation in China*. Vol. 5. Cambridge, UK: Cambridge University Press, 1976.

Williams-Garcia, Roberto. "The Ritual Use of Cannabis in Mexico." In *Cannabis and Culture*, edited by Vera Rubin. Chicago: Aldine, 1975, 133–145.

Yin-shun, Venerable. *The Way to Buddhahood: Instructions from a Modern Chinese Master*. New York: Simon and Schuster, 1998.

S

Saturday Night Live

Depictions of marijuana on NBC's late-night satirical comedy *Saturday Night Live* (*SNL*) have evolved alongside changing national attitudes about marijuana. During the show's earliest seasons from 1975 to 1979, skits often included pro-marijuana references in spite of the NBC network's policy that all drug-related content should be portrayed in a negative light. Creator and producer Lorne Michaels' former wife, comedian Rosie Shuster, referred to the inclusion of boundary-pushing content as "gonzo video guerilla" attacks on NBC policies (Stein 2013). Frequent references, for example, were made in monologues and in skits to comedian John Belushi's drug and marijuana use during the first few seasons. Similarly, toward the end of the first season, Chevy Chase reported on "Killer Weed" during a Weekend Update skit, urging viewers to help *SNL* aid the FBI in recovering marijuana by mailing samples directly to "Chevy Chase, Apt. 12, 827 W. 81 St. NYC, 10053." While the address was fictitious, some samples were sent to the *SNL* set on the seventeenth floor of the NBC building; additionally, NBC executives were unaware that the joint displayed in the skit contained actual marijuana (Hill and Weingrad 2011).

Another skit that pushed the boundaries of the corporate policy concerned a fictitious American Dope Growers Union. This sketch aired during the second season and focused on delivering a tongue-in-cheek call for potheads to support American marijuana suppliers rather than buying marijuana from Mexican or Columbian importers. By purportedly moving the skit's focus from the effects of marijuana to supporting American workers, *SNL* was able to circumvent NBC's policy and avoid censorship while still normalizing marijuana use. The comedy show did not have particularly high ratings in the early years, but *SNL*'s ability to specifically draw in viewers in the 18–34 age group prized by advertisers, which no other network did at the time, made challenging these aspects of *SNL* content difficult. Actors and comedians on the show portrayed the interests and values of that age group, which included drug use, sexualized content, and satirical political representations.

Despite the failed efforts in the early seasons to eliminate drug-related content, *SNL* skits including references to marijuana dramatically decreased during the early- to mid-1980s. While national conversations about drug use focused on zero tolerance as a result of the Reagan administration's so-called War on Drug campaign, another reason for the decrease in marijuana-related content might have been congressional pressure exerted on networks to better censor drug-related content. In 1978, Ralph Daniels, vice president of broadcasting standards for

NBC, was called to testify at a special congressional hearing on drug abuse. His testimony outlined NBC's policy regarding drug-related content:

> NBC Broadcast Standards require that narcotic addiction should be presented only as a destructive habit, and "the use of illegal drugs or abuse of legal drugs shall not be encouraged or shown as socially acceptable." This requirement is consistent with the provisions of the NAB [National Association of Broadcasters] Code. (U.S. Congress 1978, 104)

Daniels went on to describe the steps NBC takes to keep prodrug content off the network, including running episode topics by the NBC Department of Broadcast Standards, which, when faced with questionable content, is empowered to approach the producer of the show and ask that the questionable content be eliminated from the program.

One notable exception to the lack of pro-marijuana references on *SNL* during the early- and mid-1980s, however, was Sam Kinison's 1986 opening monologue, in which he insinuated that marijuana was less harmful than other drugs and therefore preferable to crack cocaine. Although his comments could not be censored in the live East Coast airing of the show, NBC replaced the offending reference with a 15-second still image of the previous year's *SNL* cast in later airings of the show on the West Coast to avoid the nationwide transmission of pro-marijuana content.

The legal status of marijuana began to change in the following decades—and *SNL* treatment of marijuana changed as well. In 1989, one poll found that just 16 percent of Americans supported legalizing marijuana; that number rose to 67 percent in 2019 according to one respected polling organization (Daniller 2019). One of the first tangible indications of this shift came in 1996, when California legalized medical marijuana. In the aftermath of this milestone, *SNL* representations of marijuana in skits increasingly shifted from negative depictions of marijuana use to those depicting use as acceptable. Even before California's move, several *SNL* skits incorporated marijuana-related content under a medical guise. A 1990 skit featuring a portrayal of President George W. Bush depicts the president using tetrahydrocannabinol (THC) eye drops to treat glaucoma, while also comically emphasizing that the drops are "Doctor-prescribed!" (S15E18 1990). Glaucoma was featured again in a 2004 skit, but this time as an excuse for someone who does not actually suffer from glaucoma to gain access to medicinal marijuana (S29E12 2004).

As public support for the legalization of both medicinal and recreational marijuana began to grow, this sentiment became frequently reflected in *SNL* sketches. Comedian Zach Galifianakis, for example, held up a sign during his 2011 monologue reading "CLAP IF YOU ENDORSE LEGALIZED MARIJUANA," to which the live studio audience enthusiastically obliged. After the first states began to legalize recreational marijuana, some skits even went so far as to poke fun at those who still vehemently opposed legalization. A 2014 parody of HLN's *Nancy Grace*, a controversial nightly celebrity news and current affairs program in which host Nancy Grace embodies the role of victim rights advocate, depicted a business owner in Colorado reacting positively to the legalization of marijuana, with Nancy Grace concerned about the effects of legalization. Nancy Grace, in dramatic fashion, shouted, "What about the babies?!" suggesting babies and children would be harmed as a result of legalization (S39E11 2014).

The decriminalization of marijuana, a new middle ground in the legalization debate, has been increasingly featured in *SNL* skits. In 2014, New York state decriminalized possession of 15 grams or less of marijuana. That week, *SNL* featured a skit loosely related to a civil rights march, *New Marijuana Policy*, in which Woody Harrelson, Pete Davidson, and other stoners in New York emerged from brownstone apartment buildings, shielding their eyes from the sunlight as pot smoke followed them out into the street. Eventually, a large neighborhood crowd began celebrating that they would no longer have to hide their marijuana use since the passing of the decriminalization law. The celebration was interrupted by a police officer when one of the crowd leaders attempted to light a joint in the street. The officer remarked that public consumption of marijuana was still illegal under the new law. At that point, dejected and disappointed, Harrelson and the other stoners give up and retreat back into their dark and smoky brownstones.

While it is unclear whether depictions of marijuana use on *SNL* have a direct impact on viewer's perceptions of marijuana, or if the show simply reflects the values of their viewers, use of marijuana and other illicit drugs has long been recognized and accepted as part of the backstage culture at *SNL*. During the late 1970s, NBC officials were reportedly aware of widespread marijuana use on *SNL* sets (and even cocaine in later years) but chose to overlook the behavior (Hill and Weingrad 2011). Reports of backstage parties with marijuana smoke drifting onstage were not uncommon, as were live references to marijuana use during sketches. When reflecting on hosting *SNL* with musical guest Nirvana in 1993, former NBA player Charles Barkley claimed that he got a "contact high" from the "mushroom clouds" every time the Nirvana dressing room door opened (Barkley 2017). More recently, *SNL* comedian Pete Davidson has openly discussed his enthusiasm for marijuana for both recreational and medicinal purposes. In a 2018 interview with *People* magazine, Davison explained that while using marijuana helps manage his bipolar disorder and Crohn's disease, he smokes daily simply because he enjoys it (Merrett 2018).

Comedian and actor John Belushi was particularly well known for being pro-marijuana during his stint on *SNL* from 1975 to 1979, with guest hosts and other comedians making multiple references to his pot-smoking behavior in skits over the years. His younger brother, Jim Belushi, who was an *SNL* cast member from 1983 to 1985, currently operates a 93-acre pot farm in Oregon, where he grows a particular strain of marijuana as a tribute to the show, named "Captain Jack 'The Smell of SNL'" (Mann 2018).

Angela M. Barlow and Christopher J. Miceli

See also: *Big Lebowski, The*; *Dazed and Confused*; *Martha and Snoop's Potluck Dinner Party*; *That '70s Show*; *Weeds*.

Further Reading

Barkley, Charles. "Interview with Dan Patrick." *The Dan Patrick Show*, March 23, 2017. https://youtu.be/lOsnvfkirRA

Daniller, Andrew. "Two-thirds of Americans Support Marijuana Legalization." *Pew Research Center*, November 14, 2019. https://www.pewresearch.org/fact-tank/2019/11/14/americans-support-marijuana-legalization/

Hill, Doug, and Jeff Weingrad. *Saturday Night: A Backstage History of Saturday Night Live.* San Francisco, CA: Untreed Reads, 2011.

Mann, Damien. "Cultivating 'the Smell of SNL': Actor Jim Belushi's Happy Place Is Growing Pot Near Eagle Point, Ore." *The Mail Tribune*, October 18, 2018. https://lmtribune.com/northwest/cultivating-the-smell-of-snl/article_bdcfbdf9-01fd-5c39-8e65-7d0ef40f0a8d.html

Merrett, Robyn. "Pete Davidson Reveals His Sobriety Lasted 3 Months but Now He Smokes Marijuana Regularly." *People,* September 24, 2018.

Stein, Ellin. *That's Not Funny, That's Sick: The National Lampoon and the Comedy Insurgents Who Captured the Mainstream.* New York: W. W. Norton & Company, 2013.

U.S. Congress. House of Representatives. Select Committee on Narcotics Abuse and Control. Prevention of Drug Abuse. 95th Cong., 2d sess., 1978. https://play.google.com/store/books/details?id=oy8Op2aRfF8C&rdid=book-oy8Op2aRfF8C&rdot=1

Sexual Functioning

In some cultures, recreational marijuana is used for sexual stimulation and pleasure. Like many recreational drugs, marijuana can be viewed as an aphrodisiac that helps facilitate social-psychological responses that heighten pleasure from sexual activities. Despite the persisting cultural association between marijuana and sexuality, however, a scientific consensus on the effect of cannabis on physiological elements of sexual response has yet to be reached. Scholars of health and sexuality show that the impact of marijuana on sexual functioning and identity is shaped by a host of social factors. However, though research tells us much about the short-term sexual effects of using marijuana, we have little understanding of the long-term sexual effects.

Marijuana can have physiological effects that intensify or attenuate sexual functioning, including increasing heart rate, increasing or decreasing blood pressure, and reducing or exacerbating panic attacks. For instance, delta-9-tetrahydrocannabinol (THC) produces mild euphoria, relaxation, and enhancement of sensory experiences (Adams and Martin 1996), which can extend into an individual's sexual activities.

Research using both survey and interview methods confirms that many users think marijuana can heighten sexual enjoyment and performance. One study on the effects of regular marijuana smoking on sex found that the marijuana did not necessarily impact sexual function, such as having more orgasms or prolonging sexual activity. However, more than three-fourths of female users and 70 percent of male users stated that marijuana use had a positive effect on sexual pleasure and satisfaction. Additionally, nearly three out of five males and over one-third of females stated that marijuana use resulted in enhanced orgasms (Halikas, Weller, and Morse 1982). In addition, many marijuana users explained that marijuana had some aphrodisiac effects. Other studies have found similar results (Crenshaw and Goldberg 1996). A 2018 study, however, found that marijuana was not associated with perceived heightened sexual effects (Palamar et al. 2018).

Interestingly, many marijuana users believe that the positive effects the drug has on sexual performance diminishes with increased usage. Indeed, according to one study, 59 percent of study participants reported a belief that smoking one joint increased sexual enjoyment. But only 39 percent of individuals in the study likewise believed that sexual experiences were enhanced by smoking more than one joint (Koff 1974). There is also evidence that any potential positive effect on sexuality from marijuana use is mediated by social factors, such as the setting, age of participants, and relationship status of the sexual participants (Crenshaw and Goldberg 1996; Rosen 1991).

Existing research, on the other hand, offers limited conclusions about the long-term sexual effects of regularly smoking marijuana. One longitudinal study utilizing interviews demonstrates that marijuana users' initial perceptions of sexual enhancement resulting from the drug remained intact six to eight years later (Halikas et al. 1985). However, another study found that use of the drug is associated with inhibited orgasm and sexual excitement, as well as painful sex for women (Johnson, Phelps, and Cottler 2004). Given the limited available research on the relationship between marijuana and sexuality, few concrete answers are available; indeed, conflicting studies suggest that marijuana use can both enable and constrain sexual pleasure and functioning. Hence, additional research is needed to clarify this relationship.

Brandon Alston

See also: Maternal Reproductive Health; Neurological Effects.

Further Reading

Adams, Irma B., and Billy R. Martin. "Cannabis: Pharmacology and Toxicology in Animals and Humans." *Addiction* 91 no. 11 (1996): 1585–1614.

Crenshaw, Theresa Larsen, and James P. Goldberg. *Sexual Pharmacology: Drugs That Affect Sexual Functioning*. New York: WW Norton & Co, 1996.

Halikas, James, Ronald Weller, and Carolyn Morse. "Effects of Regular Marijuana Use on Sexual Performance." *Journal of Psychoactive Drugs* 14 nos. 1–2 (1982): 59–70.

Halikas, James A., Ronald A. Weller, Carolyn L. Morse, and Raymond G. Hoffmann. "A Longitudinal Study of Marijuana Effects." *International Journal of the Addictions* 20 no. 5 (1985): 701–711.

Johnson, Sharon D., Deborah L. Phelps, and Linda B. Cottler. "The Association of Sexual Dysfunction and Substance Use among a Community Epidemiological Sample." *Archives of Sexual Behavior* 33 no. 1 (2004): 55–63.

Koff, Wayne C. "Marijuana and Sexual Activity." *Journal of Sex Research* 10, no. 3 (1974): 194–204.

Palamar, Joseph J., et al. "A Comparison of Self-Reported Sexual Effects of Alcohol, Marijuana, and Ecstasy in a Sample of Young Adult Nightlife Attendees." *Psychology & Sexuality* 9, no. 1 (2018): 54–68.

Rosen, Raymond C. "Alcohol and Drug Effects on Sexual Response: Human Experimental and Clinical Studies." *Annual Review of Sex Research* 2 no. 1 (1991): 119–179.

Sexual Orientation

Those who do not identify as heterosexual (sexual minorities) report more substance use than their heterosexual counterparts. This includes marijuana. Research on the relationship between sexual orientation and marijuana use often splits populations by gender and level of orientation. While gender is usually a binary variable in this strain of research, sexual orientation is more complex and captures three different concepts: identity, attraction, and behavior. Attraction (who one is sexually attracted to) and behavior (who one has sex with) are typically captured through ordinal measures. Responses to sexual attraction and behavior measures range from "only women" to "only men," representing complete heterosexuality and homosexuality depending on the gender of the respondent. Identity is often measured in a more direct way with respondents simply stating how they identify (i.e., gay, straight, etc.).

A meta-analysis found that sexual minority adolescents are more likely to report recent and lifetime marijuana use in a sample of studies published between 1998 and 2006 (Marshal et al. 2008). While the analysis and other researchers address sexual minorities broadly, others look at different sexual minority subgroups and how their rates of use compare to their heterosexual counterparts. The results consistently suggest sexual minority women are more likely to use marijuana.

A 2009 study found that sexual minority women are more likely to use marijuana than heterosexual women. Bisexual women are by far the most likely to use, followed by lesbian women, and heterosexual identifying women with same-sex partners. When analyzing men, the same study found that gay men are the only sexual minorities more likely to report marijuana use than the heterosexual men (Trocki, Drabble, and Midanik 2009). Another 2009 study measured sexual orientation with identity, attraction, and behavior. Sexual minority women across all measures of sexual orientation (minus the behavior measure for women who have sex with women) are more likely to report past-year marijuana use than heterosexual women. The findings for men are less consistent, with those who self-identify as gay and "not sure" of their sexual orientation being more likely than self-identified straights to report marijuana use. Additionally, in the attraction measure of sexual orientation for men, those who are attracted to only men and those who are attracted to mostly women are more likely to use marijuana than those who report being attracted to only women. On the behavioral front, only those who report having sex with both men and women are more likely to report past-year marijuana use than men who only have sex with women (McCabe et al. 2009).

A 2018 study that looked at substance use by orientation over time found significant differences in past-month marijuana use between heterosexual and sexual minority women. The findings show sexual minority women are more likely to report past-month marijuana use than heterosexual women. Specifically, lesbian women are most likely to report past-month marijuana use, followed by bisexual women and finally heterosexual women. The same study addressed men and found no differences between sexual minorities and heterosexual men in their usage of marijuana (Watson et al. 2018).

Researchers have suggested that the stress of being a sexual minority may result in higher substance use rates (Gonzales 2020). This stress comes from societal stigmatization associated with being a sexual minority. A 2014 study tested this assumption using sibling pairs that consist of one heterosexual and one sexual minority sibling. The study found that sexual minority siblings report less maternal attachment and affection. This alienation from the maternal figure represents minority stress. Thus, the stress of being a sexual minority is a possible explanation for the higher rates of substance use among some sexual minorities as compared to heterosexuals (Rosario et al. 2014).

Aubrey D. Johnson

See also: Gender.

Further Reading

Gonzales, Gilbert. "Differences in 30-Day Marijuana Use by Sexual Orientation Identity: Population-Based Evidence from Seven States." *LGBT Health* 7, no. 1 (2020): 60–67.

Marshal, Michael P., et al. "Sexual Orientation and Adolescent Substance Use: A Meta-analysis and Methodological Review." *Addiction* 103, no. 4 (2008): 546–556.

McCabe, Sean Esteban, et al. "Sexual Orientation, Substance Use Behaviors and Substance Dependence in the United States." *Addiction* 104, no. 8 (2009): 1333–1345.

Rosario, Margaret, et al. "Sexual-Orientation Disparities in Substance Use in Emerging Adults: A Function of Stress and Attachment Paradigms." *Psychology of Addictive Behaviors* 28, no. 3 (2014): 790–804.

Trocki, Karen F., Laurie A. Drabble, and Lorraine T. Midanik. "Tobacco, Marijuana Use and Sensation-seeking: Comparisons Across Gay, Lesbian, Bisexual and Heterosexual Groups." *Psychology of Addictive Behaviors* 23, no. 4 (2009): 620–631.

Watson, Ryan J., et al. "Substance Use among Sexual Minorities: Has It Actually Gotten Better?" *Substance Use & Misuse* 53, no. 7 (2018): 1221–1228.

Single-Use Devices

A "one-use" or "single-use" device is a convenient and disposable means of smoking marijuana. This term is not commonly cited in academic literature, but is recognized colloquially. The variations of one-use devices range from the common rolling paper to the more creative manufacturing of a device through the repurposing of bottles, foil, pens, and fruit. Given the broad span of items that can be made into or considered a single-use device, it is best to conceptualize them as falling within two broad categories: common flammable support material (e.g., rolling paper) and creative devices (e.g., apples and bottles).

Smoking marijuana remains a primary mode of ingestion of the drug. A mid-2010s study found that 85 percent of students who used marijuana in the last 30 days reported that their usual mode of consumption was inhalation (Johnson et al. 2016). Much inhalation involves joints, which are considered single-use since the rolling materials used to make them are destroyed in the process of combustion when smoking. Their popularity most likely stems from the widespread availability of rolling papers and simplicity of use. Alternatively, some users purchase existing tobacco products and replace the contents of those cigars with marijuana to create "blunts," another example of a single-use device.

Other single-use devices demonstrate the ingenuity, creativity, and resourcefulness of cannabis users. Noncombustible single-use devices can be made from any item or group of items that loosely fit the following criteria: a bowl to load the marijuana into, a screen or filter to prevent the inhalation of embers, and a mouthpiece or opening to use for inhaling. A "carb"—a hole on the side of a pipe or a bong used to starve airflow until the user is ready to inhale—is optional but commonplace in most homemade single-use devices.

Creative devices vary in complexity, but most mimic the design features and functionality of pipes or bowls, bongs, and blubbers (a mix of a pipe and bong) that are found in head shops. A complex design mimicking a traditional pipe may include a water bottle with a hole cut out of the side, a metal pen cap inserted into the hole, and aluminum foil with tiny holes poked in it inserted into the pen cap. The water bottle serves as a chamber to collect smoke, the cap and aluminum foil filter out embers, and the mouth of the water bottle acts as a mouthpiece for inhalation. A more simplistic design may include an apple and a pen. This type of device is created by removing the pen cartridge and using the hollow body of the pen to core the apple from top to center and side to center. This design permits marijuana to be packed on the top of the apple and enables the user to inhale from the side of the apple.

These devices are considered single use because of the limited life span of the materials they are made with. Plastics in water bottles and pens deform after exposure to heat, aluminum foil become brittle, and fruit will rot. The short life span of these products is evident when compared to devices made of glass, ceramics, strong metals, and treated wood.

Instructions for creating these various forms of single-use devices is ubiquitous on the internet, where many online communities are dedicated to documenting and sharing processes, materials, and advice. Popular websites such as wikihow.com, instructables.com, and youtube.com also provide step-by-step instructions and advice to site visitors. Rarely do these outlets discuss safest practices, however, and critics contend that some of the instructions they provide are risky due to the potential for burns, melted plastics coming into contact with the skin, or inhaled toxins that escape from the heated single-use device (Al-Zouabi et al. 2018).

Logan Sarvey and John Stogner

See also: Blunts; Bongs and Water Pipes; Dabbing; Gravity Bongs; Vaporizers.

Further Reading

Al-Zouabi, Ihsan, John M. Stogner, Bryan Lee Miller, and Elizabeth S. Lane. "Butane Hash Oil and Dabbing: Insights into Use, Amateur Production Techniques, and Potential Harm Mitigation." *Substance Abuse and Rehabilitation* 9 (2018): 91.

Johnson, R. M., et al. "Usual Modes of Marijuana Consumption among High School Students in Colorado." *Journal of Studies on Alcohol and Drugs,* 77 no. 4 (2016): 580–588.

Soldz, S., D. J. Huyser, and E. Dorsey. "The Cigar as a Drug Delivery Device: Youth Use of Blunts." *Addiction*, 98 no. 10 (2003): 1379–1386.

Sinsemella

Sinsemella is a form of cannabis with seedless buds. In fact, sinsemella translates to "without seeds" in Spanish. To achieve seedless cannabis, male plants must be removed from the population. Seedless cannabis is thought to offer a superior smoking experience and does not require smokers to manually remove the seeds before partaking (Canna Reps 2019). It is commonly believed that sinsemella was first produced in the western United States after growers discovered that levels of the intoxicating compound in marijuana, THC, were higher in sinsemella plants than in fertilized cannabis (Way of Leaf 2020).

Sinsemella is often misidentified as a specific strain of cannabis. However, it is a catch-all name for any form of female cannabis. Female cannabis plants grow the buds that are most commonly considered marijuana. When kept separate from male cannabis plants, which contain pollen sacks, female cannabis remains free of pollen and as a result retains its seedless character. Since at least the 1970s, sinsemella has gained a reputation as a superior and more potent form of marijuana. The more intense high produced from sinsemella also stems from the denial of fertilization. Without fertilization, female cannabis plants produce a larger quantity of resins with higher concentrations of marijuana's active compounds. The growing popularity of sinsemella, coupled with advances in growing technology, has led to the production of sinsemella in steadily greater volumes over time. In particular, the use of greenhouses has allowed for the proliferation of sinsemella because female cannabis plants grown indoors cannot be inadvertently exposed to male plants (Sherrard n.d.).

Matthew Costello

See also: *High Times*; Tetrahydrocannabinol (THC).

Further Reading

Canna Reps. "Sinsemilla: Origins of Modern Cannabis." May 16, 2019. https://www.cannareps.ca/sinsemilla-origins-of-modern-cannabis/?v=7516fd43adaa

Sherrard, Melissa. "What Is Sinsemilla?" *Civilized,* n.d. Accessed August 23, 2021. https://www.civilized.life/articles/what-is-sinsemilla/

Way of Leaf. "Cannabis Basics: What Is Sinsemilla Weed?" March 26, 2020. https://wayofleaf.com/education/what-is-sinsemilla

Snoop Dogg (1971–)

Snoop Dogg (aka Snoop Doggy Dogg and Snoop Lion), whose birth name is Cordozar Calvin Broadus, Jr., is an American rapper, songwriter, actor, television personality, and business owner. Because of the inclusion of many lyrics referencing marijuana in his songs, Snoop Dogg has come to be heavily associated with marijuana. In fact, Snoop Dogg's songs have frequently appeared in articles highlighting the "greatest weed themed songs of all time" (Bienstock et al. 2018).

Snoop Dogg was born on October 20, 1971, in Long Beach, California. Early in his life, Snoop Dogg was abandoned by his father and left to be raised by his mother, who assigned him the nickname "Snoop." She chose this name because she believed he resembled the character Snoopy from the *Peanuts* comic strip; the name stuck with him into adulthood. Growing up without a father in a high-crime area, Snoop Dogg elected to join the Crips gang in the late 1980s (24SMI 2019). During the 1990s, he was arrested on cocaine charges and first- and second-degree murder charges, the latter charges of which he was acquitted (Daunt 1996).

Despite his rough upbringing and legal troubles, Snoop Dogg was eventually able to launch a massively successful hip-hop career. Beginning in the late 1980s,

Snoop Dogg began rapping with his friends Dr. Dre (Warren Griffen) and Nate Dogg (Nathaniel Hale). He impressed Dr. Dre so much that Dr. Dre included him as the featured artist on much of his first solo album, *The Chronic* (1992), which was tremendously successful. The exposure he received from his work on *The Chronic* enabled Snoop Dogg to record a rap album of his own, *Doggystyle.* The multiplatinum-selling album became the first record to ever debut at the number one spot on the Billboard 200 Chart. Snoop Dogg went on to release several more successful albums and singles and was a feature artist on a long list of successful songs. In addition to his success in hip-hop, he has also enjoyed success in other forms of entertainment media including, but not limited to, film (i.e., his guest role as a drug dealer in *Training Day*), television (i.e., *Martha and Snoop's Potluck Dinner Party*), and even in other genres of music including reggae and gospel. In 2017, Snoop Dogg's net worth was valued at $143 million.

Snoop Dogg has faced many criticisms over the years, however, pertaining to pervasive themes in his hip-hop music. His music frequently includes criminal themes related to illegal drug use, violence (including murder), misogyny, and prostitution. For example, in 1994 C. Delores Tucker, Chair of the National Political Congress of Black Women, criticized Snoop Dogg's music several times and gangsta rap in general, citing it as one reason children are "out of control" and so many Blacks are disproportionately represented in jails (Harrington 1994). Other critics alleged that instead of using hip-hop to help people who did not grow up in poor, crime-troubled inner cities understand the plight of people living in such conditions he instead glorified his gangster status—and his murder charge in particular—for profit (Hattenstone 2013).

Snoop Dogg, while wearing multiple entertainment hats, is perhaps most frequently associated with music touting the use of marijuana. Many of his songs contain lyrics championing and glorifying the use of the drug.

In addition to praising marijuana in his songs, Snoop Dogg has also not been shy in personal interviews about his affinity for marijuana, claiming in one interview that he smokes 81 blunts a day (Von Glinow 2012).

As a result, Snoop Dogg has become a weed icon of sorts, and his impact on the public's perceptions of the drug has been considerable. In a February 2019 interview, Democratic Senator Kamala Harris of California admitted on the radio show *The Breakfast Club* to smoking weed in college. When asked if she was listening to Snoop Dogg while smoking, she stated, "Oh yeah, definitely Snoop" (Jaeger 2019). Many members of the media coined Harris's admission to smoking pot as "SnoopGate." Discussing the event, the host of *The Daily Show,* Trevor Noah, said that "whenever anyone smokes weed, they hear Snoop Dogg."

Snoop Dogg's classic hip-hop music also heavily influences contemporary hip-hop, as many hip-hop artists today (i.e., Migos, 2 Chainz, Lil Pump, etc.) frequently reference using marijuana (and often more expensive forms of marijuana as a statement of wealth) as well as other recreational drugs such as Molly (Ecstasy), Percocet, and Lean (Promethazine and Codeine), among others.

Snoop Dogg has extended his love for marijuana into a business venture. In 2018, he launched a marijuana-related venture firm centered on his own personal brand of pot, "Leafs By Snoop." The company offers cannabis in a variety of forms, including "eight strains of pre-packaged flowers, concentrates and edibles, including chocolate bars, cannabis drops, gummies and peanut butter candy" (Kovacevich 2018). Snoop Dogg, recognizing Canada's lax cannabis laws relative to that of the United States, has also extended his marijuana businesses and investments into Canada (Valiante 2018). Overall, Snoop Dogg continues to profess his love for cannabis and is establishing himself as a major player in the cannabis industry. For example, Snoop Dogg's company, Merry Jane, was honored in 2017 with an Emmy nomination for its production of "Martha & Snoop's Potluck Dinner Party," a television program cohosted by the rapper and home decorating icon Martha Stewart (Rough 2017).

Allen Copenhaver

See also: Beatles, The; Monkees, The; Nelson, Willie (1933–); *That '70s Show.*

Further Reading

Bienstock, R., M. Reeves, E. Garber-Paul, and D. Epstein. "Pot Sounds: The 20 Greatest Weed-Themed Songs of All Time." *Rolling Stone,* April 19, 2018. https://www.rollingstone.com/music/music-lists/pot-sounds-the-20-greatest-weed-themed-songs-of-all-time-627951/snoop-dogg-gin-and-juice-1993-628115/

Daunt, T. "Rapper Snoop Doggy Dogg Is Acquitted of Murder." *Los Angeles Times,* February 21, 1996. http://articles.latimes.com/1996-02-21/news/mn-38322_1_rapper-snoop-doggy-dogg

Fields, K. "Today in Hip Hop History: Snoop Dogg Releases His Debut Album 'Doggystyle' 22 Years Ago." *The Source,* November 23, 2015. http://thesource.com/2015/11/23/today-in-hip-hop-history-snoop-dogg-releases-his-debut-album-doggystyle-22-years-ago/

Harrington, L.M. "On Capitol Hill, a Real Rap Session." *Chicago Tribune,* February 24, 1994. https://www.chicagotribune.com/news/ct-xpm-1994-02-24-9402240240-story.html

Hattenstone, S. "From Snoop Dogg to Snoop Lion: The Reinvention of a Gangster Rapper." *The Guardian,* April 6, 2013. https://www.theguardian.com/music/2013/apr/06/snoop-dogg-lion-interview

Jaeger, K. "Kamala Harris's SnoopGate Is What a Political Marijuana Controversy Looks Like in 2019." *Marijuana Moment,* February 12, 2019. https://www.marijuanamoment.net/kamala-harriss-snoopgate-is-what-a-political-marijuana-controversy-looks-like-in-2019/

Kovacevich, N. "Cannabis of the Rich and Famous: Celebrities Glam Up the Cannabis Market." *Forbes,* December 10, 2018. https://www.forbes.com/sites/nickkovacevich/2018/12/10/cannabis-of-the-rich-and-famous-celebrities-glam-up-the-cannabis-market/#e546aa31ab2a

Marijuana Business Daily. "Rapper Snoop Dogg's Marijuana-Related Venture firm Raises $45 Million." March 14, 2018. https://mjbizdaily.com/rapper-snoop-doggs-marijuana-related-venture-firm-raises-45-million/

Rough, L. "'Snoop & Martha' Earns the First-Ever Cannabis Industry Emmy Nomination." Leafly.com, August 26, 2017. https://www.leafly.com/news/lifestyle/snoop-martha-tv-series-earns-cannabis-industrys-first-emmy-nomination

24SMI. "Snoop Dogg." 2019. https://en.24smi.org/celebrity/55187-snoop-dogg.html

Valiante, G. "Canada's Pot Industry Gets a New Supporter: Snoop Dogg." CTV News, May 25, 2018. https://www.ctvnews.ca/business/canada-s-pot-industry-gets-a-new-supporter-snoop-dogg-1.3946132

Von Glinow, Kiki. "Snoop Lion's Reddit Chat: Rapper Admits to Smoking 81 Blunts a Day." *Huffpost*, 2012. https://www.huffpost.com/entry/snoop-lions-reddit-81-blunts-per-day_n_2249602

Social Bonding Theory/Social Control Theory

Social bonding and social control theories contend that people resort to criminal behavior when their bonds to society, such as those to other individuals and social institutions, are weakened or severed. The stronger the bond an individual has to society, the more likely they will be to conform to the law and social conventions and refrain from engaging in unlawful or delinquent acts (Hirschi 1969). Strong, healthy bonds to society can also prevent individuals from engaging in risky behaviors that are often analogous with criminal activity, such as substance abuse. It has been suggested that the premise of social bond theory is better situated to explain less severe forms of delinquent and criminal activity (e.g., Krohn and Massey 1980), such as marijuana use. Social bonding and social control theories provide a suitable theoretical framework to understand the use of marijuana, which has become the most widely available and commonly used, federally illicit drug in the United States.

According to Travis Hirschi (1969), a researcher at the forefront of social bond and social control theories, an individual's bond to mainstream society is reinforced by four interrelated, yet independent, elements: *attachment*, *commitment*, *involvement*, and *belief*. First, regarding *attachment*, it is suggested that positive relationships and emotional closeness with nondeviant others are an important source of social control. Individuals with a strong attachment will abstain from criminal behavior because they are controlled through their affectional or emotional ties with parents, friends, teachers, and others. Concerning marijuana, which is often considered a "social drug," attachment to others may influence the likelihood of engagement in the behavior. For example, while time spent with parents has been linked to a lower risk of marijuana use (Borawski et al. 2003), weak attachment to parents or poor interactions with parents can lead youth to associate with delinquent peers and thus encourage the use of marijuana (e.g., Hirschi 1969).

Second, *commitment* refers to the time, energy, and resources an individual invests in achieving personal goals, such as getting an education or stable employment. Studies have shown that marijuana can harm neurocognitive functions, such as attention, memory, and learning, and is thus likely to influence achievement potential. Individuals with a high level of social commitment would be less inclined to use marijuana and engage in such potentially risky behavior, which can threaten the pursuit of goals and self-investment. Third, *involvement* in conventional activities reinforces prosocial norms by keeping individuals occupied with activities that promote the interest of society, such as athletic events and religious practices. Participation in these prosocial activities can then limit the ability to engage in deviant activities, including the use of substances such as marijuana. The fourth element, *belief*, refers to the general acceptance of the system of values placed on one by society.

Although growing numbers of states (and the District of Columbia) have legalized marijuana for medical and/or recreational use, however, marijuana use has become much more broadly accepted among the general population. In fact, studies have shown that about two-thirds of Americans favor the legalization of marijuana in the United States (Pew Research Center 2019; McCarthy 2018). This general support for the legalization of marijuana is likely to influence an individual's likelihood to engage in the behavior. In sum, when an individual is attached to others, committed to conventional goals, and involved in prosocial activities and believes in the legitimate value system of society, he or she will be less likely to engage in criminal and other analogous activities (Hirschi 1969), including marijuana use.

Hirschi's seminal work *Causes of Delinquency* (1969) was developed to explain delinquent behavior among youth and thus emphasizes the importance of parent-child and student-teacher bonds. Over the last decade, however, marijuana use has significantly increased among all age groups in the United States (Wu, Zhu, and Swartz 2016). John H. Laub and Robert J. Sampson's (1993) work on age-graded informal social control extends the importance of social bonds throughout the life course. The authors suggest that strong social bonds to work and family function as significant events or "turning points" in an individual's life-course trajectory. Life events, such as job stability and marriage, reduce the opportunity for offending and the influence of criminal peers and, thus, criminal behavior (Laub and Sampson 1993). Even for those who have a history of illegal activity, marital and family activities will reduce the exposure to deviant peers, which in turn will reduce the opportunity of engaging in deviant activities (Warr 1998). The use of illicit substances such as marijuana, however, has been shown to inhibit or delay the development of social bonds in the life-course trajectory. For example, research has shown an association between marijuana use and the postponement of marriage, parenthood, and marital dissolution (e.g., Kandel and Logan 1984). In addition, marijuana use has been linked to job instability and unemployment (Compton et al. 2014; Lee et al. 2015).

Social bonding and social control perspectives should be taken into consideration when explaining delinquency and criminal behavior. These perspectives, however, do not account for people's motives and pay little attention to behavioral consequences. It is rather implied that all individuals are enticed to deviate and will engage in criminal behavior if given the opportunity; asserting that even though all people have the potential to become criminal, most people are controlled by their bonds to society. In other words, it is posited that law and order are achieved through social control (Hirschi 1969), not necessarily through moral values.

Rocio Paez and Samantha Davis

See also: Age; Biosocial Theories; Conflict and Labeling Theories; Differential Association Theory/Social Learning Theory; Family Life; Gender; Subcultural and Learning Theories; Theories of Use.

Further Reading

Borawski, Elaine A., et al. "Parental Monitoring, Negotiated Unsupervised Time, and Parental Trust: The Role of Perceived Parenting Practices in Adolescent Health Risk Behaviors." *Journal of Adolescent Health* 33, no. 2 (2003): 60–70.

Compton, Wilson M., Joe Gfroerer, Kevin P. Conway, and Matthew S. Finger. "Unemployment and Substance Outcomes in the United States 2002–2010." *Drug and Alcohol Dependence* 142 (2014): 350–353.

Hirschi, Travis. "A Control Theory of Delinquency." *Criminology Theory: Selected Classic Readings* 1969 (1969): 289–305.

Kandel, Denise B., and John A. Logan. "Patterns of Drug Use from Adolescence to Young Adulthood: I. Periods of Risk for Initiation, Continued Use, and Discontinuation." *American Journal of Public Health* 74, no. 7 (1984): 660–666.

Krohn, Marvin D., and James L. Massey. "Social Control and Delinquent Behavior: An Examination of the Elements of the Social Bond." *The Sociological Quarterly* 21, no. 4 (1980): 529–544.

Laub, John H., and Robert J. Sampson. "Turning Points in the Life Course: Why Change Matters to the Study of Crime." *Criminology* 31, no. 3 (1993): 301–325.

Lee, Jung Yeon, Judith S. Brook, Stephen J. Finch, and David W. Brook. "Trajectories of Marijuana Use from Adolescence to Adulthood Predicting Unemployment in the Mid 30s." *The American Journal on Addictions* 24, no. 5 (2015): 452–459.

McCarthy, J. "Two in Three Americans Now Support Legalizing Marijuana." *Gallup,* October, 22, 2018.

Pew Research Center. "Two-thirds of Americans Support Marijuana Legalization." November 14, 2019. https://www.pewresearch.org/fact-tank/2019/11/14/americans-support-marijuana-legalization/

Warr, Mark. "Life-course Transitions and Desistance from Crime." *Criminology* 36 no. 2 (1998): 183–216.

Wu, Li-Tzy, He Zhu, and Marvin S. Swartz. "Trends in Cannabis Use Disorders among Racial/Ethnic Population Groups in the United States." *Drug and Alcohol Dependence* 165 (2016): 181–190.

Sports

Marijuana is the most commonly used drug in the world—by both athletes and nonathletes. While many states have enacted legislation permitting the medicinal and recreational use of marijuana over the course of the 2010s, the use of marijuana by athletes is subjected to restrictions imposed by the governing sports federation or league in which she or he competes. These laws vary greatly by sport and location; however, marijuana use is currently prohibited by most sports federations and leagues within the United States and internationally. As such, athletes who use marijuana or its derivatives can be subjected to sanctions imposed by their governing sports body or the individual teams or clubs to which they belong. These penalties typically include fines and/or suspensions. Public support for marijuana use and research demonstrating the medicinal effects of marijuana, however, has led some athletic commissions and leagues to mull possible changes and reforms to their anti-marijuana policies.

In 1989, the International Olympic Committee (IOC) placed cannabinoids (e.g., chemicals found in cannabis) on its prohibited substances list, effectively banning the use of marijuana by any athlete interested in participating in Olympic competition. In 2017, however, the World Anti-Doping Commission (WADA) removed cannabidiol (CBD) from that list after a number of studies were published demonstrating the medical benefits associated with CBD use. Thus, WADA's 2020 banned substance list includes "natural cannabinoids (e.g., cannabis, hashish, & marijuana)" and "synthetic cannabinoids," but not CBD.

Similarly, marijuana has been included on the banned substance list of just about every professional sports league in the United States since the formation of each respective league. Each league has different policies, procedures, and penalties surrounding the use of the drug. Some leagues have adopted less punitive punishments for a positive drug test, such as the National Hockey League (NHL). The NHL no longer bans the use of marijuana by players and recommends substance use treatment for any player who tests positive for "abnormally high levels" of tetrahydrocannabinol (THC). Other leagues, though, have maintained a harder line on marijuana use. For instance, both the National Football League (NFL) and the National Basketball Association (NBA) actively screen players for marijuana use and have clauses authorizing the suspension of players who commit multiple violations. However, the successful push for legalization of medical and recreational marijuana in numerous states across the country has led some sports leagues and players within those respective leagues to revisit the topic of complete prohibition. Many leagues are now considering the possibility of permitting athletes to use marijuana and its derivatives—especially CBD, which lacks psychoactive properties and has a well-documented, and broad, medical use (Marion 2018, 165; Pacula and Smart 2017, 405).

Arguably, the first internationally reported controversy surrounding the prohibition of marijuana use in sports came at the 1998 Winter Olympics, when Canadian snowboarder Ross Rebagliati tested positive for THC and had his gold medal stripped from him. The decision was eventually overturned, however, based on his appeal of the rules, and the gold medal was officially awarded back to him. Since then, many other athletes have faced punishment for using marijuana. For example, in 2014, two members of the Pittsburgh Steelers, Le'Veon Bell and Legarrette Blount, gained national attention after they were charged by law enforcement with possession of marijuana following a routine traffic stop. In addition to the formal criminal charges, Bell was placed on a two-game suspension by the NFL and Blount was given a one-game suspension.

There have been legitimate arguments raised by proponents on both sides of the marijuana-sport prohibition debate. Some scholars have argued that marijuana use can be beneficial for athletes' health and recovery and does not unfairly enhance athletic performance. These advocates note that marijuana may provide a safer, less addictive form of pain management for athletes who are hesitant to use opioid pain pills for sports-related injuries. Further, they cite studies suggesting that chronic marijuana use may be associated with reductions in strength, endurance, lung compacity, and reaction time—traits that place users at a disadvantage in athletic competition (c.f., Kennedy 2017, 825). Conversely, others have argued that marijuana use could give athletes of certain sports an unfair advantage over others by reducing anxiety levels during competition (Campos, Yonamine, and Moreau 2003, 398). Opponents also contend that professional athletes should abstain from using marijuana because it remains illegal at the federal level.

Tyler Frye, Tyler Manger, and Nathan E. Kruis

See also: Law Enforcement Efforts, Marijuana Control; Neurological Effects.

Further Reading

Campos, Daniel R., Mauricio Yonamine, and Regina L. de Moraes Moreau. "Marijuana as Doping in Sports." *Sports Medicine* 33, no. 6 (2003): 395–400.

Hilderbrand, Richard L. "High-Performance Sport, Marijuana, and Cannabimimetics." *Journal of Analytical Toxicology* 35, no. 9 (2011): 624–637.

Hopp, Craig D., Inna Belfer, and David Shurtleff. *Cannabis (Marijuana) and cannabinoids: What You Need to Know*. Bethesda, MD: National Center for Complementary and Integrative Health. U.S. Department of Health and Human Services, November 2019.

Kennedy, Michael C. "Cannabis: Exercise Performance and Sport. A Systematic Review." *Journal of Science and Medicine in Sport* 20, no. 9 (2017): 825–829.

Marion, Nancy E. *Drug Policy and The Criminal Justice System*. 1st ed. Durham, NC: Carolina Academic Press, LLC, 2018.

Mottram, D. R., and Neil Chester. *Drugs in Sport*. 7th ed. Milton Park, Abingdon, Oxon; New York: Routledge, 2018.

Pacula, Rosalie Liccardo, and Rosanna Smart. "Medical Marijuana and Marijuana Legalization." *Annual Review of Clinical Psychology* 13 (2017): 397–419.

Shukla, Rashi K. "Inside the Gate: Insiders' Perspectives on Marijuana as a Gateway Drug." *Humboldt Journal of Social Relations* 35 (2013): 5–23.

Stoner Films

Stoner film is a comedy subgenre that features cannabis use as a primary theme, makes cannabis use a central element of the plot, and evokes references and symbols of the marijuana subculture. The stoner film template encompasses smoked-up buddies, most commonly males, encountering calamities while they seek to acquire marijuana, to complete tasks involving marijuana, and to overcome stints of marijuana-induced paranoia. The not-so-smart buddies are often challenged by comically inept authority figures, such as police officers, parents, and/or bosses who disapprove of pot and try to dissuade them from getting high.

Early depictions of smoking marijuana on the big screen were basically nonexistent and exalted as a killer "forbidden fruit." The anti-marijuana message contained in the film *Reefer Madness* (1936) was partially responsible. That film depicts smoking marijuana as the path toward addiction, insanity, violence, jail time, and imminent death via murder or suicide.

Marijuana consumption was seen as counter to mainstream norms for much of the mid-twentieth century, and pot smoking thus became an activity conducted largely out of public view. Revolutionary social movements during the countercultural era of the 1960s, however, moved marijuana out of the shadows and into mainstream music and film. During the late 1960s and 1970s, in fact, stoner films became among the most significant art forms for conveying countercultural ideas and lifestyles. Led by films such as *Easy Rider* (1969), the animated *Fritz the Cat* (1972), and a series of *Cheech and Chong* films, stoner films became increasingly popular in the 1970s and early 1980s. The subgenre's popularity continued to increase throughout the 1980s and 1990s, and by the

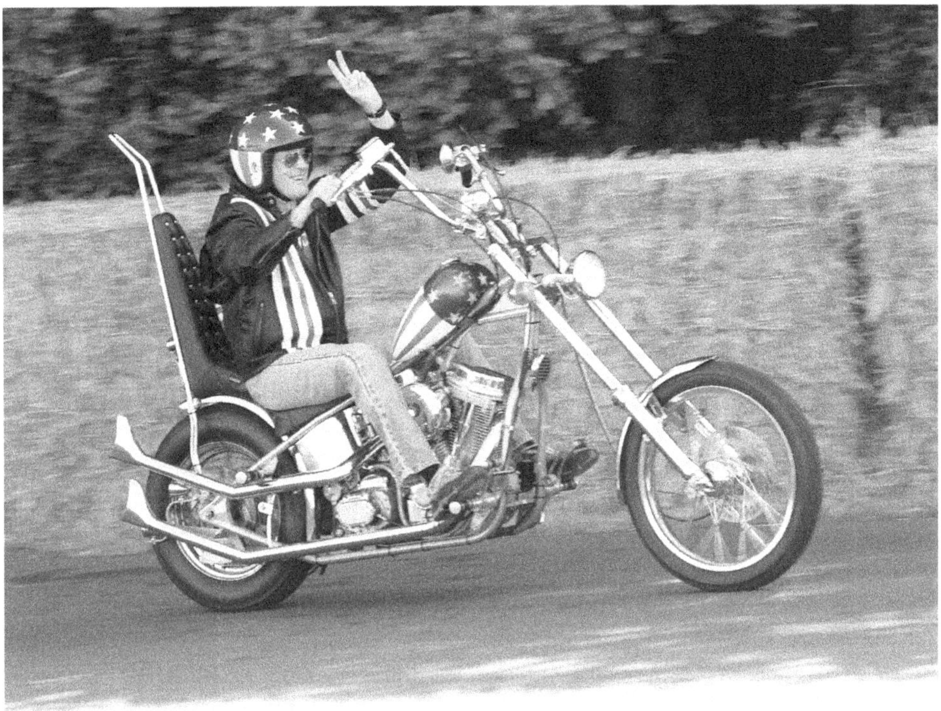

Actor Peter Fonda on an *Easy Rider* chopper. *Easy Rider* was one of many famous stoner films that center on the use of marijuana. Stoner films often glorify the use of marijuana and other drugs. They first hit the big screen in the 1960s and became increasingly popular through the 1970s and 1980s. (Chris Nolan/Dreamstime.com)

beginning of the twenty-first century, stoner films were no longer the rarity that they had once been.

The popularity of stoner films is evident from their all-star casts. For example, *Easy Rider* (1969) starred Peter Fonda, Dennis Hopper, Terry Southern, and Jack Nicholson (the latter in a supporting role that helped launch him to stardom). Similarly, *The Big Lebowski* (1998) starred Jeff Bridges, John Goodman, Julianne Moore, Steve Buscemi, and Tara Reid. Stoner films have proven so popular that they have spawned sequels. Examples include the Harold & Kumar films featuring John Cho and Kal Penn (*Harold & Kumar Go to White Castle* (2004), *Harold & Kumar Escape from Guantanamo Bay* (2008), *A Very Harold & Kumar 3D Christmas* (2011)) and Ice Cube's *Friday* (1995) franchise (*Next Friday* (2000), *Friday After Next* (2002), *Last Friday*, forthcoming). Since inception, the subgenre actors/actresses are characteristically racially and ethnically diverse and evade stereotypical portrayals of minorities. The subgenre has also become popular in crossover films such as *Puff, Puff, Pass* (2006), *Pineapple Express* (2008), and *We're the Millers* (2013) and television shows such as *Saturday Night Live*, *That '70s Show*, and *Weeds*.

Courtney B. Ross

See also: *Big Lebowski, The*; Cheech and Chong; *Saturday Night Live*; *That '70s Show*; *Weeds*.

Further Reading

Gunasekera, Hasantha, Simon Chapman, and Sharon Campbell. 2005. "Sex and Drugs in Popular Movies: An Analysis of the Top 200 Films." *Journal of the Royal Society of Medicine* 98, no. 10 (2005): 464–470.

Meltzer, Marisa. "Leisure and Innocence: The Eternal Appeal of the Stoner Movie." *Slate.com*, June 26, 2007. https://slate.com/news-and-politics/2007/06/the-eternal-appeal-of-the-stoner-movie.html

Sears, Cornelia, and Jessica Johnston. "Wasted Whiteness: The Racial Politics of the Stoner Film." *M/C Journal* 13, no. 4 (2010). https://doi.org/10.5204/mcj.267

Strain Theories

Strain theories have long been integrated into the study of the sociology of crime and other forms of social deviance (Durkheim 1897; Merton 1938), arguing that human behaviors such as marijuana use are a function of either exterior factors from general society or individual-level experiences that result in the loosening of social norms. An important early study of strain affecting deviant behavior at a macro level was made by Emile Durkheim in the nineteenth century. A century later, scholar Robert Merton made influential observations about potential linkages between strain and lawbreaking (Durkheim 1897; Merton 1938). Their bodies of work focused broadly on society and the stressors that influence large-scale human behavior. Since then, however, general strain theory (GST) has emerged as a leading model for explaining individual motivations for deviant behavior such as drug use.

All primary forms of strain theory argue that criminal behavior (such as marijuana use in locations where local and state laws restrict or outlaw such behavior) is rooted in the presentation of negative stimuli that cause stress for certain groups in society or individuals in society (Miller and Miller 2014). Merton claimed that stress is generated as a result of the inconsistency between desired goals and legitimate means of attaining those goals in society. Individuals in lower socioeconomic positions pursue the same goals that animate most other members of American society, such as monetary and material success and upward mobility. Individuals in lower social positions, however, are much more likely to lack the legitimate means of attaining those goals—such as obtaining the necessary educational credentials for careers in certain fields.

Strain theory (anomie theory) argues that individuals who suffer from the challenge of legitimately reaching desired goals will respond with one of several *modes of adaptation* (Miller, Schreck, and Tewksbury 2014; Miller and Miller 2014). These modes are conformity, innovation, ritualism, retreatism, and rebellion. Of the five modes, retreatism and rebellion are often cited as explanations for negative behaviors such as illegal marijuana consumption, as individuals may use marijuana due to its "counterculture" trappings and lingering status (in some societal circles) as an act of rebellion against prevailing cultural norms.

Drug laws have been a primary sector of the criminal justice system, and as a consequence, rebellious individuals have found that using marijuana is a representation of rebellion both through symbolism and through actual physical behavior. Additionally, individuals who retreat from or fail to invest time or energy in meeting society's goals and norms may use marijuana as a way to consciously establish distance between the individual and wider society (Miller and Miller 2014).

General strain theory presents strain as the result of one (or more) of the following three conditions: (1) removal of positive stimuli, (2) introduction of negative stimuli, or (3) failure to achieve positively valued goals (Agnew 1992). All three conditions cause strain that can equate to criminal or deviant behavior. However, the theory set forth by Agnew cautions that individuals suffering from strain can react in a multitude of ways to alleviate strain. Some may rely heavily on marijuana use, while others will not indulge in marijuana use at all. Agnew also notes that a person's behavioral coping mechanism is a key factor in evaluating whether or not the conditions of strain will lead to a person behaving negatively to manage their stress (Agnew 1992).

Research on the relationship between drug use and strain has primarily experimented with the ideas put forth by Agnew. Some of these studies have documented significant linkages between marijuana consumption and personal strain (loss of loved ones, economic stressors, parental punishment and other forms of family conflict, etc.).

Nathan D. Coleman and J. Mitchell Miller

See also: Conflict and Labeling Theories; Differential Association Theory/Social Learning Theory; Theories of Use.

Further Reading

Agnew, Robert. "Foundation for a General Strain Theory of Crime and Delinquency." *Criminology* 30, no. 1 (1992): 47–88.

Akers, Ronald L., and John Cochran. "Adolescent Marijuana Use: A Test of Three Theories of Deviant Behavior." *Deviant Behavior* 6, no. 4 (1985) 323–346.

Durkheim, Emile. *Suicide*. New York: The Free Press, 1897.

Merton, Robert K. "Social Structure and Anomie." *American Sociological Review* 3, no. 5 (1938): 672–682.

Miller, J.M., and H.V. Miller. "Sociological Criminology and Drug Use." In *The Nurture Versus Biosocial Debate in Criminology: On the Origins of Criminal Behavior and Criminality*, edited by Kevin M. Beaver, James Christopher Barnes, and Brian B. Boutwell. Thousand Oaks, CA: Sage, 2014, 315.

Miller, J.M., H.V. Miller, and T.L. Claxton. "Theorizing Novel and Emerging Drug Use: A Motivational Typology." *Deviant Behavior* 40, no. 9 (2018): 1–14.

Miller, J.M., C.J. Schreck, and R. Tewksbury. *Criminological Theory: A Brief Introduction*. Essex, UK: Pearson Higher Ed, 2014.

Street Crime

The relationship between marijuana and street crime has been meticulously studied for decades. Much of the current research on marijuana and street crime focuses on the effect of marijuana legalization on street crime. Although marijuana is still criminalized on the federal level, many states have legalized recreational use of marijuana (Pacula and Smart 2017).

Some research suggests that marijuana dispensaries act as "magnets for crime," enticing criminal offenders to the areas surrounding these dispensaries with valuable commodities and significant sums of cash (Hughes et al. 2020). Exploring this possibility, researchers found that while Denver, Colorado, has experienced a decline in murder and auto theft since the legalization of recreational marijuana, there has been a rise in various types of neighborhood crime and disorder, including alcohol and drug offenses, burglary, aggravated assault, robbery, public disorder, and theft from a motor vehicle (Hughes et al. 2020), although it is worth mentioning that there may be a host of other factors as well that could be at work here. Another study indicates that crime in Washington and Oregon, two states where recreational marijuana is legal, is decreasing. Indeed, instances of rape, property crimes, alcohol use (including binging), and other types of drug use have all decreased since the legalization of recreational marijuana (Dragone et al. 2019). On the other hand, another study found a reduction in property and violent crime rates in states where recreational marijuana is legal, relative to states where it remains illegal—but also found that the differences are not statistically significant (Maier, Mannes, and Koppenhofer 2017). Other researchers report a correlation between increased rates of marijuana-specific crimes and the density of marijuana outlets in spatially adjoining local Census block groups. Yet, there is a lack of a correlation between marijuana outlets and violent and property crime rates (Freisthler et al. 2017). There is also evidence that the legalization of marijuana for medicinal purposes did not affect rates of homicide, rape, robbery, assault, burglary, larceny, or auto theft. In fact, some researchers have suggested a correlation between medical marijuana legalization and a reduction in homicide and assault rates (Morris et al. 2014).

Overall, data suggest a downward trend in both violent and property crimes following marijuana legalization. Even so, some works suggest the nature of the relationship is still not clear. While some works suggest there has been a decrease in certain types of violent and property offenses, other works point in the opposite direction, suggesting that more research is needed to determine the best policies for reducing crime in states where marijuana is legal.

Lucas Maness

See also: Incarceration for Marijuana Offenses; Law Enforcement Resources; Trafficking.

Further Reading

Dragone, Davide, Giovanni Prarolo, Paolo Vanin, and Giulio Zanella. "Crime and the Legalization of Recreational Marijuana." *Journal of Economic Behavior & Organization* 159 (2019): 488–501.

Freisthler, Bridget, et al. "From Medical to Recreational Marijuana Sales: Marijuana Outlets and Crime in an Era of Changing Marijuana Legislation." *The Journal of Primary Prevention* 38, no. 3 (2017): 249–263.

Hughes, Lorine A., Lonnie M. Schaible, and Katherine Jimmerson. "Marijuana Dispensaries and Neighborhood Crime and Disorder in Denver, Colorado." *Justice Quarterly* 37, no. 3 (2020): 461–485.

Maier, Shana L., Suzanne Mannes, and Emily L. Koppenhofer. "The Implications of Marijuana Decriminalization and Legalization on Crime in the United States." *Contemporary Drug Problems* 44, no. 2 (2017): 125–146.

Morris, Robert G., Michael TenEyck, James C. Barnes, and Tomislav V. Kovandzic. "The Effect of Medical Marijuana Laws on Crime: Evidence from State Panel Data, 1990–2006." *PloS One* 9, no. 3 (2014). https://doi.org/10.1371/journal.pone.0092816

Pacula, Rosalie Liccardo, and Rosanna Smart. "Medical Marijuana and Marijuana Legalization." *Annual Review of Clinical Psychology* 13 (2017): 397–419.

Subcultural and Learning Theories

In that marijuana is a highly social drug, scholars often employ differential association-based and social learning theories that primarily analyze socialization and equate problematic and risky behaviors to antisocial social learning processes (Sutherland 1947). Differential association (relationships with peers affecting behavior), criminal perceptions and ways of thinking, and replication of illegal conduct all can become heightened when they become normalized and internalized through daily observed behavior (Akers 1998; Miller and Miller 2014). Delinquent peer association or interacting with friends who have deviant behavioral patterns offers environmental exposure to marijuana and popular marijuana use practices. Also informed by social learning theory, marijuana consumption brings with it substantial nonsocial and social reinforcements that vary in their specifics, depending on the group in question. For example, many young people are seen as more open to the idea of using marijuana because so many of their peers are willing to also consume marijuana—a reality increasingly bolstered by more liberal drug control policies across the nation (Miller et al. 2009). Of course, condemnation norms are changing with increasing decriminalization, legalization, and medicinal terminology, so definitions and understanding of use are rapidly changing, suggesting that web-based knowledge and faceless influencers may be more vital to onset and use behavior than in the past.

Further, the field of neuroscience has demonstrated that in young people, some areas of the brain such as the orbitofrontal cortex (a reward-seeking sector of the brain) are highly active in the company of their peers (Steinberg 2007; 2008). Given that technology stimulates cognitive activity, virtual peer influence—messaging received through social media and popular entertainment—may well influence use behavior, especially given how pervasive these elements are in the daily life of many people.

Supports of the theory of cultural transmission clearly view marijuana consumption as learned behavior (Miller and Miller 2014). Such subcultural theories, however, evaluated shared definitions and values of positively perceived behavior of social groups (Cohen 1955; Miller 1958; Ohlin 1960). Depending on the social group or environment an individual is in, behaviors such as marijuana consumption may be perceived as normal, valued, or at least excused behavior. In these settings, shared marijuana consumption can solidify group stability and personal ties over time. This is especially the case in youth subcultures in which pot use is common.

Walter B. Miller's lower-class focal concerns theory is a subcultural analysis that is recorded as one of the initial attempts at this approach (Miller 1958). In this perspective, Miller identified six focal concerns to explain why crime primarily focused in lower socioeconomic groups (Miller 1958). The characteristics he discussed are *trouble, toughness, smartness, excitement, fate*, and autonomy. Lloyd Ohlin's differential opportunity theory (1960) offers another historical subcultural-based explanation for the youthful consumption of marijuana and other drugs. Ohlin focused on differences in marijuana use within different types of juvenile gangs (Ohlin's 1960). The criminal subculture refers to the areas where crime exist and the potential for advancement through a criminal hierarchy. The conflict subculture refers to the disputes that occur between varying groups in low socioeconomic areas and its normalcy. The last adaptation (retreatism) directly addresses drug use among youth otherwise rejected both in conventional society and criminal subcultures with use indicating societal withdrawal into drug culture that may or may not be in conflict with the larger society—but, if so, in terms of morality but seldom violent or property offenses.

Another analysis, Elijah Anderson's *Code of the Street* (1999), directed attention to the urban underclass—the African American lower social class—in his study of illegal, violent, and other behavioral issues within the inner city that can be attributed to drug use (Anderson 2000). Anderson's ethnography mainly explains violence within youth groups but also speaks to high levels of marijuana use in inner cities. Anderson dichotomizes inner city society into two types of citizens—street and decent, with "street" families rejecting middle-class values and subsequently embracing the tolerance and endorsement of crime and deviance with heavy and often glorified marijuana use.

Nathan D. Coleman and J. Mitchell Miller

See also: Biosocial Theories; Conflict and Labeling Theories; Control Theories; Cultural Identity Theories; Differential Association Theory/Social Learning Theory; Moral Panics; Social Bonding Theory/Social Control Theory; Strain Theories; Theories of Use.

Further Reading

Anderson, Elijah. *Code of the Street: Decency, Violence, and the Moral Life of the Inner City*. New York: W. W. Norton & Company, 2000.

Akers, Ronald. *Social Learning and Social Structure: A General Theory of Crime and Deviance*. London, UK: Routledge, 1998.

Cohen, Albert. K. *Delinquent Boys: The Culture of the Gang*. Glencoe, IL: Free Press, 1955.

Miller, Holly Ventura, Wesley G. Jennings, Lorna L. Alvarez-Rivera, and Lonn Lanza-Kaduce. "Self-control, Attachment, and Deviance among Hispanic Adolescents." *Journal of Criminal Justice* 37, no. 1 (2009): 77–84.

Miller, J.M., and H.V. Miller. "Sociological Criminology and Drug Use." In *The Nurture Versus Biosocial Debate in Criminology: On the Origins of Criminal Behavior and Criminality*, edited by Kevin M. Beaver, James Christopher Barnes, and Brian B. Boutwell. Thousand Oaks, CA: Sage, 2014, 315.

Miller, Walter B. "Lower Class Culture as a Generating Milieu of Gang Delinquency." *Journal of Social Issues* 14, no. 3 (1958): 5–19.

Ohlin, Lloyd E. *Delinquency and Opportunity: A Theory of Delinquent Gangs*. New York: Free Press, 1960.

Steinberg, Laurence. "Risk Taking in Adolescence: New Perspectives from Brain and Behavioral Science." *Current Directions in Psychological Science* 16, no. 2 (2007): 55–59.

Steinberg, Laurence. "A Social Neuroscience Perspective on Adolescent Risk-taking." *Developmental Review* 28, no. 1 (2008): 78–106.

Sutherland, Edwin H. *Principles of Criminology*. 4th ed. Philadelphia: J.B. Lippincott, 1947.

Synthetic Cannabinoids

In the mid-2000s, an array of products containing synthetic cannabinoids became commercially available via internet retailers and head shops in Europe and the United States. Marketed and sold as "incense blends," these products contained plant matter that had been prepared with synthetic cannabinoids and that users smoked to achieve effects similar to those associated with marijuana.

Up until 2012, these products were sold and promoted as "legal highs" under popular brands such as "Spice" and "K2" in locations throughout the United States (Khey, Stogner, and Miller 2014). Because of their availability, legal status, and the inability of urine screens to accurately detect the substances, synthetic cannabinoids became widely used until more restrictive regulations were adopted in the United States and abroad (Khey et al. 2014). For many years, synthetic cannabinoids were sold via "gray markets." The word "gray" has two interrelated meanings. Although online and in-person retailers sold these products that were purportedly manufactured and labeled for one use (e.g., incense), many were aware of how these products were actually being used. Furthermore, the regulations involving synthetic cannabinoids were unclear, which made it possible for these markets to operate in a regulatory gray area. Although these are no longer available via many of these markets, synthetic cannabinoids continue to be used by individuals who want to achieve the psychoactive effects associated with marijuana while reducing the risk that their use will be detected by urinalysis.

Naturally occurring phytocannabinoids found in species of *echinacea* and *cannabis* (among others) produce psychoactive effects because they bind to cannabinoid receptors in the endocannabinoid system (Gertsch, Pertwee, and Di Marzo 2010). However, during the 1990s, John W. Huffman led a team of research scientists to synthesize the most extensive and well-known series of synthetic cannabinoids (JWH compounds). This research sought to further our understanding of the endocannabinoid system and potential therapeutic uses of cannabinoids (Castaneto et al. 2014). However, entrepreneurs used these research findings to bring cannabinoids to market for recreational use (Castaneto et al. 2014). For example, the JWH-018 compound was the first to be identified in products in Europe, although many compounds were subsequently found in products throughout the West (Vardakou, Pistos, and Spiliopoulou 2010). These compounds typically have greater binding affinity for the CB_1 receptor than phytocannabinoids such as Δ^9-tetrahydracannabinol (THC) found in many *cannabis* strains. Therefore, synthetic cannabinoids are often orders of magnitude more potent than the cannabinoids found in *cannabis* (Castaneto et al. 2014).

The increased potency of synthetic cannabinoids also leads to the potential for greater adverse health effects. Synthetic cannabinoid use has been associated with acute cardiovascular events such as hypertension, tachycardia, chest pain, stroke, and heart attack; renal failure; and psychiatric consequences such as anxiety, psychosis, suicidal ideation, and cognitive impairment (Castaneto et al. 2014; Pacher et al. 2018). However, because of the novelty of synthetic cannabinoid preparations, the long-term effects of use are not well understood (Pacher et al. 2018). Understanding the short- and long-term consequences of synthetic cannabinoid use is further complicated by the fact that the compounds used in products is constantly changing (Dresen et al. 2010; Frinculescu et al. 2017). This makes it difficult for users to know what they are consuming or how much to administer to achieve the desired effects.

Similar to other novel substances such as *Salvia divinorum*, state prohibitions in the United States preceded federal action (Khey et al. 2014). Initial regulations targeted the most common compounds (e.g., JWH-018, JWH-250, HU-210, and CP-47,497), but producers quickly substituted these compounds, creating second- and even third-generation products (Dresen et al. 2010, Frinculescu et al. 2017). Additionally, since the 1986 U.S. Federal Analog Act only regulated substances that were intended for human consumption, producers bypassed these regulations by including the warning that the products were "not for human consumption" (Khey et al. 2014). Later legislation regulated synthetic cannabinoids using broader criteria such as their structural classification and psychoactive effects, but also provided legal mechanisms by which newly discovered compounds could be added to drug schedules. At the federal level, the DEA initially placed five of the most prevalent compounds into Schedule I of the Controlled Substances Act on an emergency basis; soon after, the Food and Drug Administration Safety Innovation Act placed any cannabinoid receptor type 1 agonist into Schedule I and enabled the DEA to schedule new cannabinoids as they emerged (Khey et al. 2014). While many of these products are no longer available via brick-and-mortar retailers, producers continue to market similar products on the internet.

C. Cory Lowe and Bryan Lee Miller

See also: Cannabis Oils; Edibles; Head Shops.

Further Reading

Castaneto, Marisol S., et al. "Synthetic Cannabinoids: Epidemiology, Pharmacodynamics, and Clinical Implications." *Drug and Alcohol Dependence* 144 (2014): 12–41.

Dresen, Sebastian, et al. "Monitoring of Herbal Mixtures Potentially Containing Synthetic Cannabinoids as Psychoactive Compounds." *Journal of Mass Spectrometry* 45, no. 10 (2010): 1186–1194.

Frinculescu, Anca, et al. "Variation in Commercial Smoking Mixtures Containing Third-Generation Synthetic Cannabinoids." *Drug Testing and Analysis* 9, no. 2 (2017): 327–333.

Gertsch, Jürg, Roger G. Pertwee, and Vincenzo Di Marzo. "Phytocannabinoids Beyond the Cannabis Plant—Do They Exist?" *British Journal of Pharmacology* 160, no. 3 (2010): 523–529.

Khey, David, John Stogner, and Bryan L. Miller. *Emerging Trends in Drug Use and Distribution.* Vol. 12. New York: Springer International Publishing, 2014.

Pacher, Pal, et al. "Cardiovascular Effects of Marijuana and Synthetic Cannabinoids: The Good, the Bad, and the Ugly." *Nature Reviews Cardiology* 15, no. 3 (2018): 151.

Vardakou, Ioanna, Constantinos Pistos, and Ch Spiliopoulou. "Spice Drugs as a New Trend: Mode of Action, Identification and Legislation." *Toxicology Letters* 197, no. 3 (2010): 157–162.

T

Taxation

States have commonly sought to increase revenue by taxing goods and activities that in the past were viewed by many Americans as sinful and that even today are seen in some quarters as societal negatives. Examples include alcohol, gambling, tobacco, and—most recently—marijuana. In some states that have legalized medical marijuana, taxes are paid on the product by consumers, growers, or sellers (Trumble and Kasai 2017). These taxes usually take the form of either state sales or excise taxes, and the revenue generated from these taxes can either go into a general state fund or be earmarked for specific initiatives such as regulation and research of the medical marijuana industry (Trumble and Kasai 2017).

States have also sought to capitalize on the rise of recreational marijuana within their borders by imposing taxes on both operators and the products they produce. In 2012, Colorado and Washington became the first states to legalize the recreational use of marijuana. Over the next seven years, these early adopters were followed by the District of Columbia and nine additional states. The most recent adopter is Illinois, which began the process of legal sales in 2020. In some instances, initial passage of recreational marijuana did not allow for sales of the drug and only entitled legal adults to possess and grow the drug in restricted quantities. For instance, as of the beginning of 2020, the District of Columbia is prevented by federal law from legally selling or cultivating the drug, and Vermont has yet to finalize legislation for opening a marketplace for the regulation and taxation of marijuana.

In those states that currently allow for the regulation and sale of marijuana, a varied tax structure exists with state lawmakers setting different parameters and paths for the generation of revenue from marijuana. Some states, such as Alaska and California, require cultivators to pay a tax per ounce or pound on the flowers, stems, and leaves of the marijuana plants they sell (Federation of Tax Administrators [FTA] 2020). In other states, such as Colorado and Nevada, an excise tax is placed on the sale of marijuana between growers and distributors as a percentage of the transaction price (Tax Policy Center Urban Institute & Brookings Institution n.d.). Outside of placing taxes on cultivators, in most states (though not quite all), consumers are also taxed when they purchase marijuana legally through the marketplace. These taxes can take the form of excise ("sin") taxes or of retail sales taxes or some combination thereof. These tax rates range from a state sales tax of 6 percent in Michigan to a 37 percent tax on retail sales in Washington (FTA 2020). It is also permissible for localities to add additional taxes on to the sale of marijuana in some states (FTA 2020).

The tax revenue generated from the sale of marijuana is earmarked to go toward a wide array of programs, and each state sets its own priorities. Often, funds are used to support publicly popular initiatives in order to garner support from citizens who might only get behind legalization if they approve of where the revenue is going. For instance, in California, the income generated from the sale of marijuana has been used to support drug prevention programs, environmental protections, and industry research and regulation (Fimrite 2018). In Nevada and Oregon, revenue from marijuana goes to support education programs, and Nevada also sets funds aside for use during times of fiscal hardship (Tax Policy Center Urban Institute & Brookings Institution n.d.). Alternatively, Colorado has focused on using its marijuana tax revenue to support youth literacy along with mental health and anti-bullying programs (Julig 2019).

When establishing a marketplace for recreational marijuana, states tend to make projections on the amount of money they will receive from the new taxes being generated. Revenue projections can be hampered by unknown factors or events such as demand on the part of consumers, the actions of neighboring states, and the potential for changes in federal policy regarding marijuana. In some states, these revenue forecasts have been accurate or have even underestimated the potential revenue stream (Becker 2019). For instance, in Illinois, recreational sales began in January 2020. Despite difficulties with product availability, the state took in over $10 million in tax revenue from the industry in just one month (Marotti 2020). Despite the positive returns in Illinois, not all states have met their revenue projections, and in these states, the legal market has not been able to overtake the black market for the drug (Becker 2019).

Outside of difficulties in forecasting demand for marijuana, the states must also grapple with banking complications. In the United States, most financial institutions are unwilling to accept currency involved in the sale of marijuana or to provide checking accounts, business loans, or credit cards to marijuana retailers, dispensaries, producers, and other industry participants. These banks are resistant to offering their financial services out of fear of prosecution from the federal government given the illegal status of marijuana at the federal level (Stinson 2015). Without these services, the industry is susceptible to criminal activity, such as theft and robbery, and to a lack of ease or transparency in the accounting and auditing of the industry (Stinson 2015). Although Congress has worked on legislation to address the issue (referred to as the Secure and Fair Enforcement (SAFE) Banking Act), it has yet to pass into law as of the fall of 2020 (Krane 2020).

Rhonda Wrzenski

See also: Decriminalization; Online Marijuana Markets; Pricing.

Further Reading

Becker, Bernie. "Cannabis Was Supposed to Be a Tax Windfall for States. The Reality Has Been Different." *Politico,* October 14, 2019. https://www.politico.com/agenda/story/2019/10/14/marijuana-tax-revenue-001062/

Federation of Tax Administrators (FTA). "State Marijuana/Cannabis Taxes – 2020." March 5, 2020. https://www.taxadmin.org/assets/docs/Research/Rates/marijuana.pdf

Fimrite, Peter. "Marijuana Tax Revenue Falls Short in California." *Governing,* May 11, 2018. https://www.governing.com/topics/finance/tns-california-marijuana-taxes-fall-far-short-of-projections.html

Julig, Carina. "Marijuana Tax Revenue Surpasses $1 Billion in Colorado." *Governing,* June 13, 2019. https://www.governing.com/topics/finance/tns-colorado-1-billion-marijuana-tax-revenue.html

Krane, Kris. "Is the SAFE Banking Act on the Ropes? And Other Federal Updates." *Forbes,* February 24, 2020. https://www.forbes.com/sites/kriskrane/2020/02/24/is-the-safe-banking-act-on-the-ropes-and-other-federal-updates/#249cfe321e15

Marotti, Ally. "Recreational Marijuana Sales in Illinois Generated More Than $10 Million in Tax Revenue in January." *Chicago Tribune,* February 25, 2020. https://www.chicagotribune.com/marijuana/illinois/ct-biz-illinois-legal-weed-tax-revenue-20200224-iorl7m53qfburbrh7lv7gzszhm-story.html

National Conference of State Legislatures. "Marijuana Overview." 2019. https://www.ncsl.org/research/civil-and-criminal-justice/marijuana-overview.aspx

Stinson, Jeffrey. "The Trouble with Legal Marijuana: Banks." *Governing,* January 5, 2015. https://www.governing.com/topics/finance/trouble-with-legal-marijuana-banks.html

Tax Policy Center Urban Institute & Brookings Institution. "How Do Marijuana Taxes Work?" In *Tax Policy Center Briefing Book: The State of State (and Local) Tax Policy.* n.d. Accessed August 23, 2021. https://www.taxpolicycenter.org/briefing-book/how-do-marijuana-taxes-work

Trumble, Sarah, and Nathan Kasai. "How States Tax Medical Marijuana." *Third Way,* March 23, 2017. https://www.thirdway.org/one-pager/how-states-tax-medical-marijuana

Tetrahydrocannabinol (THC)

There are over 400 unique compounds estimated to be present in marijuana (or cannabis), but tetrahydrocannabinol or THC is the most well known and studied of them (Maroon and Bost 2018). THC is thought to be primarily responsible for the psychoactive effects of marijuana consumption, with other cannabinoids present in the plant having other, less pronounced, effects. There are various routes available for consuming THC, including smoking the plant or ingesting marijuana or its extracts in edibles. The route of administration of THC affects its rate of absorption, metabolism, and excretion.

THC is consumed by smoking the marijuana leaves, or by extracting THC from the cannabis plant and incorporating it into various consumables, such as foods (e.g., cookies, candies, and butters), beverages, and concentrates. THC can also be applied topically to the skin or administered sublingually (under the tongue). THC is highly soluble in lipids (fats) and alcohol, which means it adheres to or combines well with these substances. Thus, some common methods of preparation utilize fats (such as butter) or alcohol to extract the THC from the leaves.

When smoked, nearly all the THC inhaled is absorbed through the lungs and enters the bloodstream. Psychoactive effects begin to occur within seconds to minutes. When ingested (i.e., absorbed through the stomach by eating or drinking), only about 25–30 percent of the THC that would have been absorbed by smoking an equivalent dose enters the bloodstream, and the psychoactive effects begin much later (between 30 minutes and a few hours). However, the duration of these psychoactive effects is much longer when THC is ingested, because it is absorbed gradually through the blood vessels in the stomach lining rather than immediately through the lungs when it is inhaled (Ashton 2001).

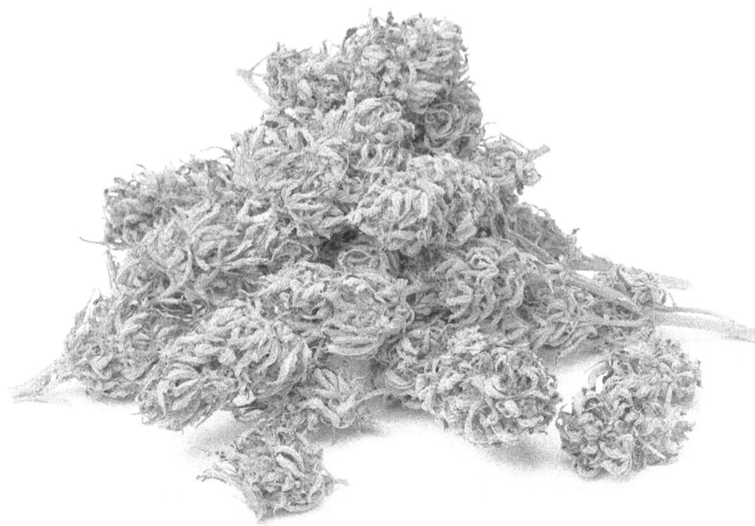

Dried marijuana buds with visible Tetrahydrocannabinol (THC). Buds of marijuana are from the plant's flowering tops. Marijuana leaves are also smoked. THC is the primary psychoactive ingredient in cannabis. (Pipa100/Dreamstime.com)

THC activates the cannabinoid receptors (Pertwee 1997; Maroon and Bost 2018). When THC binds to the CB1 receptor, it results in the blockade of voltage-gated calcium channels, the inhibition of adenylyl cyclase, and the inhibition of the release of various neurotransmitters. This inhibition has downstream effects on other neurotransmitter systems, including monoamines. There are several other biological mechanisms not discussed here, and nuances to these effects are discussed in greater detail elsewhere (e.g., see Onaivi 2002). These inhibitory effects result in the mediation of several neurotransmitter systems.

THC is metabolized in the liver by fatty acid amid hydrolase (FAAH) and monoacyl-glycerol lipase (MAGL) (Silver 2019). The endogenous cannabinoids (naturally present) anandamide and 2-AG are also metabolized by these enzymes. FAAH metabolizes anandamide and both FAAH and MAGL metabolize 2-AG, although metabolism is primarily through MAGL. THC is first metabolized into 11-hydroxy-THC (THC-OH) and then THC-OH is metabolized into 11-carboxy-THC (THC-COOH), which is then metabolized into glucuronide. THC-OH is considered an active metabolite and may be responsible for some of the psychoactive effects of marijuana. Following consumption, 25 percent of THC and its metabolites are excreted in urine, whereas 65 percent is reintroduced into the digestive system and reabsorbed. THC remains in the fat cells for several days following use. Positive drug test results in urine can be found for up to one month or longer (Ashton 2001).

THC is very lipid soluble (fat soluble) and thus remains in the fat cells of humans who have consumed it for a period of time (which varies somewhat between individuals). Not all of the THC is metabolized before it is excreted. Thus, some THC is excreted unchanged in urine and stool, along with its metabolites THC-OH, THC-COOH, and THC-A. Differences in excretion are present between THC and its metabolites. For example, the greatest proportion of THC presence can be found in blood and oral fluid, whereas the greatest proportion of THC-A presence can be found in blood and urine. Additionally, THC-COOH has the longest window of detection, at approximately 24–48 hours in blood and 16 hours to over 1 month in urine. Chronic users show longer detection windows relative to more occasional users. Presence in excreted urine or other bodily fluids is also dependent upon individual metabolism and food/water intake.

Marissa Turturici

See also: Butane Hash Oil; Cannabichromene (CBC); Cannabidiol (CBD).

Further Reading

Ashton, C. Heather. "Pharmacology and Effects of Cannabis: A Brief Review." *British Journal of Psychiatry* 178, no. 2 (2001): 101–106.

Maroon, Joseph, and Jeff Bost. "Review of the Neurological Benefits of Phytocannabinoids." *Surgical Neurology International* 9, no. 1 (2018): 91.

Onaivi, Emmanuel S., ed. *The Biology of Marijuana: From Gene to Behavior*. Boca Raton, FL: CRC Press, 2002.

Pertwee, Roger G. "Pharmacology of Cannabinoid CB1 and CB2 Receptors." *Pharmacology & Therapeutics* 74, no. 2 (1997): 129–180.

Silver, Robert J. "The Endocannabinoid System of Animals." *Animals* 9, no. 9 (2019): 686.

That '70s Show

That '70s Show is a television series that was broadcast on the Fox television network from 1998 to 2006. The program was set in the fictitious Point Place, Wisconsin, a sleepy suburban town outside of Milwaukee. The series begins in the year 1976, as the antiestablishment counterculture of the 1960s was becoming mainstream. The show is centered around Eric Forman (Topher Grace), a somewhat nerdy but ordinary teenager, and his five friends: Steven Hyde (Danny Masterson), the cynical stoner who was once described by his second-grade teacher as "destined to be the smartest man in his cell block" (Season 2, Episode 5, "Halloween"); Michael Kelso (Ashton Kutcher), the dimwitted ladies' man; Jackie Burkhart (Mila Kunis), the spoiled and self-absorbed youngest member of the group; Fez (Wilmer Valderrama), the foreign exchange student whose country of origin is never revealed; and Donna Pinciotti (Laura Prepon), the feminist girl-next-door who becomes Eric's girlfriend. Red (Kurtwood Smith) and Kitty (Debra Jo Rupp) Forman are parents to Eric and his older sister, Laurie (Lisa Robin Kelly), a promiscuous college dropout. Red is a blue-collar, quick-tempered, conservative veteran of the U.S. military and Kitty is a high-strung homemaker and nurse who has a soft spot for Eric and his friends despite a prickly relationship with her own daughter. Although they are often exasperated with the endless antics of six disorderly teenagers, Red and Kitty often act as parental figures to their son's friends—they even take Hyde to raise as their own when his mother abandons him (Season 1, Episode 24, "Hyde Moves In").

Red rules the house with a stern fist, while Kitty is more compassionate and acts as a buffer when Red gets angry. Their dynamic mix of parenting styles is what guides the series' contradictory messages about the drug scene.

That '70s Show is known for documenting the stoner subculture and marijuana use of the time. Most often, the teen group's marijuana smoking takes place in the basement at the Forman residence. The basement, in all its unimpressive glory, is a sacred place for Eric and his friends. It is because of the safe refuge provided by the basement that they can circle up, burn incense, and smoke a joint. While television censorship rules prevented them from ever showing explicit images of the cast smoking *actual* weed in these scenes, it is made abundantly clear via the work-arounds and context clues that these gatherings serve a specific purpose. The cast is seated in a circle with a camera in the middle that rotates to reflect the passing of a joint from one person to the next as a cloud of smoke floats in the background.

While in the circle, Eric and his friends discuss a wide range of topics—some of them shallow, but other times exploring subjects such as family, relationships, love, heartbreak, religion, culture, and careers. Eric and Kelso frequently turn to the circle for wisdom regarding dating, sex, breakups, betrayal, and overcoming their own insecurities. The circle is depicted on the show as a sacred place, a trusted source of advice, and an escape from the pressures of the world.

Despite an extensive list of hints and clues about the enthusiasm that Eric and his peers have for pot, the show makes few direct, explicit references to marijuana or the consumption of it. That is not to say marijuana is never pictured or identified, but it is usually done so through innuendos such as "special brownies" or code words like "stash." Even though smoking weed is a major element of the show, the various storylines surrounding the drug reveal opposing attitudes.

In perhaps one of the heaviest episodes of the series, Jackie buys a bag of weed to impress Hyde, who takes the fall for her and gets himself arrested when the cops show up (Season 2, Episode 26, "Moon Over Point Place"). To protect Hyde from the wrath of Red for marijuana possession, Eric throws himself in the line of fire by boldly admitting that he also smokes (Season 3, Episode 1, "Reefer Madness"). At first, Red is unusually quiet. Then he decides to lay down the law and installs smoke detectors, sets strict curfews, and bans all of Eric's friends from the house (Season 3, Episode 2, "Red Sees Red"). He even goes so far as to nail Eric's bedroom window shut. Meanwhile, Kitty takes a different approach, proposing the radical idea that they do not dole out punishment and instead forgive him. Offended at the thought, Red facetiously asks if she intends to act like it never happened. Kitty hesitatingly confirms that, yes, that is indeed what she means. To top it all off, they *commend* Hyde for his noble act of sacrifice when they learn that he took responsibility for the bag of weed to protect Jackie from getting arrested. This contradictory message exemplifies the Formans' delicate balancing act between condoning and condemning the consumption of marijuana.

This paradox is illustrated again when Kitty brings home a bag of condoms from the hospital and delivers them to an embarrassed Eric, who hides them in his sock drawer next to the stash of weed Hyde asked him to hide since he knows Red has been snooping around in his room recently (Season 4, Episode 13, "Jackie Says Cheese"). When Eric catches his dad rifling through his sock drawer, he becomes paranoid that Red has found the bag of weed, but his parents mistake his defensive reaction for embarrassment. Eventually, Kitty sits them both down to clear the air. They can tell their son is hiding something, but aren't sure what it is exactly. Wanting to assert their disapproval without showing their hand, they ground Eric for a week. Once Eric has left the room, Kitty asks Red if he thinks there really could have been anything suspicious in Eric's drawer. To which Red answers, "*Who cares?*" This exchange sends a clear message that not only are Red and Kitty more comfortable talking about sex than marijuana, but they would rather not have to know what Eric and his friends are up to in their free time, as long as they maintain the *appearance* of respect for the Formans' household rules and disciplinary decisions.

Perhaps the best way to explore the portrayal of marijuana in *That '70s Show* is to compare it to how the show handled other traditionally forbidden subjects, such as sex, cigarettes, and underage drinking. The Formans were more permissive about drinking alcohol than any other behavior. When Eric comes home drunk from a Christmas party at Hyde's house, his parents' biggest concern was why Hyde's father left the boys alone with a keg of beer in the first place (Season 3, Episode 9, "Hyde's Christmas Rager"). Occasionally, the boys and Red even drink together: Red takes Eric out for a beer when a breakup with Donna leaves him devastated (Season 4, Episode 2, "Eric's Depression"); the boys also join Red for a few beers after he is laid off from his job (Season 2, Episode 2, "Red's Last Day"); and in an act of desperation after his heart attack leads Kitty to ban all alcohol from the house, Red sneaks down to the basement and asks Hyde to share his stockpile of beer (Season 6, Episode 2, "Join Together"). So, while they have to sneak around to smoke marijuana, alcohol can be enjoyed in the company of one's parents.

Conversely, smoking cigarettes and cigars is depicted as *more* harmful than marijuana. Those who smoke cigarettes are shamed and reminded of how unhealthy it is (Season 2, Episode 9, "Eric Gets Suspended"). Even though Kitty quits smoking, she seeks out Eric's friends and the basement as a safe space to savor one last cigarette (Season 1, Episode 10, "Sunday, Bloody Sunday"). Tobacco products are undesirable, even among the teenagers who smoke marijuana on a regular basis. As they smoke cigars for the first time, Hyde describes the experience by saying, "This is way worse than what we usually do in the circle. Tastes disgusting, smells rank, doesn't even make stuff funny. *THIS* should be illegal!" (Newman and Trainer 2004, Season 7, Episode 3, "(I Can't Get No) Satisfaction").

The series also featured many frank discussions about sex. Overall, the tone of the show is sex positive, despite the problematic slut-shaming targeted toward promiscuous female characters. When Eric and Donna get caught having sex in the back of his Vista Cruiser and a police officer escorts them home, they have to come clean to their parents about the fact that they are sleeping together (Season 2, Episode 19, "Parents Find Out"). Red and Kitty's reactions differ radically as to their response to his confession of smoking marijuana (Season 3, Episode 1, "Reefer Madness"). Rather than doling out punishment, Kitty is deeply saddened at the thought of her youngest son growing up and mourns his loss of innocence (Season 2, Episode 19, "Parents Find Out"). Red tries to reason with her by calmly stating that they knew this would happen eventually, especially since Kitty has been having frank discussions about sex since Eric was six years old. This time, Red has the more relaxed approach and Kitty expresses negative emotions. Still, both parents are more permissive than punitive.

Later, Red and Kitty sneak away to have a romantic weekend at a hotel, only to find Eric and Donna in the room next door (Season 3, Episode 16, "Romantic Weekend"). When Red realizes what is happening, he makes a deal with Eric in order to avoid ruining his weekend with Kitty, telling him to expect serious punishment on Monday, but for the time being they will both forget they ever saw each other. Again, the message is clear—Red and Kitty tolerate the kids' apparent deviance, as long as they can *pretend* not to know about it. This approach is best illustrated in Kitty's response to Hyde's umpteenth poorly disguised insult to Laurie's sexual history, which was "Steven, if you keep doing that, it's going to be really hard for me to pretend I don't know what you're talking about" (Mettler and Trainer 2003, Season 6, Episode 5, "I'm Free"). Much like the way marijuana consumption is never *actually* seen on the show, deviance is permitted, as long as it can be obscured from view.

Over 8 seasons and 200 episodes, *That '70s Show* softened the image of marijuana users and introduced the 1970s stoner subculture to a new generation. Its unique approach delivered conflicting perspectives through the lens of comedy, offered discourse on controversial topics, and allowed the audience to feel like they, too, were welcome in the circle.

Kristin Richardson

See also: Age; Hippies; Monkees, The.

Further Reading

Goldstein, Michael. "TV's Greatest [Bong] Hits." *LA Weekly*, April 12, 2012. https://www.laweekly.com/tvs-greatest-bong-hits/

Hedash, Kara. "*That '70s Show*: 'The Circle' was Used to Battle Network Censorship." *ScreenRant*, February 15, 2020. https://screenrant.com/that-70s-show-circle-trope-gag-battle-network-censorship-drug-use-explained/

Meslow, Scott. "How TV Fell in Love with Marijuana." *The Atlantic*, April 20, 2012. https://www.theatlantic.com/entertainment/archive/2012/04/how-tv-fell-in-love-with-marijuana/256169/

Mettler, G., and D. Trainer. 2003. "I'm Free." In *That '70s Show*, edited by M. Carsey, T. Werner, and C. Mandabach. Studio City, CA: Carsey-Werner.

Newman, K., and D. Trainer. 2004. "(I Can't Get No) Satisfaction." In *That '70s Show*, M. Carsey, T. Werner, and C. Mandabach. Studio City, CA: Carsey-Werner.

Taroy, Daniel. "How TV Learned to Stop Worrying and Love Its Weed." *Fast Company*, October 20, 2016. https://www.fastcompany.com/3064589/how-tv-learned-to-stop-worrying-and-love-its-weed

Theories of Use

Substance abuse has been examined from a number of medical, social science, and professional school disciplines resulting in a range of theories purporting to explain use (Petraitis, Flay, and Miller 1995). As noted in Miller and Miller

(2014), marijuana use theorizing derives from a number of disciplines, including medical sociological epidemiology (patterns and extent of marijuana use), drug ethnography (symbolic meaning and social functions of use), econometrics (societal implications of economic theory applied to licit and illicit substance exchange markets), and criminology (social origins, dynamics, and functions of use and regulation).

Criminological-based marijuana research has been primarily focused on illicit substance consumption and less focused on individuals and groups in locales with more tolerant drug control policies regarding cannabis. Given the short history of marijuana legal reform, the extant knowledge base on open and legal use is still forming, so the literature on the topic has been almost inseparable from crime and deviance. Thus, *social origins* and *social context* are leading themes in sociological research on marijuana as evidenced by indications of increased interest in the history of marijuana prohibition, the manifest and latent functions of use, enforcement realities, correlates of use and abuse, treatment, and symbolic effects influencing culture more generally (Faupel, Horowitz, and Weaver 2003; Miller 2000).

Nathan D. Coleman and J. Mitchell Miller

See also: Social Bonding Theory/Social Control Theory; Subcultural and Learning Theories.

Further Reading

Faupel, C.E., A.M. Horowitz, and G. Weaver. *The Sociology of American Drug Use*. New York: McGraw-Hill Humanities/Social Sciences/Languages, 2003.

Miller, J. Mitchell. "Marijuana as Social Common Denominator: Reconsidering the Use and Academic Success Relationship." *Humanity & Society* 24, no. 4 (2000): 338–347.

Miller, J. M., and H.V. Miller. "Sociological Criminology and Drug Use." In *The Nurture Versus Biosocial Debate in Criminology: On the Origins of Criminal Behavior and Criminality*, edited by Kevin M. Beaver, James Christopher Barnes, and Brian B. Boutwell. Thousand Oaks, CA: Sage, 2014. 315.

Petraitis, John, Brian R. Flay, and Todd Q. Miller. "Reviewing Theories of Adolescent Substance Use: Organizing Pieces in the Puzzle." *Psychological Bulletin* 117, no. 1 (1995): 67.

Trafficking

Marijuana trafficking in the United States continues to evolve in response to changes in legislation governing its legality. Trafficking has become complex as it is now occurring in both licit and illicit markets as states enact and reform legislation to allow medicinal and/or recreational marijuana use. Marijuana remains the most commonly used illicit drug in the United States. It can be produced domestically by growers for medical or personal use markets or drug trafficking organizations (DTOs), but it is also grown internationally, often by DTOs, and trafficked into the country.

Offenders carrying out drug trafficking and production activities vary from low-level, independent, and loosely organized networks of individuals to more structured and organized groups (see DEA 2019; Natarajan and Belanger 1998;

Natarajan, Zanella, and Yu 2015). The increased public and legal approval of marijuana use, coupled with the ease of access, has attracted diverse networks to become involved with illegal marijuana cultivation and distribution in the United States. In addition to the involvement of Mexican DTOs, which has resulted in a significant number of marijuana seizures along the border over the past several decades, smaller quantities of the drug are also seized along the border with Canada and at access points to and from Caribbean nations (DEA 2019). Additionally, Asian DTOs are known to operate indoor marijuana grow houses in states with legal personal-use marijuana laws (DEA 2019).

Traditionally, the U.S. marijuana markets have been controlled by Mexican DTOs (United Nations Office on Drugs and Crime (UNODC) 2010, 2014). However, significant changes to marijuana legislation in the form of state laws permitting marijuana production, sales, and use for medical or recreational purposes have spurred significant increases in domestic production. Despite decreased seizure amounts, Mexico remains the most significant foreign source for the drug. Most of the marijuana trafficked into the United States occurs at ports of entry along the borders. In 2018, the U.S. Customs and Border Protection (CBP) seized nearly 300,000 kilograms of marijuana in approximately 9,000 incidents along the southwest border (DEA 2019). Cartels routinely employ U.S. citizens to traffic drugs across the border, with the United States Sentencing Commission (2017) reporting half of the marijuana trafficking offenders in 2017 identified as such. In line with declining seizures, from 2013 to 2017, the number of marijuana trafficking offenders has decreased by 43.2 percent, down to 2,710 from 4,768 offenders (United States Sentencing Commission 2017).

Trafficked product is often hidden and transported in plain sight. Domestically produced marijuana is typically transported across state lines, from states allowing the cultivation of marijuana to, or through, states that have not legalized pot production. Drug traffickers utilize diverse forms of transportation, including automobiles, trains, buses, and aircrafts (DEA 2019; NDIC 2011). Additionally, large quantities of marijuana produced internationally are smuggled into the country via tunnels, boats, drones, and even catapults (DEA 2019). In contrast to plant forms of the drug, the compact nature of concentrated forms of marijuana allows them to be concealed in envelopes and flattened parcels through commercial parcel services such as the United States Postal Service or FedEx (DEA 2019).

Traffickers have proven adaptive in attempts to evade detection and circumvent control efforts to traffic drugs to profitable markets. The production and trafficking of marijuana are likely to continue to evolve as states adopt and modify legislation pertaining to the drug. Traffickers are currently utilizing legitimate means (e.g., vehicles, wooden furniture) and transporting illicit products with new technologies (e.g., drones). The networks of producers and traffickers operating at various levels service the dynamic marijuana market. Although declining, Mexico-produced marijuana continues to enter the United States in larger quantities. Individuals, businesses, and criminal organizations alike are exploiting the varying degrees of legality of marijuana from state to state to establish and maintain a presence in states without state-approved marijuana.

Danielle M. Stoneberg

See also: Drug Cartels; Drug Enforcement Administration (DEA); Law Enforcement Efforts, Marijuana Control; Law Enforcement Resources.

Further Reading

Drug Enforcement Administration (DEA). *2019 National Drug Threat Assessment.* Arlington, VA: Drug Enforcement Administration, 2019. https://www.dea.gov/sites/default/files/2020-01/2019-NDTA-final-01-14-2020_Low_Web-DIR-007-20_2019.pdf

Natarajan, Mangai, and Mathieu Belanger. "Varieties of Drug Trafficking Organizations: A Typology of Cases Prosecuted in New York City." *Journal of Drug Issues* 28 (1998): 1005–1026.

Natarajan, Mangai, Marco Zanella, and Christopher Yu. "Classifying the Variety of Drug Trafficking Organizations." *Journal of Drug Issues* 45, no. 4 (2015): 409–430.

National Drug Intelligence Center (NDIC). *National Drug Threat Assessment 2011.* Johnstown, PA: National Drug Intelligence Center, 2011.

United Nations Office on Drugs and Crime (UNODC). *World Drug Report 2010.* Vienna, Austria: United Nations, 2010. http://www.unodc.org/documents/wdr/WDR_2010/World_Drug_Report_2010_lo-res.pdf

UNODC. *World Drug Report 2014.* Vienna, Austria: United Nations, 2014. www.unodc.org/documents/data-and-analysis/WDR2014/World_Drug_Report_2014_web.pdf

United States Sentencing Commission. *Quick Facts on Marijuana Trafficking Offences.* Washington, DC: United States Sentencing Commission, 2017. https://www.ussc.gov/sites/default/files/pdf/research-and-publications/quick-facts/Marijuana_FY17.pdf

Trump, Donald (1946–)

Donald J. Trump (1946–) was the forty-fifth president of the United States from January 2017, when he was inaugurated, to January 2021. In many ways, Trump's position on marijuana was a reversal from that of his immediate predecessor, Barack Obama, and represented a reversion to earlier approaches to marijuana legislation. In general, the Trump administration was against the recent trend of relaxing the enforcement of federal law that criminalizes marijuana under the Comprehensive Drug Abuse Prevention and Control Act. Federal law currently defines marijuana as a Schedule I controlled substance with high potential for abuse, no currently accepted medical use in the United States, and no accepted safety standard for use under medical supervision. As a Schedule I drug, marijuana is illegal at the federal level, and the Trump administration supported continuing this classification, despite the legalization of medical and recreational marijuana use in numerous states and federal policies that curbed the federal government's interference in these states' marijuana laws.

When Trump assumed office in January 2017, medical marijuana was legal in 28 states and the District of Columbia, and recreational marijuana use was legal in 8 states and the District of Columbia. Toward the end of Obama's second term, federal prosecutors were directed to not prosecute violations of federal marijuana laws in states where medical or recreational marijuana was legal under state laws. Trump had appeared to support this approach while running for office; however, early in his tenure as president, the Trump administration issued statements indicating they would reconsider that approach in states where recreational marijuana was legal (Wagner and Zapotosky 2017). Shortly after announcing this change in policy approach, the Trump administration began taking action to roll back the more lenient approach that had allowed the legal marijuana industry to flourish in numerous states (Rogers 2017).

First, Trump's 2017 omnibus appropriations bill included a signing statement that directed federal agencies to disregard the Rohrabacher-Blumenauer amendment. This amendment, passed in 2014, prohibited federal funds from being used to prosecute those using medical marijuana in jurisdictions that allowed it (Olorunnipa 2017). Similarly, in January 2018, Attorney General Jeff Sessions formally overturned the Department of Justice's position that had adopted an approach of noninterference in states where marijuana was legal (Gurman 2018). In 2019, the administration issued a memo stating that engaging in cannabis-related "activities" such as using it or working for a dispensary made immigrants ineligible for citizenship, even if these activities occurred in states where such businesses and activities were legal (Jaeger 2020). Finally, in the 2021 fiscal budget, President Trump proposed lifting restrictions on the use of federal funds to prosecute medical marijuana use in states that permit it. In addition, the proposed budget includes a rider prohibiting the use of local taxes to regulate the legal sale of marijuana in Washington, D.C. (Bures 2020).

Despite this stance, Trump did indicate that he would sign the Strengthening the Tenth Amendment through Entrusting States (STATES) Act, which would eliminate many federal marijuana penalties in states that had legalized cannabis, if Congress passed it. This act would amend the Comprehensive Drug Abuse and Prevention Act to prevent federal prosecution of individuals or corporations for marijuana offenses, provided they were in compliance with state and local laws. The STATES Act, however, had yet to come up for a vote in Congress before President Trump left office in 2021.

Overall, while President Trump implemented a number of actions that reversed Obama-era guidelines on marijuana prosecutions, his administration did not pursue a full-scale crackdown on marijuana in states where it is legal. He also expressed support for modest reform of marijuana legislation and signed federal law that legalized hemp production (Jaeger 2020).

James Hawdon

See also: Comprehensive Drug Abuse Prevention and Control Act (1970); Incarceration for Marijuana Offenses; Incarceration Rates; Medical Marijuana and the Law; Nixon Administration "War on Drugs"; Obama, Barack (1961–); Reagan Administration "War on Drugs"; Recreational Marijuana Laws.

Further Reading

Bures, Brendan "Trump Administration Doubles Down on Anti-marijuana Position." *Chicago Tribune,* February 21, 2020. https://www.chicagotribune.com/marijuana/sns-tft-trump-anti-marijuana-stance-20200221-jfdx4urbb5bhrf6ldtfpxleopi-story.html

Gurman, Sadie. "Sessions Terminates US Policy That Let Legal Pot Flourish." *Associated Press*, January 4, 2018. https://apnews.com/article/19f6bfec15a74733b40eaf0ff9162bfa

Jaeger, Kyle. "Where President Donald Trump Stands on Marijuana." *Marijuana Moment,* September 29, 2020. https://www.marijuanamoment.net/where-president-trump-stands-on-marijuana/

Olorunnipa, Toluse. "Trump Questions Legal Binds on His Spending in Signing Statement." *Bloomberg News*, May 6, 2017. https://www.bloomberg.com/news/articles/2017-05-06/trump-questions-legal-binds-on-his-spending-in-signing-statement

Rogers, Kate. "Marijuana Entrepreneurs Try to Stay Calm after Spicer Comments on Weed." *CNBC Make It,* February 24, 2017. https://www.cnbc.com/2017/02/24/marijuana-entrepreneurs-try-to-stay-calm-after-spicer-comments-on-weed.html

Wagner, John, and Matt Zapotosky. "Spicer: Feds Could Step up Enforcement against Marijuana Use in States." *Washington Post,* February 23, 2017. http://washingtonpost.com/news/post-politics/wp/2017/02/23/spicer-feds-could-step-up-anti-pot-enforcement-in-states-where-recreational-marijuana-is-legal/

V

Vaporizers

A vaporizer is a product that heats unprocessed cannabis, cannabis wax, or cannabis e-liquid to produce cannabinoid vapors. During this process, which avoids combustion through temperature control, toxic compounds that result from the combustion of cannabis are avoided. When using a vaporizer, users achieve the delivery of cannabinoids and their effects through aerosol inhalation while minimizing the risks associated with cannabis smoke inhalation. Handheld vaporizers (also known as e-cigarettes) were first produced in China in the early 2000s, and by 2007, the products reached the United States. Following introduction to the United States market, e-cigarettes saw rapid growth. While early versions of e-cigarettes typically focused on the delivery of nicotine, the products are now increasingly used for the delivery of cannabinoids in therapeutic and recreational contexts. From e-cigarettes to large tabletop designs, these tools come in many forms and offer discreteness and effectiveness (Hazekamp et al. 2006).

Vaporizers come in three types: those that use unprocessed cannabis plant material, those that use cannabis wax, and those that use cannabis e-liquids. All of these products produce a cannabinoid-containing vapor that is inhaled by the user. The simplest are the vaporizers that use unprocessed plant material. These vaporizers are referred to as herbal vaporizers. To use an herbal vaporizer, cannabis is ground and placed in a dry herb cartridge. The cartridge is loaded, the cannabis is heated, and the resulting vapor is inhaled (Giroud et al. 2015).

Cannabis wax, known as butane honey oil or butane hash oil (BHO), can be used in a similar way to plant material. Specifically, both products can be smoked or vaped. While these products are used similarly, their production differs. Like using plant material, the first step in producing cannabis wax is drying harvested plants and having them ground into small pieces. However, when producing BHO, the ground plant is carefully heated in a process that converts the acid forms of cannabinoids to their nonacid counterparts. For example, nonpsychoactive tetrahydrocannabinolic acid (THCA) can be converted to psychoactive tetrahydrocannabinol THC and cannabidiolic acid (CBDA) can be converted to cannabidiol (CBD). The final step in BHO creation is extraction and purification, which leads to a wax-like substance with a high concentration of the desired cannabinoids. The wax is then loaded into a vaporizer, heated, and the resulting vapors are inhaled.

Cannabis e-liquids can be created and used in vaporizers by taking the cannabis wax production process a step further. To prepare an e-liquid, the wax-like concentrate is combined with propylene glycol (PG) or a combination of polyethylene glycols and PG to create an e-liquid that can be used in a vaporizer. Researchers have raised concerns about some THC-containing e-liquids. Investigations of vape-related lung illnesses in the late 2010s led some to conclude that vitamin E acetate (used to thicken or dilute THC e-liquid) and other chemical additives such as diacetyl were contributors to the illnesses. These findings have led some jurisdictions to ban the additives (Boudi et al. 2019).

Though concerns exist, vaporizers remain a popular method of cannabis consumption for a variety of reasons. Vaporizers can filter out nonessential and potentially dangerous by-products found in cannabis smoke. Thus, vaporizers are harm-reduction tools that effectively deliver cannabinoids as opposed to water pipes, blunts, and joints that use combustion and expose users to tars and toxins. Because of the reduction of harm and the convenience of prepackaged e-liquids, vaporization is useful in therapeutic settings (Varlet et al. 2016). Vaporizers also differ from traditional smoking methods because, in some cases, flavoring can mask the taste and smell. This offers users who wish to avoid the appearance, taste, and smell of cannabis smoke a greater measure of anonymity and a more appealing experience (Lee et al. 2016).

Aubrey D. Johnson

See also: Blunts; Bongs and Water Pipes; Cannabidiol (CBD); Dabbing; Gravity Bongs; Tetrahydrocannabinol (THC).

Further Reading

Boudi, F. Brian, Sonia Patel, Ava Boudi, and Connie Chan. "Vitamin E Acetate as a Plausible Cause of Acute Vaping-related Illness." *Cureus* 11, no. 12 (2019): 1–5.

Giroud, Christian, et al. "E-Cigarettes: A Review of New Trends in Cannabis Use." *International Journal of Environmental Research and Public Health* 12 (2015): 9988–10008.

Hazekamp, Arno, et al. "Evaluation of a Vaporizing Device (Volcano®) for the Pulmonary Admiration of Tetrahydrocannabinol." *Journal of Pharmaceutical Sciences* 95, no. 6 (2006): 1308–1317.

Lee, Dustin C., et al. "Online Survey Characterizing Vaporizer Use Among Cannabis Users." *Drug and Alcohol Dependence* 159 (2016): 227–233.

Varlet, Vincent, et al. "Drug Vaping Applied to Cannabis: Is 'Cannavaping' a Therapeutic Alternative to Marijuana?" *Scientific Reports* 6, no. 25599 (2016): 1–13.

Vermont

Vermont approved the use of marijuana recreationally in 2018. However, Vermont is unique relative to prior adopters of pro-recreational marijuana laws in that recreational usage was approved by lawmakers within the state legislature and signed into law by the state governor—rather than through a ballot proposition introduced by citizens and adopted by voters within the state (National Conference of State Legislatures 2019). Historically, legalization of the recreational use of marijuana has been a policy change driven by voters taking advantage of state laws that provide for legally binding public referendums on various issues of the day.

When the Vermont state legislature approved the use of recreational marijuana, however, it placed several restrictions on the practice. The language contained in House Bill 511 mandated that only citizens of legal age (those over 21) could lawfully possess and consume marijuana and that possession could only be up to one ounce. If individuals exceed these limits, they can still be subject to penalties and prosecution by the state. The legislation set the parameters for these penalties ranging from $500 to $500,000 and no jail time to 15 years. Citizens can also face fines or jail time if they attempt to sell or dispense marijuana to other individuals (particularly those under 21), if they consume marijuana in public places such as on public sidewalks or in public parks, if they drive while under the influence of marijuana, or if they have an open container containing alcohol or marijuana in their vehicle. In addition, the state legislature mandated that citizens could also grow marijuana in their private homes as long as they limit the number of plants in their residencies to no more than two mature and four immature plants and keep marijuana growing efforts out of the view of the public (McCullum 2018; Vermont General Assembly House 2018). If citizens are not the primary homeowners and are renting their property, the law requires that tenants obtain the consent of their landlord prior to growing marijuana and allows for landlords to ban the possession of marijuana on their premises (McCullum 2018; Vermont General Assembly House 2018). The law also allows for employers to prohibit their employees from consuming, possessing, transporting, selling, or growing marijuana in the workplace (Vermont General Assembly House 2018). In addition, school administrators can impose their own penalties for anyone in possession of marijuana on school grounds, and the use or possession of marijuana is not permitted at any licensed childcare facility within the state (Vermont General Assembly House 2018).

At the time of passage in 2018, House Bill 511 did not specify parameters for the sale and taxation of marijuana. Thus, the sale of marijuana remained illegal within the state. However, state lawmakers have subsequently crafted and voted on legislation that would permit the sale, regulation, and taxation of marijuana starting in 2022 (Barton 2020). In the fall of 2020, Vermont Governor Phil Scott allowed Senate Bill 54 to pass and become state law without his signature (Herrington 2020). This legislation establishes an executive commission to oversee the licensing of various entities that would cultivate, test, or sell marijuana, such as retailers, manufacturers, and laboratories (Barton 2020; Marijuana Policy Project 2020). The legislation also equips the commission to put rules in place concerning packaging, storing, labeling, advertising, and lab testing of marijuana (Marijuana Policy Project 2020). Suppliers will have to adhere to legal limits on the potency of their products, and retailers will be required to post warnings crafted by the health department. In addition, the proposed legislation creates a recommended tax structure, along with licensing fees, and requires police officers to receive training in order to recognize drivers who are under the influence of marijuana (Marijuana Policy Project 2020). According to assessments by *Marijuana Business Daily*, if marijuana sales are legalized in the state of Vermont, the state could see an increase in revenue, ranging from $130 to $160 million within five years of initiation (Smith 2020).

Rhonda Wrzenski

See also: Alaska; California; Colorado; Decriminalization; Taxation; Washington D.C.; Washington State.

Further Reading

Barton, April. "Vermont House Passes Bill to Regulate Marijuana Sales: What Comes Next for S.54?" *Burlington Free Press,* February 26, 2020. https://www.burlingtonfreepress.com/story/news/2020/02/26/vermont-legislature-passes-cannabis bill-governor-veto/4878860002/

Herrington, A.J. "Vermont Legalizes Recreational Marijuana Sales." *High Times,* October 8, 2020. https://hightimes.com/news/vermont-legalizes-recreational-marijuana-sales/

Marijuana Policy Project. "Summary of S.54, the Bill to Regulate and Tax Cannabis in Vermont." 2020. https://www.mpp.org/states/vermont/summary-of-s-54-the-bill-to-regulate-and-tax-cannabis-in-vermont/

McCullum, April. "Vermont's Legal Marijuana Law: What You Should Know." *Burlington Free Press,* January 22, 2018. https://www.burlingtonfreepress.com/story/news/politics/government/2018/01/22/vermonts-legal-marijuana-law-what-you-should-know/1045478001/

National Conference of State Legislatures (NCSL). "Marijuana Overview." 2019. https://www.ncsl.org/research/civil-and-criminal-justice/marijuana-overview.aspx

Smith, Jeff. "Vermont House Gives Initial OK to Recreational Cannabis Sales, Putting State on Track to $160M Market." *Marijuana Business Daily,* February 26, 2020. https://mjbizdaily.com/vermont-house-gives-initial-ok-to-recreational-cannabis-putting-state-on-track-to-160m-market/

Vermont General Assembly House. An Act Relating to Eliminating Penalties for Possession of Limited Amounts of Marijuana by Adults 21 Years of Age or Older. H.511 (Act 86), 2018. https://legislature.vermont.gov/Documents/2018/Docs/ACTS/ACT086/ACT086%20As%20Enacted.pdf

W

Washington D.C.

As of February 26, 2015, the District of Columbia (DC) decriminalized the possession of up to 2 ounces of marijuana by adults at least 21 years of age under the Legalization of Possession of Minimal Amounts of Marijuana for Personal Use Initiative of 2014. The initiative formally legalized certain circumstances under which adults at least 21 years of age may possess marijuana in the district. However, criminal charges may still result from marijuana possession in some circumstances.

Voters in the District of Columbia approved the Legalization of Possession of Minimal Amounts of Marijuana for Personal Use Initiative (D.C. Law 20-153; 62 DCR 880)—better known as Initiative 71—in November of 2014. The new law became effective on February 26, 2015. As of February 26, 2015, adults at least 21 years of age in the district can possess up to 2 ounces of marijuana; transfer up to 1 ounce of marijuana to another adult at least 21 years of age as long as there is no exchange of payment, goods, or services; cultivate up to six marijuana plants in their residence (no more than three may be mature); possess marijuana paraphernalia (e.g., bongs, cigar wrappers, rolling papers) associated with up to 1 ounce of marijuana; and use marijuana on private property.

Although these provisions were legalized, several actions remain criminal violations. Examples include the possession of marijuana by an individual less than 21 years of age, possession of more than 2 ounces of marijuana, the sale of marijuana to another person, and the operation of a vehicle or boat under the influence of marijuana. Additionally, ingesting marijuana (smoking, eating, drinking) in any public space, including any place to which the public is invited, remains illegal. The list of prohibited public spaces is extensive and includes any street, sidewalk, alley, park, or parking area (whether in or out of a vehicle). The carrying or holding of any lit smoking equipment (e.g., joint or similarly wrapped paper, bong, pipe) filled with marijuana in any public space, including any place to which the public is invited; any street, sidewalk, alley, park, or parking area; or in any vehicle on any street, alley, park, or parking area, also remains illegal.

Consequences for violations vary. If a person under 21 years of age is found to be in possession of up to 2 ounces of marijuana by a Metropolitan Police Department (MPD) officer, the MPD officer will seize the marijuana but will not issue a ticket or make an arrest. If a person at least 21 years of age cannot prove his/her age, the MPD officer will issue a warning ticket and seize the marijuana. After 24 hours but less than 21 days from the seizure, the person can bring the warning ticket and proof of age to the police station in the police district in which the seizure occurred to retrieve the seized marijuana.

In additional to recreational marijuana, possession of medical marijuana is permitted in the District of Columbia in certain circumstances. The District Department of Health issues medical marijuana cards to qualified individuals; these cards permit holders to possess up to 2 ounces of medical marijuana per month. However, similar to recreational use, medical marijuana use in public is a criminal offense. While the district decriminalized the possession of marijuana in certain circumstances, the possession or use of any amount of marijuana is still prohibited by federal law. Federal law enforcement officers are thus empowered to arrest anyone for possession or use of any amount of marijuana in the District of Columbia.

Julie Marie Baldwin

See also: Alaska; California; Colorado; Decriminalization; Taxation; Vermont; Washington State.

Further Reading

District of Columbia Law 20-153. *Legalization of Possession of Minimal Amounts of Marijuana for Personal Use Initiative of 2014.* n.d. Accessed August 23, 2021. http://lims.dccouncil.us/Download/33230/B20-1064-SignedAct.pdf

Government of the District of Columbia. *Facts on Marijuana in DC.* n.d.-a Accessed August 23, 2021. https://mayor.dc.gov/sites/default/files/dc/sites/mayormb/release_content/attachments/I-71Factsheet.pdf

Government of the District of Columbia. *Facts on Marijuana in DC (Infographic).* n.d.-b Accessed August 23, 2021. https://mayor.dc.gov/sites/default/files/dc/sites/mayormb/release_content/attachments/I-71Infograph.pdf

Government of the District of Columbia. *Initiative 71 and DC's Marijuana Laws: Questions and Answers.* n.d.-c Accessed August 23, 2021. https://mayor.dc.gov/sites/default/files/dc/sites/mayormb/release_content/attachments/I-71-FAQ.pdf

Metropolitan Police District of Columbia. *Know the Facts About Marijuana in DC.* 2015a. https://mpdc.dc.gov/sites/default/files/dc/sites/mpdc/page_content/attachments/Marijuana%20Fact%20Card_FEB2015.pdf

Metropolitan Police District of Columbia. *SO-15-07: Legalization of Possession of Minimal Amounts of Marijuana for Personal Use Initiative of 2014 (Initiative 71).* 2015b. https://go.mpdconline.com/GO/SO_15_07.pdf

Office of the Mayor. *Bowser Administration Outlines Changes in District Marijuana Laws.* 2015. https://mayor.dc.gov/release/bowser-administration-outlines-changes-district-marijuana-laws

Washington State

Marijuana is legal in the state of Washington for both medicinal and recreational purposes. This status stems from more than three decades of legalization efforts by advocates and reformers, as well as a gradual but steady change in acceptance of marijuana by the citizens of the state.

In 1979, the Washington Court of Appeals recognized that a medical necessity defense for the possession of cannabis existed in specific circumstances. However, medical marijuana patients did not yet have an avenue for legally obtaining cannabis. This legal route did not occur until 1998, when Initiative 692 passed in

Washington, decriminalizing medical marijuana. Physicians were now allowed to recommend marijuana to their patients if they suffered from a terminal or debilitating illness. Patients who qualified for medical marijuana were permitted to possess a 60-day supply of cannabis, which was defined as 24 ounces of marijuana and no more than 15 plants. Dispensaries popped up all around Washington, and especially in major cities such as Seattle and Spokane. Although Initiative 692 did not explicitly allow for dispensaries, law enforcement typically adopted a lax approach toward such establishments (Washington State Department of Health n.d.).

After the passage of Initiative 692, support for legalized recreational marijuana began to increase in Washington. After several failed initiatives, Initiative 502 moved to the general ballot and was approved in 2012. Initiative 502 legalized the use of cannabis for adults over the age of 21, making Washington the first state to legalize marijuana for recreational use. The bill also afforded the Washington State Liquor Control Board the right to regulate and tax cannabis sales and also set maximum tetrahydrocannabinol (THC) content levels that individuals can have in their bloodstream while driving. The 2012 law legalized the possession of up to 1 ounce of marijuana, 16 ounces of marijuana-infused edibles in solid form, 72 ounces in liquid form, and 7 grams of marijuana concentrate for adults. It did not allow for the personal cultivation, sale, or gifting of marijuana, though. Buying and selling marijuana is only legal at state-licensed retail stores in Washington. Additionally, marijuana cannot be used in public view in Washington, and it is also illegal to drive while intoxicated on marijuana or to transport marijuana outside of Washington.

While medicinal and recreational marijuana is popularly supported in Washington, cannabis legalization is not without controversy. In particular, a sizable black market for cannabis has sprung up in Washington. Mexican drug cartels, increasingly under scrutiny from U.S. border agents, have started to grow their crops inside the United States. The amenable climate in Washington has made it a popular location for Mexican drug cartels. Concerns over crime related to the illegal drug trade, as well as environmental degradation, have led to opposition to the legality of marijuana in Washington.

In spite of the controversies, marijuana remains popular in Washington. In fact, marijuana use in Washington is significantly higher than average usage in the rest of the country. In addition, several marijuana-themed events, including the annual Seattle Hempfest and Olympia Hempfest, as well as the Cannabis Farmers Market held in Seattle, are well-attended. Originating in Tacoma, the Cannabis Farmers Market is the first and largest legal medical cannabis farmer's market in the world (McNertHney 2007; Nierenberg 2016). Marijuana sales have also offered a tax revenue boon to Washington. Indeed, during the first year of legalization, sales revenue from cannabis peaked at $260 million. By 2016, sales topped $1 billion. In 2017, tax revenue from the sale of marijuana was roughly $15 million (Washington State Liquor and Cannabis Board n.d.-b.).

Matthew Costello

See also: Alaska; California; Colorado; Decriminalization; Taxation; Vermont; Washington D.C.

Further Reading

Drug Enforcement Agency. "Washington 2005." n.d. Accessed August 23, 2021. https://web.archive.org/web/20050729090644/http://www.usdoj.gov/dea/pubs/states/washington.html

McNerthney, Casey. "Where There's Smoke, There's Hempfest." *Seattle PI*, August 17, 2007. https://www.seattlepi.com/local/article/Where-there-s-smoke-there-s-Hempfest-1247028.php

Nierenberg, Jacob. "Hempfest Approaches 25th Anniversary, but Financial Outlook is Hazy." *The Seattle Times*, August 15, 2016. https://www.seattletimes.com/entertainment/events/hempfest-approaches-25th-anniversary-but-financial-outlook-is-hazy/

Washington State Department of Health. "Medical Marijuana." n.d. Accessed August 23, 2021. https://www.doh.wa.gov/YouandYourFamily/Marijuana/MedicalMarijuana/LawsandRules/HistoryinWashington

Washington State Liquor and Cannabis Board. "Know the Law." n.d.-a. Accessed August 23, 2021. https://lcb.wa.gov/mj-education/know-the-law

Washington State Liquor and Cannabis Board. "Marijuana Dashboard." n.d.-b. Accessed August 23, 2021. https://data.lcb.wa.gov/stories/s/WSLCB-Marijuana-Dashboard/hbnp-ia6v/

Weed and Seed Programs

The Weed and Seed Program was a federal effort to reconnect police and local communities suffering from high levels of crime with the goals of revitalizing neighborhoods by reducing violence, poverty, and other societal disruptions associated with the illegal drug trade. With each site having its own set of factors and priorities driving their operations, this multifaceted agency strategy gradually expanded to improve the lives of community members in over 300 sites around the country.

The Weed and Seed Strategy, now the Weed and Seed Program, began with the opening of three sites in 1991 during the administration of Republican President George H. W. Bush (1989–1993). Designed by the U.S. Department of Justice (DOJ), the Executive Office for Weed and Seed (EOWS) managed the program with the support of the Bureau of Justice Assistance and the U.S. Attorney's Office (USAO) (Trudeau et al. 2010, 25). In 2004, the EOWS became the Community Capacity Development Office (CCDO) under the DOJ. The CCDO continued to manage the program until 2011 when its funding was not renewed (The United States Department of Justice 2018).

The process to select site applicants to join the Weed and Seed Program was detailed. One requirement included developing site plans alongside local government officials following national guidelines. Once the site became official, it received continued evaluation-based funding. These recognized participating sites fostered an opportunity for decreasing crime, especially by reducing violent and drug-related offenses. Before being defunded, there were "256 . . . active (funded and graduated) [Weed and Seed Program sites] in 46 states and 2 territories" (Trudeau et al. 2010, 26). Graduated sites are those that continue to follow the approved program strategy but are not funded by the Weed and Seed Program.

The Weed and Seed Program was a strategy to implement measures for the control and reduction of crime in high-crime areas. It did so by providing the community agency with resources not only to report crime but also to facilitate improvement to the daily lives and school experiences of community members (Bridenball and Jesilow 2005, 66). The Weed and Seed Program strategy reflects a two-phase approach—"weeding" and "seeding"—focused on four fundamental principles: collaboration, coordination, resident participation, and leveraging resources (Trudeau et al. 2010, 12).

The "weeding" portion sought to remove people responsible for major criminal activity from the community through the help of law enforcement and participating community members. In specific sites, this meant the District Attorney worked with law enforcement to identify and prosecute members of the community engaged in major criminal activity, such as dealing illegal drugs (Lilley 2015, 441–442; Bridenball and Jesilow 2005, 66). With their absence, the community has an opportunity to reconstruct their neighborhoods. Thus, the second phase of the program, "seeding," was designed to provide social and economic resources alongside continued law enforcement to reconstruct the area with an eye toward both public safety and community/business investment (Bridenball and Jesilow 2005, 66).

The Community Capacity Development Office (CCDO) required sites to collect data and evaluate their sites locally. They also conducted national evaluations through requested agencies. In 2003, the Justice Research and Statistics Association (JRSA) with the Office for Weed and Seed (OWS) conducted a national evaluation. They collected information on 98 sites with a range of program participation data. The most that was collected for a particular site was six years of data. The national pattern analysis from the JRSA's 2004 report reflected crime issues with drugs affected 61.2 percent of the sites (O'Connell, Perkins, and Zepp 2004, 3). For the Weed and Seed Program, specific drug types were not disclosed or shown to be analyzed separately. However, marijuana falls under the illicit drug category. For the JRSA pattern study, drugs were ranked first in crime issues by type of offense for the sites. JRSA identified a pattern with the data collected and found an increase in illicit drug activity during years one and two, followed by a decline in year three. These attributed site fluctuations of an increase in year one and two reflect being in areas of more significant drug activity (that already had a higher rate of drug activity than other jurisdictions), followed by the decrease in year three with the implementation of increase in policing and an increase in community reporting.

In contrast, *the Independent Evaluation of the National Weed and Seed Strategy, 2010 Final Report* conducted by RTI International provided a study that included 200 plus participating sites, personnel, community members, local data collection, and key stakeholders (Trudeau et al. 2010, 13). The pattern found in drug arrests also had a similar appearance to the 2004 study in that arrests in both studies decreased after the third year.

While some locations did see a decline in crime, not all were able to stay funded or funded long enough to stabilize the seed phase of the program. Destabilization was often due to the participating local and national agencies being unsuccessful in balancing their efforts in the proposed two-step process. Often, these programs lost their funding upon not meeting program expectations pertaining to community participation and support (Bridenball and Jesilow 2005, 66–68). A significant recommendation for improvement and federal funding retention by the 2010 Final Report was to provide equal amounts for each phase and, if necessary, to reduce the number of new sites to provide adequate funding to implement the program properly. Thus, the need for reflection on adequate support to reconstruct communities was necessary. If community members lacked proper support to change and retain the culture and structure of their community, they would fail to retain the program or to sustain its new status after it was defunded (Bridenball and Jesilow 2005, 68). The 2010 Final report also noted that the empirical significance for these national evaluation studies is challenging to generalize due to the individual complexities of each site, data collection focus, and community participants' perceptions. However, despite the fact the study was able to provide sufficient success to warrant the continued funding of the Weed and Seed Program in 2010 (Trudeau et al. 2010, 24; Lilley 2015, 442), the program was terminated.

Arlett S. Lomelí

See also: Drug Enforcement Administration (DEA); Street Crime; Trafficking.

Further Reading

Bridenball, Blaine, and Paul Jesilow. "Weeding Criminals or Planting Fear: An Evaluation of a Weed and Seed Project." *Criminal Justice Review* 30, no. 1 (2005): 64–89.

O'Connell, Jack, Matthew Perkins, and Jim Zepp. "Weed and Seed Crime Pattern Data Analysis." Justice Research and Statistics Association, May 3, 2004. https://www.jrsa.org/pubs/reports/jrsa-crime-pattern.pdf

Lilley, David. "The Weed and Seed Program: A Nationwide Analysis of Crime Outcomes." *Criminal Justice Policy Review* 26, no. 5 (2015): 423–447.

Trudeau, James, Kelle Barrick, Jason Williams, and Jan Roehl. "Independent Evaluation of the National Weed and Seed Strategy: Final Report September 2010." Research Triangle Institute. RTI Project Number 0210717.001.410. https://www.jrsa.org/projects/WnS_Final_Evaluation_Report.pdf

The United States Department of Justice. "Operation Weed and Seed." 2005. https://www.ncjrs.gov/pdffiles1/205894.pdf

The United States Department of Justice. "Weed and Seed." Last modified October 5, 2018. https://www.justice.gov/usao-ndca/weed-and-seed

Weeds

Weeds is a drama-comedy that broadcast on the Showtime network from 2005 to 2012 about Nancy Botwin, a widowed mother (played by Mary-Louise Parker) in suburbia who turns to selling pot to support herself and her two sons. The show became notable for mixing dark and suspenseful plot elements with the traditional "silly" vibes for which marijuana use is notorious. Variously described as cutting edge, irreverent, cheeky, and barrier breaking, *Weeds* ignited a conversation about marijuana and legalization by providing a storyline television had never seen before.

The series creator, Jenji Kohan, attributed some of the show's popularity to its marijuana-oriented plotlines and exploration of marijuana use. "There's a pot smoker in every family—it crosses all social, religious, economic, political, and racial lines." Kohan successfully depicted this idea by including various types of people, situations, and backgrounds. Due to the relatability and freethinking the show encouraged, *Weeds* became one of the most watched shows on showtime. Furthermore, public opinion on legalization and decriminalization of marijuana evolved immensely while the show was on the air. When *Weeds* first aired in 2005, the medicinal use of marijuana was legal in only 10 states. By the time the series ended in 2012, the number of states that had legalized (and decriminalized) marijuana use for both medical and recreational use had nearly doubled.

The show's central character is Botwin, who loses her husband unexpectedly to a heart attack a few weeks before the series begins. Finding herself in debt, with 15-year-old Silas (Hunter Parrish) and 10-year-old Shane (Alexander Gould) to support, she turns to a business of growing and selling marijuana. Due to the premise of the show, *Weeds* is a fitting title. More interesting are two other explanations for the title. First, the term "widow's weeds" originated during the Victorian era and was used to describe black clothing worn by a widow in mourning. Second, weeds are plants with a well-deserved reputation for being tough and hardy and for thriving even in gardens and sidewalk cracks where they are not wanted.

The first three seasons of the show take place in a fictional suburb called Agrestic, located near Los Angeles, California, which is populated by middle- and upper-class citizens. During these seasons, each episode opens with the song "Little Boxes" (written and composed by Malvina Reynolds), a song that mocks the conformist lifestyle suburbia holds, where "all the boxes look the same" (i.e., houses, people, occupations, hobbies). However, Agrestic also harbors a "high" population of secretive, unconventional marijuana users. Buyers range from soccer moms and teachers to city commissioners. As the show progresses, Nancy's drug-running operation takes off, and she becomes the self-proclaimed "suburban baroness of bud." It is important to note that Nancy rarely gets high on her supply; the same cannot be said about many of the other regular cast members. For example, Nancy's brother-in-law, Andy Botwin (Justin Kirk), is a lovable airhead who helps Nancy throughout the series; his knowledge of the business comes mostly from his long history of buying and consuming pot.

As Nancy's commerce increases, so does her number of reckless decisions until disaster strikes. Guillermo (Guillermo Diaz), a "frenemy" of Nancy's who is also the leader of a band of Mexican dealers, sets fire to a competitor's marijuana field. Soon the brush fire engulfs the town of Agrestic creating a doomsday-like scenario reported as the "Majestic Inferno." So, what does an ambitious drug dealer with a crumbling business do? Dowse her house in gasoline, hit the road, and relaunch her marijuana business in Ren Mar, another fictional town located between San Diego and Mexico.

The change of setting also marked a darker turn for the show, which incorporates themes of hard drug trafficking and human trafficking. These episodes also show how the trafficking of illegal drugs and the trafficking of humans are often correlated, with trafficking victims used to smuggle drugs across the border. After relocating to Ren Mar, Nancy marries Esteban Reyes (Demián Bichir), the mayor of Tijuana and leader of the Tres Seis, an organization that exports cocaine and sex workers to the United States. Nancy also becomes pregnant with Esteban's child, Stevie. When Shane commits murder, Nancy flees once again with her sons. Despite traveling across the country, the drug lords find Nancy. To avoid being killed by the traffickers, she turns herself in to authorities, confesses to Shane's crime, goes to jail, and is released after three years—whereupon she turns back to the marijuana trade once again.

The Botwin family dynamic is unique, to say the least. A carpooling, iced coffee-sipping mom switches to the role of a ruthless drug lord, who in time employs her two sons and brother-in-law (who essentially takes over the father-figure role). In addition to the pain and anger associated with losing their father, the brothers are dealing with a mother who is constantly distracted and detached due to her "extended" family of drug dealing colleagues. It becomes obvious that their mother is up to something behind the scenes, and eventually, the boys find out about her profession. Silas is eager to join the game, and although Nancy is initially hesitant to include him in her marijuana-selling activities, he quickly shows his skills and passion for the trade. In the middle of the series, he studies plant cultivation and eventually opens a medical marijuana dispensary. Silas's relationship with his mother is tumultuous, but much of it stems from a business standpoint. In contrast, Shane is more affected by the neglect at home and chaos of their family's work. He copes by abusing alcohol and drugs and pursuing sexual encounters. Shane's behavior becomes increasingly erratic, violent, and sociopathic over the course of the series—a descent that culminates with his murder of a woman with a croquet mallet after overhearing her verbally threaten his family. After the act, Shane shows no remorse and calmly states that he used the mallet because "I couldn't find a golf club."

The series comes to an end after skipping several years into the future, to a time when marijuana is legal and the Botwin family is thriving. Nancy gives up her criminal lifestyle and starts a legitimate business of marijuana shops that become so successful Starbucks wants to buy it. Nancy finally has money and success, but her relationship with her family remains damaged. In the final scene, however, the originals of the group—Nancy, Andy, Silas, Shane, and Doug—gather on Nancy's front porch and enjoy a joint together, giving viewers hope that the family can someday be reconciled.

Mackenzie McBride

See also: Family Life.

Further Reading

Drug Policy Alliance. "Marijuana Legalization and Regulation." n.d. Accessed August 23, 2021. http://www.drugpolicy.org/issues/marijuana-legalization-and-regulation

Pirnia, Garin. "10 Facts About *Weeds*." MentalFloss.com, November 8, 2017. http://mentalfloss.com/article/503233/facts-about-weeds

Raymond, Chris. "The Origins and History of Widow's Weeds." Verywellhealth.com, March 15, 2020. https://www.verywellhealth.com/what-are-widows-weeds-113195

Stanley, Alessandra. "Life in the Suburbs, Where the Grass Is a Little Greener." *New York Times*, September 1, 2006. https://www.nytimes.com/2006/09/01/arts/television/01weed.html

Woodstock

Staged over the course of three days in the summer of 1969, the Woodstock rock music festival became one of the most significant cultural and musical events of the 1960s. The festival, which organizers touted as "three days of peace and music," was held from August 15 to 18 on a farm in Bethel, New York, about 40 miles from the town of Woodstock. An estimated 250,000–750,000 concertgoers attended the festival during the course of the three days, during which time more than 30 nationally recognized artists and bands performed (Helfrich 2010). Not only was this event influenced by the culture of the time, it also bred a new counterculture around music festivals and those who attended them (McKean 2006). The event was documented in the 1970 film *Woodstock*, was celebrated in a Joni Mitchell (1943–) song with the same title, and has emerged as an iconic symbol of the 1960s' countercultural movement. The event is also regarded as a pivotal event in music history, and several Woodstock anniversary concerts have been held to commemorate the original festival.

While live rock music was the organizing foundation and main attraction of the Woodstock festival, the experience of concertgoers was also heavily influenced by the presence of drugs. In fact, Woodstock is regarded as a pivotal event not only for music history but also for the history of the drug subculture.

The number of young people using marijuana increased steadily during the latter half of the 1960s because of its relatively low risk of physical harm and addiction and its growing symbolism as both an expression of freedom and a rejection of "mainstream" values. By the time of Woodstock, marijuana was the primary drug of choice of drug-using youth, and marijuana was the drug of choice for most concertgoers at Woodstock. Despite concerns from members of the Bethel community that the festival would attract hordes of destructive, drug-addled hippies, the policing of marijuana (and drugs in general) was not a priority for law enforcement at the festival (McKean 2006; Helfrich 2010). Police were reluctant to arrest people who smoked marijuana because there was not enough room in the county jails to hold all those who were using drugs. The relative lack of policing also allowed drugs to be widely available. With little fear of being arrested, festivalgoers smoked marijuana freely throughout the festival. Marijuana was also commonly used as a currency between people to trade for food or other amenities (Aydlette 2019).

While marijuana was the most commonly and frequently used drug at the festival, LSD use was also common and attracted much more attention. Over 5,000 medical cases were reported during the festival, and over 800 of these were drug related. Of these latter cases, LSD was the main culprit (Kelly 2010). By contrast, the extensive use of marijuana was credited by many observers for "keeping the peace" even though the festival was tremendously overcrowded and rocked by periods of rain and storms (Musto 1991, 46). Fortunately, festival organizers alerted local hospitals and flew in over 80 medical professionals from nearby areas to manage drug-related and other health issues occurring during the three days. While there were two documented deaths during the festival, only one of these was possibly drug related (Kelly 2010).

Jordan Y. Marth

See also: Hippies.

Further Reading

Aydlette, Larry. "The Mud, the Music, the Memories. Readers Recall their Magical and Messy Journey through Rock's Most Famous Festival." *The Palm Beach Post*, August 2019: 1–4.

Collier, B. L. "Tired Rock Fans begin Exodus." *The New York Times*, August 1969: 1–25.

Gfroerer, Joseph and Marc Brodsky. "The Incidence of Illicit Drug Use in the United States, 1962–1989." *Journal of Addiction* 87, no.1 (1992): 1345–1351.

Helfrich, Ronald. "What Can a Hippie Contribute to Our Community? Culture Wars, Moral Panics, and the Woodstock Festival." *New York History* 91, no. 3 (Summer 2010): 221–244.

Kelly, Jack. "EMS at Woodstock." *Journal of Emergency Medical Services* 5, no.25 (April 2010): 2–12.

McKean, Sean. "Beyond the Myth: A Deeper Look at the 1969 Woodstock Festival." *Woodstock Preservation Archives* (2006): 1–7.

Milsten, Andrew M., et al. "Mass-Gathering Medical Care: A Review of Literature." *Prehospital and Disaster Medicine* 17, no. 3 (July–September 2002): 151–162.

Musto, David F. "Opium, Cocaine and Marijuana in American History." *Scientific American* 265, no. 1 (July 1991): 40–47.

Schowalter, Daniel F. "Remembering the Dangers of Rock and Roll: Toward a Historical Narrative of the Rock Festival." *Critical Studies in Media Communication* 17, no. 1 (March 2000): 85–102.

Weiner, Rex, and Deanne Stillman. *Woodstock Census: The Nationwide Survey of the Sixties Generation.* New York: Viking Press,1979.

About the Editors and Contributors

THE EDITORS

James Hawdon
Professor and Director of the Center for Peace Studies and Violence Prevention
Department of Sociology
Virginia Tech

Bryan Lee Miller
Associate Professor and Graduate Coordinator
Department of Sociology, Anthropology and Criminal Justice
Clemson University

Matthew Costello
Assistant Professor
Department of Sociology, Anthropology and Criminal Justice
Clemson University

THE CONTRIBUTORS

Brandon Alston
Graduate Student
Department of Sociology
Northwestern University

Katherine Ayers
Graduate Student
Department of Sociology
Virginia Tech

Julie Marie Baldwin
Research Professor
Department of Justice, Law & Criminology
American University

Daisy Ball
Assistant Professor
Department of Public Affairs
Roanoke College

Angela M. Barlow
Associate Professor
Department of Criminal Justice Studies
Keene State University

Jonathan F. Bastian
Graduate Student
Department of Criminal Justice
University of Louisville

Virginia Benefield
Graduate Student
Department of Criminal Justice Administration
Middle Tennessee State University

John H. Boman, IV
Associate Professor
Department of Sociology
Bowling Green State University

Amanda M. Burroughs
Graduate Student
Department of Sociology
Virginia Tech

Lyla Byers
Graduate Student
Department of Sociology
Virginia Tech

Jason T. Callahan
Graduate Student
Department of Sociology
Virginia Tech

Nathan D. Coleman
Graduate Student
Department of Criminal Justice
University of Central Florida

C. Cozette Comer
Evidence Synthesis Librarian
University Libraries
Virginia Tech

Nicholas Copeland
Associate Professor
Department of Sociology
Virginia Tech

Allen Copenhaver
Assistant Professor and Criminal Justice Program Coordinator
Department of Criminal Justice
Lindsey Wilson College

Samantha Davis
Student
Department of Sociology and Criminology
University of Arkansas

Joao Fasolino De Menezes
Criminal Justice Research Alliance

Craig A. Depken, II
Professor
Department of Economics
University of North Carolina at Charlotte

John M. Eassey
Research Professor
Department of Justice, Law & Criminology
American University

Alex Espinoza-Kulick
Graduate Student
Department of Sociology
University of California, Santa Barbara

Mario Alberto V. Espinoza-Kulick
Lecturer
Ethnic Studies Department
California Polytechnic State University

Tyler Frye
Student
Department of Criminal Justice
Penn State Altoona

Margot Gage Witvliet
Assistant Professor
Department of Sociology
Lamar University

Marc D. Glidden
Assistant Professor
Department of Criminology and Justice Studies
California State University, Northridge

Alexandria Goldstein
Graduate Student
Department of Sociology and Criminal Justice
Kennesaw State University

O. Hayden Griffin, III
Associate Professor
Department of Criminal Justice
University of Alabama at Birmingham

Jonathan A. Grubb
Assistant Professor
Department of Criminal Justice & Criminology
Georgia Southern University

Antonio Paniagua Guzmán
Lecturer
Department of Sociology
University of Wisconsin–Milwaukee

Ezekiel Hall
Graduate Student
Department of Criminal Justice Administration
Middle Tennessee State University

Meghan Harrigan
Student
Department of Criminal Justice
Penn State Altoona

Rhys Hester
Assistant Professor
Department of Sociology, Anthropology and Criminal Justice
Clemson University

Melody Hicks
Graduate Student
Department of Criminal Justice Administration
Middle Tennessee State University

Aleksi Hupli
Graduate Student
School of Social Sciences and Humanities
Tampere University

Zachary Hutchinson
Investigative Specialist
HireRight

Shelby I. Ingalls
Graduate Student
Department of Sociology, Anthropology and Criminal Justice
Clemson University

Veronyka James
Associate Professor
Department of Criminology and Criminal Justice
Shenandoah University

Eric Jardine
Assistant Professor
Department of Political Science
Virginia Tech

Aubrey D. Johnson
Graduate Student
Department of Sociology, Anthropology & Criminal Justice
Clemson University

Sitinga Kachipande
Instructor
Department of Sociology
Virginia Tech

Paige Kennett
Law Student
Virginia School of Law
University of Virginia

Stan Korotchenko
Adjunct Instructor
Department of Criminal Justice
University of Central Florida

Stephanie M. Koskinen
Graduate Student
Department of Criminology and Criminal Justice
University of North Florida

Nathan E. Kruis
Assistant Professor
Department of Criminal Justice
Penn State Altoona

Andrew M. Lindner
Associate Professor
Sociology Department
Skidmore College

Arlett S. Lomelí
Assistant Professor
Department of Sociology
University of Texas Rio Grande Valley

Gabrielle L. Lory
Graduate Student
Department of Sociology
West Virginia University

D. Tyler Love
Graduate Student
Department of Sociology, Anthropology and Criminal Justice
Clemson University

C. Cory Lowe
Graduate Student
Department of Sociology and Criminology & Law
University of Florida

Lucas Maness
Graduate Student
Department of Criminal Justice and Criminology
University of North Carolina at Charlotte

Tyler Manger
Student
Department of Criminal Justice
Penn State Altoona

Jordan Y. Marth
Graduate Student
Department of Sociology
Virginia Tech

Mackenzie McBride
Instructor
Department of Criminology and Criminal Justice
Georgia Southern University

Katherine McCarthy
Research Assistant
Anti-Defamation League, Center on Extremism

Christine McCown
Instructor
Department of Sociology
Virginia Tech

Jenae McGill
Student
Department of Criminal Justice
Penn State Altoona

Christopher J. Miceli
Graduate Student
Department of Sociology
Virginia Tech

J. Mitchell Miller
John A. Delaney Presidential Professor
Department of Criminology and Criminal Justice
University of North Florida

Rocio Paez
Visiting Assistant Professor

Department of Sociology and Criminology
University of Arkansas

Anne McNutt Patrick
Graduate Student
Department of Sociology
Virginia Tech

Robert Perdue
Assistant Professor
Department of Sociology and Anthropology
Elon University

Thomas J. PlaHovinsak, II
Assistant Professor
College of Business & Economics
Longwood University

Chad Posick
Associate Professor and Graduate Coordinator
Criminal Justice & Criminology
Georgia Southern University

Jebadiha E. Potterf
Instructor
Department of Sociology
Colorado State University

Cori Pryor
Graduate Student
Department of Sociology
Bowling Green State University

Salvatore J. Restifo
Associate Professor
Department of Sociology
University of Texas Rio Grande Valley

Kristin Richardson
Lecturer
Department of Sociology and Public Health
Roanoke College

Courtney B. Ross
Instructor
Department of Sociology
Virginia Tech

Bienvenido Ruiz
Associate Professor
Department of Sociology
University of Texas Rio Grande Valley

Logan Sarvey
Business Systems Analyst
LPL Financial

Iina Savolainen
Postdoctoral Researcher
Information Technology and Communication Sciences
Tampere University

Olivia P. Shaw
Graduate Student
Department of Criminal Justice and Criminology
University of North Carolina at Charlotte

Kristen N. Sobba
Assistant Professor
Department of Criminal Justice, Social Work and Sociology
Southeast Missouri State University

Chelsea Starr
Associate Professor and Department Chair
Department of Sociology
Eastern New Mexico University

Ben Stickle
Associate Professor
Department of Criminal Justice Administration
Middle Tennessee State University

John Stogner
Associate Professor
Department of Criminal Justice and Criminology
University of North Carolina at Charlotte

Danielle M. Stoneberg
Graduate Student
Department of Sociology
West Virginia University

Richard Stringer
Assistant Professor
Department of Sociology and Criminal Justice
Kennesaw State University

Jose Torres
Assistant Professor
Department of Sociology
Louisiana State University

Steve Trost
Virginia Tech University

Marissa Turturici
Independent Scholar

Shanyn Viars
American Rivers

Anastasia S. Vogt Yuan
Associate Professor
Department of Sociology
Virginia Tech

Lauren Waldrop
Graduate
Department of Criminal Justice and Department of Global Cultures and Languages
Southeast Missouri State University

Rhonda Wrzenski
Associate Professor
Department of Political Science
Indiana University Southeast

Index

Note: Page numbers in **bold** indicate the location of main entries.

www.ingramcontent.com/pod-product-compliance
Ingram Content Group UK Ltd.
Pitfield, Milton Keynes, MK11 3LW, UK
UKHW051451290926
15471UKWH00008B/1146

9 798216 494713